Tracheostomies
The Complete Guide

Linda L. Morris, PhD, APN, CCNS, FCCM, is the clinical nurse specialist for respiratory care and tracheostomy specialist at Northwestern Memorial Hospital in Chicago, Illinois. She is also assistant professor of clinical anesthesiology at Northwestern University Feinberg School of Medicine. With many years of experience in critical care, Dr. Morris has also held positions in clinical education and academia. Current research interests include quality of life and body image perception with tracheostomy patients, outcomes of an exercise program with newly tracheostomized patients, and awareness during resuscitation from cardiac arrest.

M. Sherif Afifi, MD, FCCM, FCCP, is an associate professor of anesthesiology and surgery, and Chief of the Anesthesiology Critical Care Division at Northwestern University Feinberg School of Medicine, Chicago, Illinois. The scope of his clinical practice is centered on the perioperative care of cardiac, thoracic, and transplant patients. His postgraduate medical training started with a research fellowship in respiratory physiology and drug safety and efficacy at the Duke University Hyperbaric Center and completed with clinical residency and fellowship training at the Cleveland Clinic Foundation. He served on the faculty at the Cleveland Clinic, Yale University School of Medicine, and was interim residency program director at the Advocate Masonic Medical Center in Chicago, Illinois. He has mentored and consulted in the United States and internationally, and is the recipient of awards from national societies and specialty international medical centers.

Tracheostomies

The Complete Guide

Linda L. Morris, PhD, APN, CCNS, FCCM
M. Sherif Afifi, MD, FCCM, FCCP
Editors

SPRINGER PUBLISHING COMPANY
New York

Copyright © 2010 Springer Publishing Company, LLC

All rights reserved.

No part of this publication may be reproduced, stored in a retrieval system, or transmitted in any form or by any means, electronic, mechanical, photocopying, recording, or otherwise, without the prior permission of Springer Publishing Company, LLC, or authorization through payment of the appropriate fees to the Copyright Clearance Center, Inc., 222 Rosewood Drive, Danvers, MA 01923, 978–750–8400, fax 978–646–8600, info@copyright.com or on the web at www.copyright.com.

Springer Publishing Company, LLC
11 West 42nd Street
New York, NY 10036
www.springerpub.com

Acquisitions Editor: Allan Graubard
Project Manager: Julia Rosen
Cover Design: Mimi Flow
Composition: Apex CoVantage, LLC

E-book ISBN: 978-08261-0518-9

10 11 12/5 4 3 2 1

The author and the publisher of this Work have made every effort to use sources believed to be reliable to provide information that is accurate and compatible with the standards generally accepted at the time of publication. Because medical science is continually advancing, our knowledge base continues to expand. Therefore, as new information becomes available, changes in procedures become necessary. We recommend that the reader always consult current research and specific institutional policies before performing any clinical procedure. The author and publisher shall not be liable for any special, consequential, or exemplary damages resulting, in whole or in part, from the readers' use of, or reliance on, the information contained in this book. The publisher has no responsibility for the persistence or accuracy of URLs for external or third-party Internet Web sites referred to in this publication and does not guarantee that any content on such Web sites is, or will remain, accurate or appropriate.

Library of Congress Cataloging-in-Publication Data

Morris, Linda, 1954–
   Tracheostomies : the complete guide / Linda Morris, M. Sherif Afifi.
     p. ; cm.
   Includes bibliographical references and index.
   ISBN 978-0-8261-0517-2 (alk. paper)
  1. Tracheotomy. I. Afifi, M. Sherif. II. Title.
   [DNLM: 1. Tracheostomy. 2. Tracheotomy. WF 490 M877t 2009]
   RF517.M67 2009
   617.5'33—dc22   2009043752

Printed in the United States of America by Hamilton Printing Company.

To my parents, Louise Hostert Morris and the late Bernard Franklin Morris, who have inspired my inquisitive nature and supported all of my endeavors....

L.L.M.

Contents

Contributors xi
Preface xiii
Acknowledgments xv

Chapter 1   Functional Anatomy of the Airway 1
M. Sherif Afifi

     The Upper Airway 2
     The Lower Airway 11
     Comparative Anatomy of the Adult and Infant Airways 13
     Conclusion 14
     Key Points 14

Chapter 2   Tracheotomy Procedure 17
Michiel J. Bové and M. Sherif Afifi

     Indications for Tracheotomy 18
     Timing of Tracheotomy 19
     Preoperative Management 20
     Anesthesia Management 21
     Surgical Technique 25
     Postoperative Care 37
     Summary 38
     Key Points 38

Chapter 3   Types of Tracheostomy Tubes and Related Appliances 41
Linda L. Morris

     Parts of a Tracheostomy Tube 42
     General Types of Tracheostomy Tubes 47
     Special Use Tracheostomy Tubes 75
     Tracheostomy Accessories and Appliances 103
     Summary 112
     Key Points 112

Chapter 4	Fitting and Changing a Tracheostomy Tube 115
	Linda L. Morris
	Considerations When Fitting a Tracheostomy Tube 115
	Tracheostomy Tube Changes 145
	Fitting a Tracheostomy Button 154
	Summary 157
	Key Points 157
Chapter 5	Special Considerations for the Tracheostomy Patient 159
	Linda L. Morris
	The Critically Ill Patient on Mechanical Ventilation 160
	Retained Secretions 163
	Cuff Leaks 164
	Pistoning 169
	Cuff Changes at Altitude 169
	Cuff Changes With Anesthesia 172
	The Complex Tracheostomy Wound 173
	Tracheostomy as a Lived Experience 175
	Defective Tracheostomy Tubes 177
	Missing Parts 177
	Summary 178
	Key Points 178
Chapter 6	Phonation With a Tracheostomy 181
	Linda L. Morris
	General Principles of Voice Restoration 181
	Patients Who Do Not Require Mechanical Ventilation 183
	Patients Who Require Intermittent Positive-Pressure Ventilation 196
	Patients Who Require Continuous Mechanical Ventilation 197
	Summary 207
	Key Points 208
Chapter 7	Care of the Tracheostomy Patient 211
	Linda L. Morris
	Maintenance of the Tracheostomy Tube 211
	Mobilization of Secretions 221
	Oral Care 229
	Other Tracheal Appliances 229
	Nutrition 232
	Care of the Patient at Home 232
	Summary 236
	Key Points 236
Chapter 8	Special Considerations for the Child With a Tracheostomy 243
	Linda Sue Van Roeyen
	Indications for Tracheostomy in Children 244

Outcome of Children With Tracheostomies 244
Procedural Steps in the Care of the Child
    With a Tracheostomy 246
Management of the Child With a Tracheostomy
    in the Community 251
Developmental Issues 255
Summary 262
Key Points 262

Chapter 9 Special Considerations for the Patient With a Laryngectomy 265
Jeri A. Logemann

Types of Laryngectomy 266
Swallowing After Laryngectomy 268
Speech After Laryngectomy 270
Ventilator-Dependent Tracheostomized Patients 272
Quality of Life 273
Summary 274
Key Points 275

Chapter 10 Complications and Emergency Procedures 277
Michiel J. Bové and Linda L. Morris

Intraoperative Complications 280
Early Postoperative Complications 285
Late Postoperative Complications 291
Summary 299
Key Points 299

Chapter 11 Downsizing and Decannulation 303
Linda L. Morris

Factors to Consider Prior to Decannulation 304
Determining Readiness for Decannulation 309
Decannulation Protocol 311
After Decannulation 318
Summary 319
Key Points 319

Chapter 12 Rehabilitation and Recovery 323
John Parson and Linda L. Morris

Discharge Disposition of Patients With Tracheostomies 323
Tracheostomy in Acute Rehabilitation 324
Adapting Choice of Tracheostomy Tube and
    Care Plans to Clinical Settings 329
Providing Phonation for Patients Who Require
    Positive-Pressure Ventilation 331
Evaluating the Need for Relief of Upper Airway Obstruction 335
Considerations for Transitioning Tracheostomy Tubes 337
Discharge to Home 339

Care for Patients at Home 341
Clinical Follow-Up................................. 347
Summary 347
Key Points.. 347

Index.. 351

Contributors

Michiel J. Bové, MD
Assistant Professor of Otolaryngology
Northwestern University Feinberg School of Medicine
Chicago, Illinois

Jeri A. Logemann, PhD, CCC-SLP, BRS-S
Ralph and Jean Sundin Professor
Department of Communication Sciences and Disorders
Northwestern University
Evanston, Illinois

John Parson, BA, RRT
RIC Administrator, Respiratory Care
Rehabilitation Institute of Chicago
Chicago, Illinois

Linda Sue Van Roeyen, MS, CSN, CCRP, CFNP
Nurse Practitioner, Pulmonary Habilitation Program, Transitional Care Unit
Department of Critical Care
Children's Memorial Hospital
Chicago, Illinois

Preface

The first edition of this clinical resource is written for health care professionals of all disciplines who care for patients with tracheostomies. The nature of compartmentalized care in medicine today does not allow for a clear overview of the continuum of care for a patient with a tracheostomy. Surgeons are skilled in the procedure of placing a tracheostomy but are often unaware of the myriad of tubes available and the advantages and disadvantages of each. Intensivists make decisions every day regarding the optimal time to place a tracheostomy but may not have the opportunity to follow the complete process of downsizing and decannulation. Nurses routinely do tracheostomy care but may not realize its significance in preventing complications. Respiratory therapists are experts in managing the ventilator but may not be comfortable with other aspects of care such as vocalization. In this book, we provide the fine details of the daily care of patients with tracheostomies to help health care practitioners make appropriate decisions and educate their patients.

Some medical centers have the benefit of a tracheostomy specialist to manage these patients, but it frequently falls to junior residents or others who are often unaware of the available options and necessary precautions. We hope the reader will come to appreciate the importance of this work as we describe in detail the art and science of caring for the patient with a tracheostomy. The book spans the entire spectrum of care—from surgical placement, to choices and fitting of tubes, to restoration of voice, and, finally, to rehabilitation and recovery. Because care of the tracheostomy patient involves many disciplines, chapter authors have been chosen to share their unique perspectives and expertise.

We are certain the reader will find this book a useful clinical reference and refer to it again and again. We invite comments, questions, and alternative approaches and techniques to trachs@yahoo.com, or visit our Web site at www.TrachResource.com. Perhaps a future edition can include any omissions.

Acknowledgments

The editors thank the many people who contributed to this work, including the chapter authors; the editorial assistance of Allan Graubard, Brian O'Connor, and colleagues at Springer; Mary Zemaitis and the team of medical illustrators at Publication Services, Inc., who brought life to our words; the copy editors at Apex CoVantage; the tracheostomy manufacturers for providing photographs and information about their products; and Alberto de Hoyos for his bronchoscopic images of a percutaneous dilatational tracheotomy (in chapter 2).

Tracheostomies
The Complete Guide

Functional Anatomy of the Airway

M. Sherif Afifi

Normal air passages start from the nose and end at the bronchioles of the lung. They are vital to the delivery and modification of respiratory gas to and from the alveoli, which are the center of gas exchange. For descriptive purposes, the airway is divided into the upper airway, which includes the nose, mouth, pharynx, and larynx, and the lower airway, which includes the trachea, bronchi, and the subdivisions of the bronchi. Each of these parts has its own independent structural constitution, vascular supply, and nerve supply, all of which serve to facilitate different and coordinated functions. The functions of the airway include olfaction, deglutition (swallowing), phonation, and, of course, gas exchange. Any interruption to the normal anatomy of the constituents of the airway results in altered function of its various organs. As such, this chapter will review the anatomical landmarks of the upper and lower airways, identify the airway's vascular and nerve supplies, and review the function of its various parts. A comparison of changes in the airway from infancy to adulthood will also be provided.

The Upper Airway

The upper airway is composed of the nose, mouth, pharynx, and larynx. Besides providing a natural conduit for gas exchange, the structures of the upper airway have additional functions in humidification of gases, protection of the lower airway, deglutition, and phonation.

The Nose

The external nose consists of a bony vault and a cartilaginous vault. The bony vault comprises the nasal bones, the frontal processes of the maxillae, and the nasal portion of the frontal bone. The cartilaginous vault is formed by the upper lateral cartilages, which meet the cartilaginous portion of the septum in the midline. The cavities of each nostril are continuous with the nasopharynx posteriorly. The nasal airway is between the laterally placed inferior turbinate, the septum, and the floor of the nose. The nasal cavities are bounded posteriorly by the nasopharynx. The adenoids are located posteriorly in the nasopharynx just above the nasal surface of the soft palate. The soft palate rests on the base of the tongue during quiet nasal respiration, sealing the oral cavity.

Functional Anatomic Relevance

- The nose provides moisture to approximately 10,000 liters of ambient air that pass through the nasal airway every day (Grande, Ramanathan, & Turndorf, 1988). The moisture is constituted from transudated fluid through the mucosal epithelium as well as secretions from glands and goblet cells. These secretions have bactericidal properties.
- The floor of the nose is tilted slightly downward at approximately 10 to 15 degrees. Thus, when a nasal tube or fiberscope is inserted through the nose, it should be directed slightly inferiorly to follow this major channel.
- The nasal mucosa is exquisitely sensitive to topically applied vasoconstricting medications such as phenylephrine, epinephrine, or cocaine. Cocaine has the added advantage of providing profound topical anesthesia and is the only local anesthetic agent that produces vasoconstriction; the others cause vasodilatation.
- The contiguity of the paranasal sinuses with the nasal cavity leads to infections of the paranasal sinuses with prolonged nasotracheal intubation. Surveillance for infected paranasal sinuses is important with long-term placement of airways or nasogastric tubes in the nasal passages.

The Mouth

The mouth, or oral cavity, is divided into two parts: the vestibule and the oral cavity proper. The vestibule is the space between the lips and the cheeks externally and the gums and teeth internally. The oral cavity proper is bounded anterolaterally by the alveolar arch, teeth, and gums; superiorly by the hard and soft palates; and inferiorly by the tongue. Posteriorly, the oral cavity communicates with the palatal arches and pharynx.

The Tongue

The tongue is a noncompressible muscular structure. The tongue is attached to the symphysis of the mandible anteriorly and anterolaterally and the stylohyoid process and hyoid bone posterolaterally and posteriorly, respectively. The posterior limit of the tongue corresponds to the position of the hyoid bone. The sensory and motor innervations of the tongue include different sources. Sensory fibers for the anterior two-thirds are provided by the lingual nerve. Taste fibers are furnished by the chorda tympani branch of the nervus intermedius. Sensory fibers for the posterior third come from the glossopharyngeal nerve (IX). Some sensory innervation is provided by the superior laryngeal nerve. The major motor supply is from the hypoglossal nerve (XII).

Functional Anatomic Relevance

- During laryngoscopy, the tongue is ordinarily displaced to the left and into the mandibular space; thus, the larynx is exposed for intubation under direct vision. Also, encroachment of the mandibular space by a large tongue, a small mandible, infection (e.g., Ludwig's angina), or masses limits displacement of the tongue into this space and, thus, makes orotracheal intubation difficult or impossible.
- A forward jaw-thrust maneuver pulls the mandible and tongue forward to open the upper airway and alleviate upper airway obstruction. Normally, the mandibular condyles articulate within the temporomandibular joint for the first 30 degrees of mouth opening. Beyond 30 degrees, the condyles translate out of the temporomandibular joint anteriorly into the zygomatic arches. The jaw-thrust maneuver can prove life saving for many patients with upper airway obstruction, and it facilitates ventilation with a face mask as well as the insertion of orogastric tubes.

The Pharynx

The pharynx is a U-shaped musculo-membranous tube that extends from the base of the skull to the inferior border of the cricoid cartilage anteriorly and the lower border of the sixth cervical vertebra (C6) posteriorly. It is approximately 15 cm long and, in the adult, has its widest point at the level of the hyoid bone and its narrowest at the lower end, where it joins the esophagus. Anteriorly, it opens into the nasopharynx, oropharynx, and laryngopharynx (see Figure 1.1). The pharynx is the common pathway for food and respiratory gases.

Functional Anatomic Relevance

- Oropharyngeal muscle tone keeps the upper airway open during quiet breathing. Respiratory distress is associated with pharyngeal muscular activity attempting to open the airway further. Sedative hypnotic and opiate agents may attenuate some of this tone and precipitate partial or total airway obstruction.

1.1

Anatomy of pharynx and larynx.

Labels: Epiglottis, Vestibule of the larynx, False vocal cord, Thyroid cartilage, Cricoid cartilage, Hyoid bone, Aryepiglottic fold, Vocal cord, Infraglottic space, Trachea

- The pharynx defends against pathogens through the presence of lymphoid tissue at its base. Inhaled micro-particles are removed by impaction as they pass in the posterior pharynx. An inhaled airstream changes direction sharply by 90 degrees at the nasopharynx, thus causing some loss of momentum of the suspended particles. The particles are then trapped by a circular array of lymphoid tissue located at the entrance of the respiratory and gastrointestinal tracts. The ring includes the tonsils, which, if infected or enlarged, often impede the passage of endotracheal tubes. Abscess formation, hemorrhage, or tumor growth may cause airway obstruction.
- Patency of the pharynx is a critical component for proper gas exchange. Upper airway obstruction in patients who are sedated or anesthetized (with or without an endotracheal tube) or who have altered levels of consciousness is caused by a tongue with loss of muscle tone falling back against the posterior pharyngeal wall. Shorten, Opie, Graziotti, Morris, and Khangure (1994) used magnetic resonance imaging (MRI) to demonstrate a different mechanism for upper airway obstruction in patients sedated with midazolam. A decrease in the anterior-posterior dimension at the level of the soft palate and epiglottis occurred while

sparing the tongue. Thus, the soft palate and epiglottis may have a more important role than muscle tone in the development of upper airway obstruction.

- Obstructive sleep apnea (OSA) results from a reduction in the size of the pharynx, among other causes. Normally, the longer axis of the pharyngeal airway is transverse; however, in OSA patients the anterior-posterior axis is predominant. It is believed this orientation is less efficient for airway muscle function. Imaging studies using MRI, computed tomography (CT), nasopharyngoscopy, fluoroscopy, and acoustic reflections divulged differences in anatomical structure between awake and asleep males (Ayappa & Rapoport, 2003). In awake males with OSA, CT demonstrated a reduced airway caliber at all levels of the pharynx when compared with normal patients, with the narrowest point posterior to the soft palate (Haponik et al., 1983). The application of continuous positive airway pressure (CPAP) increases the cross-sectional area, and thus volume, of the oropharynx, especially in the lateral axis (Schwab, Gefner, Pack, & Hoffman, 1993).

The Larynx

The larynx is the organ of phonation and is located in the anterior portion of the neck. It extends from its oblique entrance formed by the aryepiglottic folds, the tip of the epiglottis, and the posterior commissure between the arytenoids cartilages (interarytenoid folds) through the vocal cords to the cricoid ring (see Figure 1.2). It is a boxlike structure, 4 to 5 ml in volume, and is

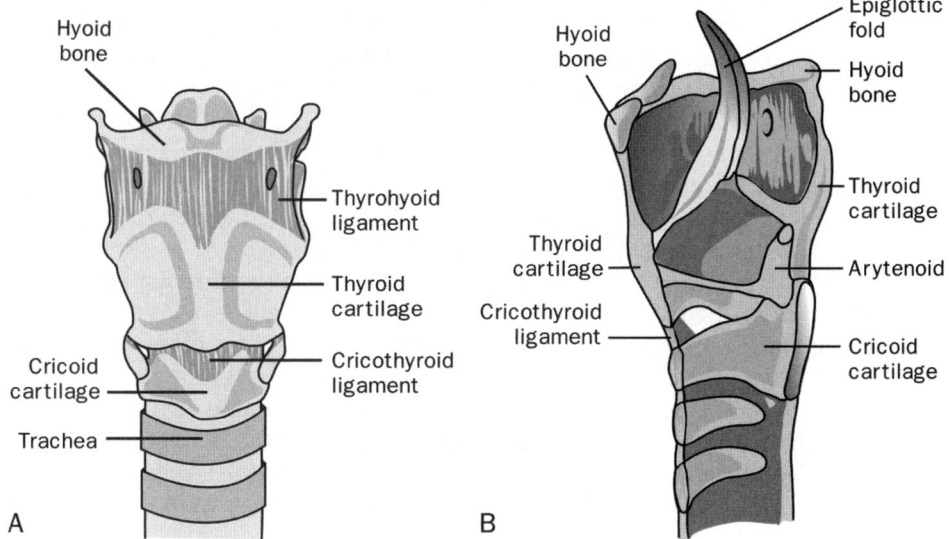

Anatomy of larynx: (A) anterior view; (B) sagittal view.

made up of cartilages, ligaments, muscles, and mucous membrane. In adults, it is situated in the anterior portion of the neck at the level of C3 through C6. The larynx is shorter in women and children and is situated at a slightly higher level. The larynx consists of three single cartilages—the epiglottis, the thyroid, and the cricoid—and three paired cartilages—the arytenoids, the corniculates, and the cuneiforms. The laryngeal cavity is a space between the true vocal cords and the arytenoid cartilages and is known as the rima glottidis. It divides the larynx into two parts: the upper compartment extends from the laryngeal outlet to the vocal cords and contains the vestibular folds and the sinus of the larynx; the lower compartment extends from the vocal cords to the upper portion of the trachea. The piriform sinus is the space between the epiglottis and the aryepiglottic folds medially and the hyoid bone, thyrohyoid ligament, and thyroid cartilage laterally (known as the piriform fossa).

The larynx is innervated by two branches of the vagus: the superior laryngeal and the recurrent laryngeal nerves. The superior laryngeal nerve reaches the internal side of the larynx. It divides into an external (motor) branch that descends to supply the cricothyroid membrane and upper and lower branches that supply the mucous membrane of the base of the tongue, pharynx, epiglottis, and larynx. The superior laryngeal branch of the vagus nerve supplies sensation to the undersurface of the epiglottis, all of the larynx to the level of the false vocal cords, and the pyriform recesses posterolaterally to either side of the larynx.

The recurrent laryngeal nerve (RLN) arises from the vagus nerve and loops around the subclavian artery on the right and the aortic arch on the left. After ascending between the trachea and esophagus, it passes behind the thyroid gland and innervates all the intrinsic muscles of the larynx except the cricothyroid. In addition, it supplies sensory branches to the mucous membranes of the larynx below the vocal cords.

Functional Anatomic Relevance

- The larynx is the most heavily innervated sensory structure in the body, followed closely by the carina. Stimulation of the unanesthetized larynx during intubation causes tremendous reflex sympathetic activation, with significant elevation in heart rate, blood pressure, and intracranial pressure (particularly in patients with loss of autoregulation). This elevation of heart rate and blood pressure may precipitate marked increase in myocardial oxygen demand and significant afterload that could potentially lead to large vessel dissection or rupture (e.g., injured or dissected carotid artery, thoracic aorta, or abdominal aorta).
- The pyramidal arytenoid cartilages sit on the posterior aspect of the larynx. The intrinsic laryngeal muscles cause them to swivel, opening and closing the vocal cords. An endotracheal tube that is too large may, over time, compress these structures, causing mucosal and cartilaginous ischemia and resulting in permanent laryngeal damage. A traumatic intubation may dislocate these cartilages posteriorly (most commonly from a MAC, or curved, blade) or anteriorly (most commonly from a Miller, or straight, blade). Early diagnosis and intervention may avoid permanent hoarseness.

- The larynx bulges posteriorly into the hypopharynx, leaving deep recesses on either side called pyriform recesses or sinuses. Foreign bodies (e.g., plastic, glass, or fish bones) occasionally become lodged there.
- During active swallowing, the larynx is elevated and moves anteriorly, the epiglottis folds down over the glottis to prevent aspiration, and the bolus of food passes midline into the esophagus. When not actively swallowing (e.g., the unconscious patient), the larynx rests against the posterior hypopharynx such that a nasogastric tube must traverse the pyriform recess to gain access to the esophagus and stomach.
- The cricothyroid membrane extends between the upper anterior surface of the cricoid cartilage to the inferior anterior border of the thyroid cartilage. Its height tends to be about that of the tip of the index finger in both male and female adults. Locating the cricoid cartilage and the cricothyroid membrane quickly in an airway emergency is crucial. It is usually easily done in men because of their obvious laryngeal prominence (Adam's apple).
- Clinical examination of the vocal cords (VC) with laryngoscopy and fiberoptic bronchoscopy determines their position, mobility, and structure as well as their pathology and dysfunction during inspiration, expiration, and phonation. Under normal conditions, the vocal cords meet in the middle in the production of phonation. On inspiration, they part from each other and then return to midline during expiration, leaving a small opening between them (see Figure 1.3). A reflexive, forceful contraction of all laryngeal muscles, as commonly occurs when a foreign body lodges in the larynx, is referred to as a laryngospasm. When laryngospasm occurs, both true and false VC lie tightly in the midline.
- VC palsies result from interrupted innervations of the larynx. The RLN may be traumatized during surgery (commonly thyroid or parathyroid

1.3

Vocal cord position during phonation and inspiration.

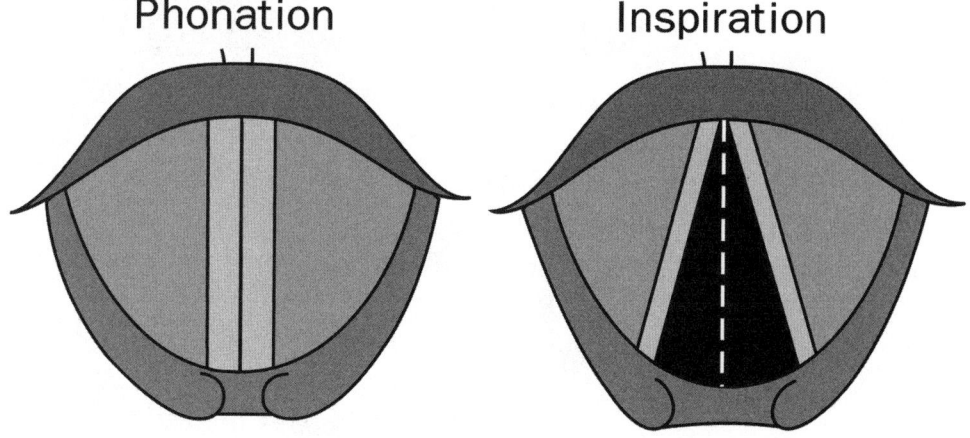

procedures), damaged from a tumor growth or trauma in the neck, or stretched due to pressure from an endotracheal tube (ETT) (Ellis & Feldman, 1993). The left RLN is more likely to be paralyzed than the right because of its close proximity to many intrathoracic structures, making it liable to injury from neoplasms, organ enlargement (aortic aneurysm or left atrial dilation), ice-cold solutions, or erroneous surgical ligation.

- The RLN carries both abductor and adductor fibers to the vocal cords. The abductor fibers are more vulnerable, and moderate trauma causes a pure abductor paralysis, whereas severe trauma causes both abductor and adductor fiber injury. In pure unilateral abductor palsy, both VC meet in midline during phonation because adduction can still occur on the affected side. However, only one cord abducts during inspiration: the unaffected one. By contrast, in complete unilateral RLN palsy both abductors and adductors are affected, and the affected VC lies in a paralyzed position midway between complete abduction and complete adduction. During phonation, the unaffected VC crosses the midline to meet the paralyzed cord (see Figure 1.4). On inspiration, the unaffected

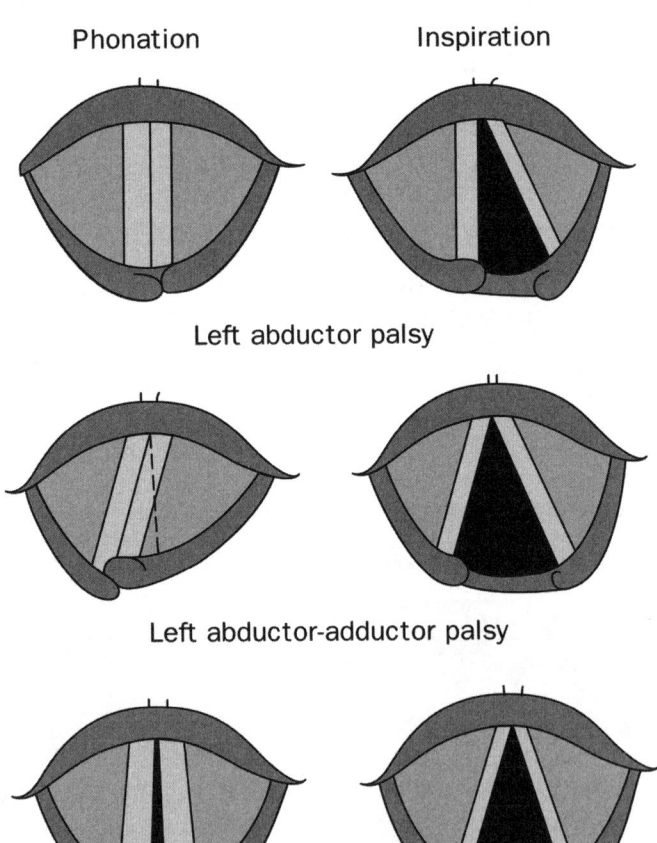

1.4 Vocal cord position during phonation and inspiration in the presence of nerve palsies. Top: left abductor palsy; middle: left abductor–adductor palsy; bottom: bilateral recurrent laryngeal palsy.

cord moves to full abduction. Bilateral RLN palsy produces a different result. In incomplete bilateral abductor damage to the RLN, the adductor fibers draw the VC toward each other, and the glottis opening is reduced to a thin slit, which leads to significant respiratory distress. By contrast, in complete bilateral palsy of the RLN each VC lies midway between adduction and abduction, producing a moderate glottis opening. Therefore, bilateral incomplete RLN palsy is more life threatening than complete bilateral palsy (Redden, 2000).

The Epiglottis

The epiglottis is shaped like a leaf, with its lower end attached to the thyroid cartilage by the thyroepiglottic ligament and its upper, rounded part free and posterior to the tongue. The epiglottis is attached to the hyoid bone anteriorly by the hyoepiglottic ligament. Small depressions on either side of this ligament are referred to as the valleculae.

Functional Anatomic Relevance

- During swallowing, as the laryngeal muscles contract, the downward movement of the epiglottis and the closure and upward movement of the glottis prevent food from entering the larynx.
- When the epiglottis becomes acutely inflated and swollen (acute epiglottitis), a life-threatening airway obstruction may occur.

Physiology of Swallowing

- Normal swallowing consists of three phases: oral preparatory and transport, pharyngeal, and esophageal. The **oral preparatory phase** consists of opening and closing the mouth, moistening food, masticating, preparing an appropriate size bolus with the movement of the tongue and cheek muscles. The **oral transport** (or "buccal") **phase** lasts 1 second and begins with the compression of the food bolus against the hard palate. Next, the tongue retracts in a posterior direction to force the bolus to the oropharynx. Then, the posterior tongue is lifted by the styloglossus and palatoglossus muscles, which also elevate the uvula and seal the nasopharynx to prevent nasal aspiration. This phase is *voluntary* and involves important cranial nerves: V (trigeminal), VII (facial), and XII (hypoglossal). In the **pharyngeal phase** (1 second), the bolus is advanced from the pharynx to the esophagus through the sequential contraction of the constrictor muscles. The soft palate is elevated to the posterior nasopharyngeal wall through the action of the levator veli palatini. The palatopharyngeal folds on each side of the pharynx are brought close together through the superior constrictor muscles so that only a small bolus can pass. Then the larynx and hyoid are elevated and pulled forward to the epiglottis to relax the cricopharyngeus muscle. This passively shuts off its entrance and pulls the vocal cords close together, narrowing the passageway between them. This phase is passively controlled reflexively and involves cranial nerves V, X (vagus), XI (accessory), and XII (hypoglossal). The respiratory center of the medulla is directly inhibited by the swallowing center for the very brief time it takes to swallow. This means it is briefly impossible to breathe during this phase of swallowing, and the moment where breathing is prevented is known as *deglutition apnea*. The bolus moves through the pharynx at a speed of 25 feet per second (8 m/s). During the **esophageal phase** (8–20 seconds), the upper esophageal sphincter relaxes to let food past, after which various striated constrictor muscles of the pharynx as well as the peristalsis and relaxation of the lower esophageal sphincter sequentially push the bolus of food through the esophagus into the stomach.

Neural Regulation of Swallowing

- Swallowing is initiated by sensory impulses transmitted as a result of stimulation of receptors on the fauces, tonsils, soft palate, base of the tongue, and posterior pharyngeal wall.
- Sensory impulses reach the brainstem primarily through the 7th, 9th, and 10th cranial nerves, while the efferent (motor) function is mediated through the 9th, 10th, and 12th cranial nerves. The cricopharyngeal sphincter opening is reflexive; relaxation occurs when the bolus reaches the posterior pharyngeal wall prior to reaching this sphincter.

Cranial Nerves

- CN V—Trigeminal nerve contains both sensory and motor fibers that innervate the face and is important in chewing.
- CN VII—Facial nerve contains both sensory and motor fibers and is important for the sensation of oropharynx and taste to anterior two-thirds of the tongue.
- CN IX—Glossopharyngeal nerve contains both sensory and motor fibers and is important for taste to the posterior tongue and the sensory and motor functions of the pharynx.
- CN X—Vagus nerve contains both sensory and motor fibers, provides taste to oropharynx and sensation and motor function to the larynx and laryngopharynx, and is important for airway protection.
- CN XII—Hypoglossal nerve contains motor fibers that primarily innervate the tongue.

Thyroid Cartilage

The thyroid cartilage is a shield-like structure composed of two plates that meet to form a notch. The thyroid notch is more prominent in men than in women. The prominence of the Adam's apple in males is due to the more acute angle at which the thyroid laminae meet, with a greater anteroposterior diameter. At the posterior aspect of each lamina there are horns on the superior and inferior aspects. The inferior horn has a circular facet that allows it to articulate with the cricoid cartilage.

Cricoid Cartilage

The cricoid cartilage is shaped like a signet ring. It has articular facets that attach to the thyroid cartilage and the arytenoids. It is separated from the thyroid cartilage by the cricothyroid ligament, or membrane.

- It is important to identify the cricoid cartilage because the cricothyroid membrane is contiguous with it inferiorly. In acute airway obstruction, the cricothyroid membrane may be penetrated with a needle, knife, or tube and connected to an oxygen source via a standard 15-mm connector. Cricothyrotomy is the first procedure performed to relieve asphyxiation in situations where intubation and mask ventilation are impossible. The hyoid bone, which is not part of the larynx proper, is attached to the thyroid cartilage by the thyrohyoid ligament. The inferior horn of the thyroid cartilage, joined by the cricothyroid ligaments, articulates with the cricoid cartilage bilaterally. Cricothyrotomy is performed by penetrating this ligament.

Paired Cartilage

The arytenoids are triangular structures located on the posterosuperior aspect of the cricoid cartilage.

The Lower Airway

The lower airway is composed of the trachea, two mainstem bronchi, and terminal and respiratory bronchioles. The scope of this section will be limited to the trachea and bronchi in relation to the patient with a tracheostomy.

Trachea

The trachea is a tubular structure, about 15 cm long in adults, extending from the cricoid cartilage to the bronchial bifurcation. It has an outer diameter of 2.5 cm. It consists of 16 to 20 C-shaped cartilages joined by fibroelastic tissue and closed posteriorly by the trachealis muscle. At the level of the fifth thoracic vertebra, the trachea bifurcates into right and left mainstem bronchi. The right (more than the left) mainstem bronchus appears to be a vertical continuation of the trachea; furthermore, the right upper lobe bronchus has its origin about 2 cm from the carina, compared to the left, which arises about 5 cm from the carina. For these reasons, aspiration of food, liquid, or foreign bodies is far more likely to occur on the right side, and right mainstem intubations are more common than left.

The trachea begins at the inferior border of the cricoid ring. The sensory supply to the tracheal mucosa is derived from the recurrent laryngeal branch of the vagus nerve. The trachea is between 9 and 15 mm in diameter in the adult and is 12 to 15 cm long. It may be somewhat larger in the elderly. The adult male trachea will generally easily accept an 8.5-mm inner diameter (ID) ETT; a 7.5-mm ID ETT may be preferable in women. If the patient being intubated might require bronchoscopic pulmonary toilette after admission (e.g., due to chronic obstructive pulmonary disease or airway burns), consider increasing to a 9.0-mm ID tube for men or an 8.0-mm ID tube for women.

- It is physiologically important to note that the upper part of the trachea is extrathoracic, whereas the lower half is intrathoracic. This relationship creates different behaviors during inspiration and expiration. The extrathoracic trachea, which is subject to the effects of ambient atmospheric pressure, decreases slightly in caliber during inspiration and increases during expiration. By contrast, the intrathoracic trachea undergoes expansion during inspiration as a result of negative intrathoracic pressure transmitted from the pleural cavity. During expiration, however, surrounding pleural pressure diminishes the tracheal caliber, which may be exaggerated in the setting of marked increased expiratory effort in airway obstruction.
- Forces affecting airflow through the airways can be categorized as those that facilitate airflow and those that oppose it. In general, differences in pressure drive airflow in and out of the respiratory system from areas of higher to lower pressure. The lung contains two different pressure systems, whereas the chest wall exerts a separate one. The force driving airflow is the difference between the airway opening, or mouth (Pm), and the pressure in the alveoli (Palv) and the pleural space (Ppl). The difference between these two pressures is called the transpulmonary pressure (PL, the pressure across the lung). The pressure across the chest wall (Pcw) is the difference between the pleural pressure (Ppl) and the atmospheric pressure (PB) (see Table 1.1).
- Forces opposing airflow in the airways result from elastic, flow resistive, or inertial properties of the respiratory system. Collectively, they result in pressure drops across the respiratory system. Inertance deals with the mass of the lung and the acceleration of these tissues and the linear acceleration of gas in the lung. Thus, pressure losses due to inertial forces increase progressively as respiratory frequency increases but are generally

1.1 Pressure Differences Across the Respiratory System

Airway (Paw)	Palv – Pm
Lung (PL)	Palv – Ppl
Chest wall (Pcw)	Ppl – PB
Total respiratory system (PRS)	Palv – PB

Paw: airway pressure; Palv: pressure in alveolar spaces; PB: atmospheric pressure; Pcw: pressure of the chest wall; PL: lung pressure; Ppl: intrapleural pressure (estimated at esophageal pressure); Pm: mouth pressure (or airway opening); PRS: total pressure within the respiratory system.

negligible during quiet breathing. Elastance, and its reciprocal compliance, reflect the relationship between pressure and volume when there is no airflow. Hence, these measures are static. By contrast, resistance is dependent on the rate of changes of lung volume (i.e., flow) during active breathing and are, thus, dynamic pressures.

Comparative Anatomy of the Adult and Infant Airways

The anatomical differences between the adult and infant airways include the position and shape of the larynx, tongue, epiglottis, and bronchi (see Figure 1.5). In proportion to the rest of the body, the infant's head is much larger than the adult's, so its weight forces the cervical spine to assume a more flexed position, which easily produces airway obstruction. The infant's tongue is proportionately larger than that of the adult's and with lack of muscle tone may "fall back," obstructing the flow of air during inspiration and expiration. Furthermore, the epiglottis is omega shaped, longer, and stiffer.

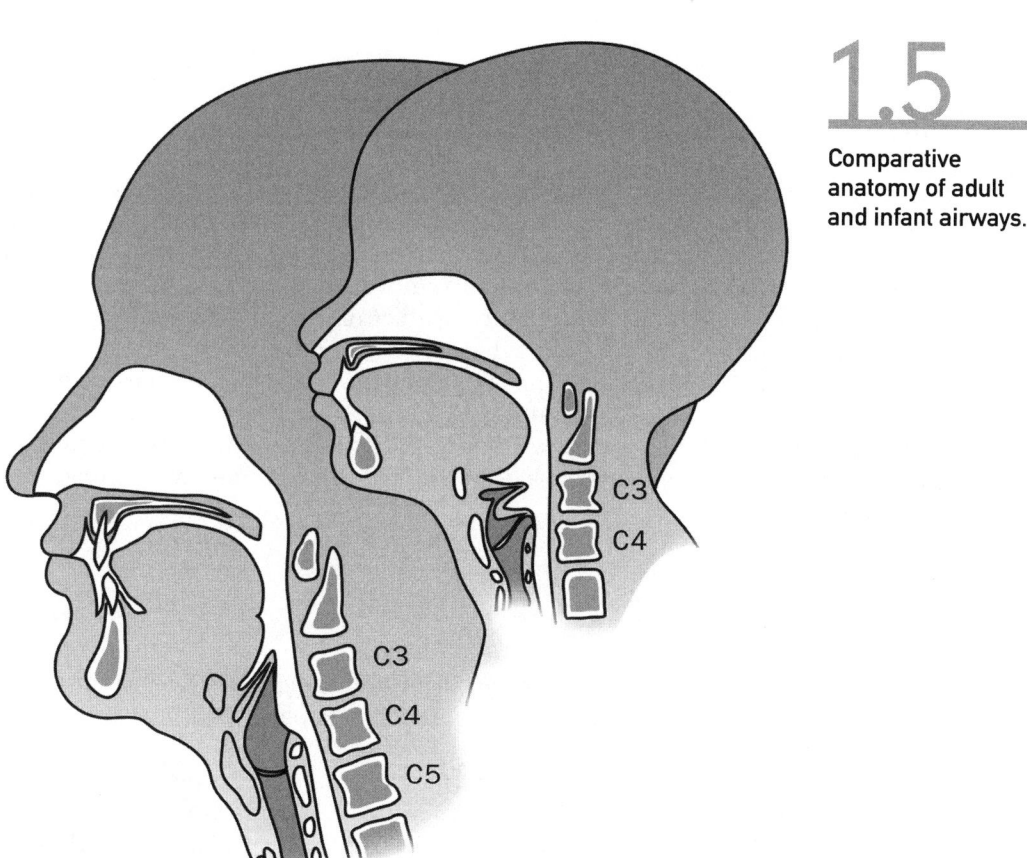

1.5

Comparative anatomy of adult and infant airways.

The larynx is situated at a higher level in relation to the cervical spine in infants. At birth, the rima glottidis lies at the level of the interspace between the third and fourth cervical vertebrae. Upon reaching adulthood, it lies one vertebra lower. The narrowest part of the infant's laryngeal airway is at the level of the cricoid cartilage, whereas that of the adult is at the rima glottidis. At age 8, the larynx of the child closely resembles that of the adult except in size. The infant's vocal cords are concave and lie more horizontally. The biggest difference between the adult and infant larynx is that the overall diameter of the adult's airway is 10 to 12 mm wider than that of the newborn. If the internal diameter of a neonate's larynx is 4 mm at the level of the cricoid cartilage, a 1-mm circumferential reduction in this diameter (caused by either trauma or infection) would reduce the overall cross-sectional area of the airway by approximately 75%. A similar reduction in the diameter of the adult airway would reduce the cross-sectional area by about 44%.

The major conducting airways are both narrower and shorter in infants, leaving less room for error in positioning endotracheal tubes. The trachea of a premature infant may be as short as 2 cm. In infants, the bifurcation of the trachea (into right and left mainstem bronchi) projects at an angle of about 30 degrees from tracheal axis, whereas the angle of the left mainstem bronchus and tracheal axis is more acute. Thus, in infants the right mainstem bronchus is less vertical than in adults (Morris, 1988).

Conclusion

Functional anatomy is important to understand when treating the patient with a tracheostomy tube. Paying attention to the nuances of anatomy in relation to technique will often mean the difference between success and failure in tracheostomy tube placement as well as removal and the host of day-to-day functions (respiratory, swallowing, and vocalization) in between. A clear understanding of the relevant anatomical structures, their blood supply, and their innervation will enhance understanding of this interdependent relationship. A study of the airway's functional anatomy will also guide the best approaches for instrumentation and intervention with each patient. It also provides a basis for understanding how complications are best avoided or, if they occur, how they may be detected.

Key Points

- The upper airway provides a natural conduit for gas exchange, it humidifies and protects the lower airway and participates in the functions of deglutition and phonation.
- Alteration of pharyngeal anatomy may lead to the development of obstructive sleep apnea (OSA) and upper airway obstruction.
- The larynx is the organ of phonation. Disruption of its highly innervated structure immediately interferes with upper airway patency and, thus, impedes respiration.

- Deglutition and phonation are highly coordinated processes between several structures of the upper airway and gastrointestinal tracts, and are dependent on intact sensory and motor innervation.
- Pediatric airway anatomy varies from that of adult anatomy in the size of the head, the position of the larynx, the shape of the epiglottis, the angle of the mainstem bronchi, and, most importantly, the diameter of the upper airway.

References

Ayappa, I., & Rapoport, D. M. (2003). The upper airway in sleep: Physiology of the pharynx. *Sleep Medicine Review, 7,* 9.

Ellis, H., & Feldman, S. (1993). *Anatomy for anaesthetists* (6th ed.). Oxford, England: Blackwell Scientific.

Grande, C. M., Ramanathan, S., & Turndorf, H. (1988). The structural correlates of airway function. *Problems in Anesthesia, 2,* 175–182.

Haponik, E. F., Smith, P. L., Bohlman, M. E., Allen, R. P., Goldman, S. M., & Bleecker, E. R. (1983). Computerized tomography in obstructive sleep apnea: Correlation of airway size with physiology during sleep and wakefulness. *American Review of Respiratory Diseases, 127,* 221.

Morris, I. R. (1988). Functional anatomy of the airway. *Emergency Medicine Clinics of North America, 6,* 639–669.

Redden, R. J. (2000). Anatomic considerations in anesthesia. In C. A. Hagberg (Ed.), *Handbook of difficult airway management* (pp. 1–13). Philadelphia, PA: Churchill Livingstone.

Schwab, R. J., Gefner, W. B., Pack, A. L., & Hoffman, E. A. (1993). Dynamic imaging of the upper airway in normal subjects. *Journal of Applied Physiology, 74*(4), 1504.

Shorten, G. D., Opie, N. J., Graziotti, P., Morris, I., & Khangure, M. (1994). Assessment of upper airway anatomy in awake, sedated, and anaesthetized patients using magnetic resonance imaging. *Anaesthesia and Intensive Care, 22,* 165.

Tracheotomy Procedure

Michiel J. Bové and M. Sherif Afifi

Despite being one of the more common surgical procedures, tracheotomy can be one of the most challenging because of the medical complexities presented by many patients requiring it. Anatomical limitations make the trachea difficult to assess in certain patients, and emergent situations and nonoperative settings provide less than ideal circumstances.

Tracheotomy was first described nearly 3,500 years ago, making it one of the earliest recorded surgical procedures. Alexander the Great was alleged to have carried out a tracheotomy in the fourth century B.C. (Frost, 1976). The first successful tracheotomy is attributed to Antonio Musa Brasavola, who published his account of the procedure in 1546 A.D. The initial indications for the procedure were limited to life-threatening airway obstruction, and associated rates of mortality were therefore extremely high. The eventual expansion of its indications as well as the standardization of its methods produced wider acceptance of the procedure. Chevalier Jackson's description of his modifications to the procedure, published in 1909, improved its efficiency and safety and reduced the mortality of tracheotomy from 25% to less than 2%. This improved procedure also reduced the incidence of tracheal stenosis, particularly in children.

Jackson's systematic analysis led him to recognize the importance of several factors, including avoiding too high an incision or dividing the cricoid cartilage, using an appropriate cannula, and providing appropriate postoperative care.

Indications for Tracheotomy

The indications for tracheotomy placement in the adult population can be grouped into four broad categories: A tracheotomy can be performed to relieve a mechanical obstruction, manage aspiration and promote bronchial hygiene maneuvers, provide long-term ventilation (while avoiding the long-term complications of translaryngeal intubation), and promote weaning from mechanical ventilator support. The indications for tracheotomy were recently defined by the American Academy of Otolaryngology—Head and Neck Surgery in the Clinical Indicators Compendium (2009) seen in Table 2.1.

The decision to perform a tracheotomy remains complex; however, a consideration of multiple factors is necessary to ensure optimal patient outcome. Relevant factors include the relative risk of tracheotomy versus alternative means of providing an artificial airway, characteristics of the patient's respiratory anatomy and physiology, the patient's specific pathologic process and prognosis, available institutional facilities, and skilled personnel.

Whenever possible, acute upper airway obstruction should be managed with endotracheal intubation while other prioritized supportive care is provided. Angioneurotic edema, temporary bilateral vocal cord paralysis, and epiglottitis are examples of acute airway obstruction in which temporary orotracheal intubation usually obviates the need for a surgical airway. Alternatively, if planned interventions such as radiation therapy or surgery predict airway obstruction, a tracheotomy can be performed prior to treatment to protect the airway. Tracheotomy is also frequently performed as part of head and neck surgical procedures involving free tissue transfer reconstruction in the oral cavity, oropharynx, hypopharynx, or larynx. In these cases, postsurgical edema may be deleterious

2.1 Indications for Tracheotomy as Defined by the American Academy of Otolaryngology—Head and Neck Surgery in the Clinical Indicators Compendium

1. Prolonged or expected prolonged intubation
2. Inability of patient to manage secretions
3. Facilitation of ventilation support
4. Inability to intubate
5. Adjunct to manage head and neck surgery
6. Adjunct to manage significant head and neck trauma

to the viability of the newly placed flap and may lead to obstruction and reintubation because of altered anatomy.

Tracheotomy may be necessary in cases of laryngotracheal trauma, facial trauma, obstructing upper aero-digestive tract neoplasm, or even severe angioneurotic edema, in which intubation may not be technically feasible. Rarely, tracheotomy is used in severe cases of obstructive sleep apnea where medical treatments have failed and other forms of surgical correction are not appropriate.

Timing of Tracheotomy

The decision about the most appropriate time to perform a tracheotomy should balance the likelihood of laryngeal injury due to the continued use of an endotracheal tube versus the likelihood of surgical or stoma-related complications following tracheotomy (see Table 2.2) (Stone & Bogdonoff, 1992).

There is no convincing evidence that endotracheal intubation should be limited to a specific time frame to prevent laryngeal dysfunction. However, many clinicians believe only patients who are unstable or unlikely to benefit from tracheotomy should be ventilated via an endotracheal tube for more than 21 days (Heffner, 1993; Plummer & Gracey, 1989). Part of the rationale is that tracheotomy improves patient comfort and communication and enhances nursing care (Bishop, 1989). A multicenter international study of 1,638 patients found that tracheotomy was performed after a median of 11 days, suggesting this view is widespread (Esteban et al., 2000).

2.2 Comparison of Tracheotomy and Endotracheal Intubation

Tracheotomy	Endotracheal Intubation
■ Reduced need for sedation	■ Easier and quicker to perform compared with tracheotomy
■ Reduced damage to glottis	■ Tolerated well for short periods
■ Reduced work of breathing (by reducing dead space)	■ Weaning more difficult after long-term placement
■ Reduced patient discomfort	■ Requires sedation
■ More invasive and complicated compared with endotracheal tube placement	■ Prevents aspiration of secretions
■ Scar formation	■ Can be used to give certain medications (e.g., adrenalin)
■ Tracheotomy site can bleed or become infected	■ Need to warm and filter gases as the nose, which would normally provide this function, is bypassed
■ Requires skill to perform the procedure	■ Improper placement can occur (e.g., esophageal placement)
■ May be associated with long-term complications (e.g., swallowing difficulties)	

Early tracheotomy has been supported by a number of studies. In a randomized trial, Rumbak and co-investigators (2004) compared early tracheotomy (within 48 hours) to late tracheotomy (14 to 16 days) in 122 medical patients with respiratory failure who were expected to require mechanical ventilation for more than 14 days. They found the early group had significantly decreased mortality (31.7% versus 61.7%), incidence of hospital-acquired pneumonia (5% versus 25%), length of intensive care unit (ICU) stay (4.8 versus 16.2 days), and duration of mechanical ventilation (7.6 versus 17.4 days). In a meta-analysis of five studies (406 patients), Griffiths, Barber, Morgan, and Young (2005) found that early tracheotomy (within 7 days) was associated with a shorter duration of mechanical ventilation as well as a shorter length of ICU stay. In a retrospective cohort study of more than 10,000 tracheotomy patients, Scales, Thiruchelvam, Kiss, and Redelmeier (2008) compared those who underwent early tracheotomy (within 10 days) with those who underwent late tracheotomy (after 10 days). The early tracheotomy group had more ventilator-free days and a significant reduction in 90-day mortality (34.8% versus 36.9%), 1-year mortality (46.5% versus 49.8%), and study mortality (63.9% versus 67.2%). Better outcomes were associated with early tracheotomy in all of the diagnostic subgroups except for patients with a history of cardiac disease, in whom early tracheotomy was associated with an increased risk of death at 90 days (relative risk 0.135, 95% CI 0.003–0.285).

Other studies argue against early tracheotomy, however. One observational study of 54 male veterans found that laryngeal pathology was significantly worse among patients who had undergone a tracheotomy 24 hours previously compared to patients who were extubated without a tracheotomy (Colice, Stukel, & Dain, 1989). There was no association between severe laryngeal complications and duration of endotracheal intubation in this study.

In a prospective, randomized study by Blot and coauthors (2008), 123 patients requiring prolonged intubation were randomized to early tracheotomy (within 4 days) versus prolonged intubation. There were no significant differences in any clinical outcome, including mortality, incidence of pneumonia acquired in the ICU, number of ventilator-free days, time in ICU, number of septic episodes, sedation requirement, and laryngeal or tracheal complications. The trial was underpowered, however, since it was terminated early due to poor recruitment.

Taking these data together, early tracheotomy (i.e., within 7 to 10 days of mechanical ventilation) appears appropriate for patients for whom weaning and extubation are not likely before day 14, provided the patient is stable. For those patients for whom early tracheotomy is not chosen, a daily evaluation of the probability that mechanical ventilator support will be needed beyond 21 days should determine the timing of tracheotomy as long as the patient is stable and benefits are anticipated.

Preoperative Management

The patient with an unstable airway represents the most acute of medical emergencies. Proper management requires the coordinated mobilization of a well-trained team of physicians, nurses, and respiratory care practitioners. Initial intervention, if feasible, should be via orotracheal intubation or rigid bronchoscopy. If these modalities are contraindicated or not possible, tracheotomy should be performed in the operating room where resources are readily available. In elective situations, however—for the stable, intubated patient—open bedside tracheotomy is performed more frequently in the ICU setting. Bedside tracheotomy has the advantages of decreased transport-related risks, operating room cost, and schedule burden. Regardless of the setting, adequate lighting (especially headlights), suction, and assistance should be available. If possible, the anesthesia team should be present during tracheotomy for intensive cardiovascular and respiratory monitoring, to assist with mechanical ventilation, and to provide any necessary cardiopulmonary resuscitation. Frequently, patients with chronic respiratory obstruction develop elevated carbon dioxide levels, leading to loss of respiratory drive after the establishment of a surgical airway. Preoperative laboratory profiles, including coagulation, hemoglobin, and electrolytes, should be reviewed. Any abnormalities should be corrected and remain stable prior to elective tracheotomy.

The patient should be optimally positioned and secured. The neck should be extended (unless contraindicated) with a shoulder roll. For tracheotomies performed in an emergency on patients in respiratory distress, optimal neck extension is usually not tolerated, and the procedure is performed with the patient in the semi-Fowlers position. The patient's face, neck, chest, and shoulders should be sterilized with prep solution. The patient's face should not be draped—both to allow easy access to the endotracheal tube as well as to avoid the collection of flammable, oxygen-enriched vapors beneath the drapes. Further, the use of alcohol-based antiseptics calls for strict adherence to the proper use of these substances, including observing the required drying time. It is also recommended that whenever electrocautery or diathermy is used on the skin, one of many aqueous-based antiseptics be used. If an alcohol-based antiseptic is used, it should be cleaned off with a dry swab before the diathermy is used.

Anesthesia Management

Typically, patients presenting for tracheostomy are either intubated patients in chronic respiratory failure, those suffering major trauma, or patients for whom tracheostomy is part of a scheduled procedure (e.g., radical neck dissection). Features of the history and physical exam that may be associated with a difficult airway include: (a) specific anatomic characteristics (e.g., bull neck, large tongue, receding jaw, limited mouth opening, difficulty visualizing posterior pharynx, diminished cervical spine range of motion, and obesity); (b) either inspiratory stridor (signifying obstruction at or above the level of the larynx) or expiratory stridor (signifying subglottic or intrathoracic obstruction); (c) hoarseness (vocal cord lesion or dysfunction); (d) tachypnea; (e) marked respiratory effort; (f) dyspnea; (g) a previous history of thyroid gland or neck surgery, trauma, or radiation therapy; (h) a history of previous difficult intubation or vocal cord paralysis; and (i) infections such as epiglottitis or Ludwig's angina (Nekhendzy, Guta, & Champeau, 2009).

Preoperative Evaluation

Patients with respiratory insufficiency may require mechanical ventilation with positive end-expiratory pressure (PEEP) to maintain adequate oxygenation.

The continued application of PEEP is important during transport from the ICU to the operating room. Based on the assessment, the anesthesiologist must decide whether to choose a direct laryngoscopy, an awake fiberoptic intubation, or a tracheotomy under local anesthesia to secure the airway. Often, these patients have a long history of smoking, with consequent chronic obstructive pulmonary disease (COPD). If symptoms of worsening pulmonary function are present, helpful preoperative testing includes pulmonary function tests (PFT) and arterial blood gases.

The most valuable cardiovascular history is exercise tolerance and the presence of any symptoms with exertion. If the patient reports incapacitating dyspnea, chest pain, or light-headedness with climbing more than two flights of stairs or on occasion at rest, then further testing is indicated, including a stress test or even a coronary angiography. Pre-existing risk factors include smoking, alcohol abuse, male gender, hypercholesterolemia, hypertension, and a family history of cardiovascular disease.

Hematologic profiles are also essential to exclude conditions of anemia or abnormal coagulation, especially in cases of malignancy or chronic disorders. Preoperative laboratory data should survey a complete blood count, prothrombin time (PT), activated thromboplastin time (PTT), and platelet count. Any existing preoperative neurologic deficits should be documented clearly. Finally, the patient should have nothing by mouth for at least 6 hours prior to the procedure. Similarly, enteral feeding via a nasogastric tube should be stopped 6 hours prior to the tracheostomy procedure (Brown, 1996).

Premedication

Standard premedication for elective cases is an anxiolytic benzodiazepine, most commonly midazolam (approximately 2 mg IV). However, premedication is best avoided if the airway is compromised or in emergency procedures.

Anesthetic Technique

The anesthetic technique of choice for tracheotomy is general anesthesia with endotracheal intubation.

Equipment and Monitoring

The ASA (American Society of Anesthesiologists) standard monitoring is used and includes continuous pulse oximetry, capnography, and electrocardiography (ECG), along with frequent blood pressure measurements (every 3–5 minutes). For patients with critical end-organ dysfunction (neurologic or cardiovascular), arterial blood pressure should be used for closer monitoring. Peripheral intravenous access must be ensured with the placement of, at minimum, a 20-gauge intravenous catheter that infuses well.

A preprocedure patient safety checklist for bedside tracheotomies in the ICU is provided in Table 2.3 for reference. Low FiO_2, which avoids airway fires when electrocautery is needed during surgery, can be maintained by using a regulator for mixing oxygen and air to target FiO_2 around 30% oxygen concentration

2.3 Bedside Tracheostomy Preprocedure Checklist

Members Present
- Surgeon: _____
- Anesthesiologist: _____
- RN: _____

Key Elements
- Patient is stable to undergo procedure at this time.
- Bipolar vs. monopolar cautery has been considered.
- Both CO_2 and ABC fire extinguishers have been located with their triggers, and the responsible person has been outlined to the team.
- Main O_2 gas shut-off valve in the ICU has been located, and the responsible person has been outlined to the team.
- Skin antisepsis: product is confirmed alcohol-free.
- Drape does not cover mouth, endotracheal tube, or ambu bag.
- FiO_2 level has been coordinated with electrocautery.
- Time Out has been performed and documented.

while ensuring the patient's blood oxygen saturation stays at a minimum of 94% or higher (see Figure 2.1).

Induction

If already intubated, preexisting sedation should be converted to general anesthesia using carefully titrated induction agents. If not intubated and no airway problems are anticipated, a standard induction may be appropriate. If airway problems are anticipated, an awake fiberoptic intubation is the method of choice. In any event, the anesthesiologist should be prepared to deal with a failed intubation and must have a surgeon immediately available to perform a tracheotomy if ventilation proves impossible.

A popular regimen is propofol for hypnosis and fentanyl for analgesia, in addition to a muscle relaxant to keep the patient immobile during the surgical procedure, particularly at the point of tracheotomy.

Induction: Propofol 1–1.5 mg/kg

Muscle relaxation: Succinylcholine 1.5–2 mg/kg if a difficult intubation is anticipated (half-life is 5 min); if a difficult intubation is not anticipated, a nondepolarizing muscle relaxant such as rocuronium can be administered at a dosage of 0.6 mg/kg (half-life is 20–30 min)

Maintenance

The simplest maintenance is to administer a hypnotic, an analgesic, and a muscle relaxant.

2.1

The O$_2$ regulator can be adjusted to dial the FiO$_2$ (in %) up or down depending on the use of electrocautery and patient oxygen requirements. An oxygen analyzer is used to calibrate the concentration of oxygen from the O$_2$ regulator. An air/O$_2$ gas mixture is delivered through a humidifier to a resuscitation ventilation bag, which the anesthesiologist uses to deliver manual breaths in concert with surgical maneuvering. A capnograph must be used as a standard monitor for tracheotomy procedures to confirm adequate ventilation and access to the upper airway.

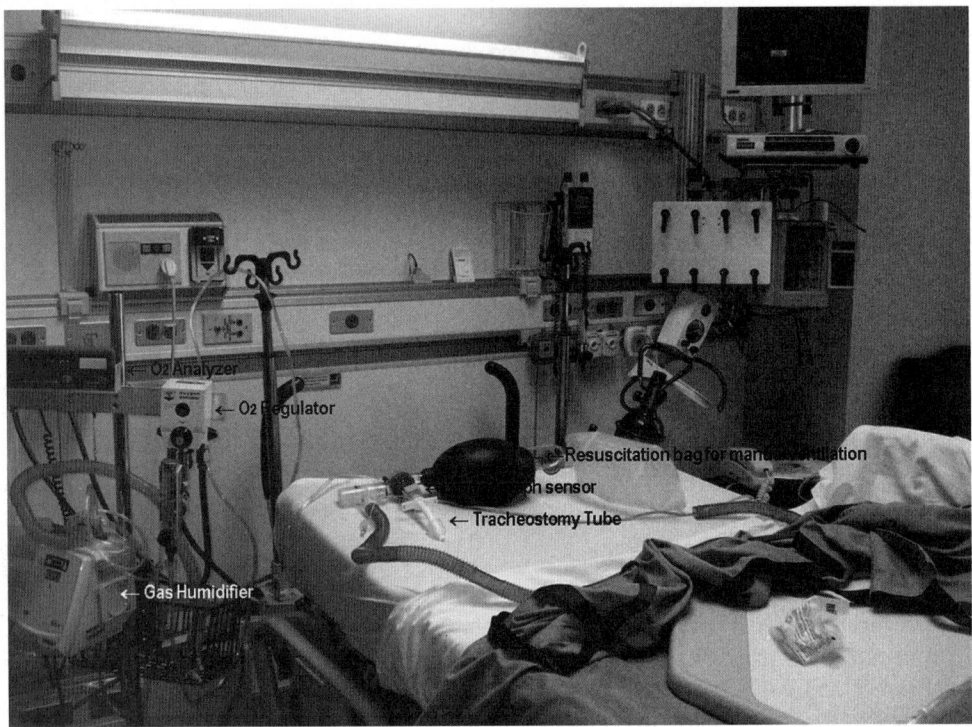

- Propofol infusion: 40–100 mcg/kg/min
- Fentanyl infusion: 3 mcg/kg/hr, or a total of approximately 250 mcg for the entire procedure (it is helpful to administer the fentanyl a few minutes before the surgeon enters the trachea, which, in general, is the time of highest stimulation); a fentanyl dose of 150–200 mcg IV can ablate a significant increase in intracranial pressure in patients with intracranial hypertension and presumed loss of autoregulation of cerebral blood flow with intracranial pathology

Fluid requirements average 1–2 ml/kg/hr for the entire procedure, and blood loss is minimal, particularly when tracheotomy is done as an isolated procedure.

A rigid bronchoscope should be available to reestablish the airway in case of a failed reintubation. Alternatively, a large-bore airway exchange catheter can be advanced through the bronchoscopy elbow adapter attached to the existing ETT prior to tracheostomy tube insertion in patients at high risk for failed reintubation. Frequently, when tracheostomy is a prelude to a more major procedure, an anode tube is inserted through the tracheostomy and sutured in place. It is replaced at the end of surgery by a cuffed tracheostomy tube.

Emergence

Besides analgesia, surgical site hemostasis, and adequate gas exchange, there are no special considerations for emergence following tracheotomy. Opioid sedation and analgesia will blunt any reactions to suctioning in the early postoperative period.

Complications

Postoperative surveillance for complications should look for pneumothorax, hemorrhage in the form of an obstructing hematoma, aspiration of blood, loss of airway requiring reintubation, difficult endotracheal tube reinsertion, and pneumomediastinum. Pneumothorax may also occur with low neck dissection. A postoperative chest radiograph will define the position of the tracheostomy tube and survey for the presence of pneumothorax or pneumomediastinum.

Surgical Technique

The surgical technique for tracheotomy has evolved throughout history. The division of the thyroid isthmus was first described by Degarengot in 1720 (Grillo, 2003). Tracheotomies continued to be performed high; because of the relative speed and ease of this approach, this practice was not altered until 1909, when Jackson described the increased rates of subglottic stenosis associated with high tracheotomy placement. Today, many variations in technique are still commonplace. Current technique can nonetheless be divided into two broad categories: the open surgical approach and percutaneous dilatational tracheotomy.

Surgical Anatomy

The sternal notch and thyroid and cricoid cartilages are usually easily palpable through the skin. A key surface landmark, the cricoids, is usually found by using the thyroid cartilage above and the sternal notch below as reference points. The cricothyroid membrane spans the anterior aspect of the thyroid and cricoid cartilages. It is identified by palpating a slight indentation in the skin inferior to the thyroid notch. The paired cricothyroid arteries traverse horizontally along the superior aspect of this membrane and anastomose in the midline.

The cricothyroid muscles arise from the anterior surface of the cricoid and extend superiorly and posteriorly to attach to the lateral surfaces of the thyroid alae. The innominate, or brachiocephalic, artery crosses from left to right, just anterior to the trachea at the superior thoracic inlet and deep to the sternal notch. Its pulsations are often felt during dissection of the anterior tracheal wall. The trachea is comprised of 18 to 22 semicircular cartilaginous rings and is posteriorly separated from the esophagus by a membranous portion. The average width of the tracheal lumen is 2.3 cm in the coronal dimension and 1.8 cm in the sagittal dimension. The average length of the adult trachea is 11 cm, with a range of 12 to 15 cm.

The thyroid gland lies anteriorly to the trachea with each thyroid lobe lying laterally, and the isthmus crosses it anteriorly at the level of the second to fourth tracheal rings. The endocrine tissue is highly vascular and must be handled carefully to prevent bleeding. The recurrent laryngeal nerves and inferior thyroid veins travel in the tracheoesophageal grooves and are out of the surgical field unless dissection strays significantly. The great vessels, too, are lateral to the intended dissection and should be avoided.

Open Tracheotomy

The open surgical tracheotomy can be performed in the operating room or at the bedside in a monitored setting such as the ICU. The procedure is most commonly performed under general anesthesia in a previously intubated patient. Occasionally, when the patient presents in acute distress, the procedure is performed in the nonintubated patient under local anesthesia, while the patient breathes spontaneously.

The patient is placed on the operating table with a bolster underneath the shoulders to extend the neck and expose the laryngotracheal landmarks (Figure 2.2A). This maneuver is contraindicated in patients with cervical spine injuries or atlantoaxial instability, as seen in Trisomy 21 syndrome, where neck extension can result in spinal cord compression. Certain patients with tenuous airways may not be able to tolerate either neck extension or even the supine position, requiring tracheotomy to be performed with the patient in a sitting position without neck extension. Patients with significant kyphoscoliosis, cervical osteoarthritis, or other conditions in which the neck cannot be hyperextended can present a significant technical challenge.

The procedure begins with the palpation of the landmarks of the neck, including the thyroid cartilage, cricoid cartilage, and sternal notch. A marking pen can be used to indicate the relative position of each of these crucial landmarks on the skin of the extended neck (Figure 2.2B). Lidocaine (usually 1% with a 1:100,000 dilution of epinephrine) is injected into the skin and subcutaneous tissues where the incision will be placed. The neck and upper chest are prepared in povidone-iodine (Betadine) solution, and the surgical site is draped to allow easy access to the oral cavity so the endotracheal tube can be easily mobilized and manipulated by the anesthesiologist during the procedure. A critical precaution involves avoiding the use of Bovie cautery in the presence of alcohol-based surgical prep solution (DuraPrep). The risk of surgical fire associated with the incomplete drying of this agent in the context of electrosurgical procedures has been described previously (Weber, Hargunani, & Wax, 2006). Particular risks are associated with head and neck operations when an oxygen-enriched atmosphere can develop under the surgical drapes. This is a significant risk during the use of oxygen-rich gas delivery from nasal cannulas or ventilation masks when the procedure is performed on the awake, spontaneously breathing patient. The use of electrocautery in these circumstances constitutes a significant hazard.

A 2–3 cm incision is carried out in a vertical or horizontal fashion (Figure 2.3). The horizontal incision provides a more cosmetically pleasing postoperative scar, as it follows the relaxed skin tension lines. This benefit decreases, however, the longer the tracheostomy remains in place. Vertical incision avoids the anterior jugular venous system, therefore minimizing cumbersome bleeding in cases of emergency tracheotomies. Vertical incisions start just below the cricoid cartilage, whereas horizontal incisions are made either two finger's breadths below the cricoid cartilage or halfway between the cricoid cartilage and the sternal notch, typically over the interspace between the second and third tracheal rings. The subcutaneous tissues are then divided with either a 15 blade or Bovie electrocautery to the level of the strap muscles. Care should be exercised at this stage to avoid damage to the anterior jugular vein, which, when identified, should be lateralized or ligated in order to avoid unnecessary bleeding. Once identified, the strap muscles should be divided vertically along their midline raphe until the thyroid isthmus is exposed (Figure 2.4).

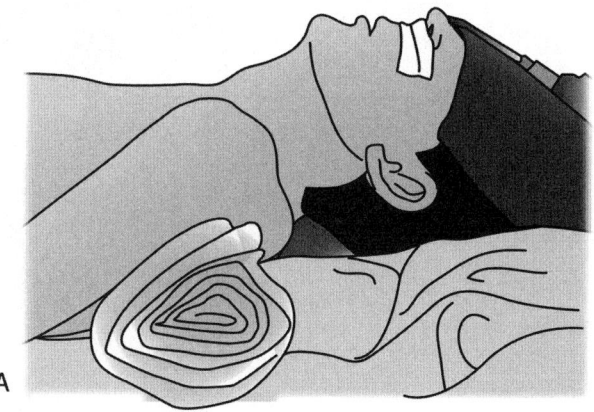

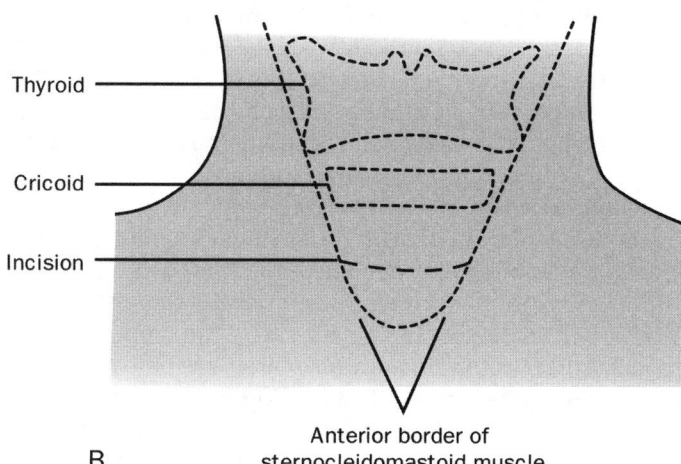

2.2

Surgical tracheotomy preparation. (A) Patient positioning with roll under shoulders. (B) Surface landmarks showing the thyroid, the cricoid, the intended location of the skin incision, and the anterior border of the sternocleidomastoid muscle.

2.3

Surgical tracheotomy procedure. (A) Initial incision. Note the anterior border of the sternocleidomastoid muscle. (B) Incision with spreaders.

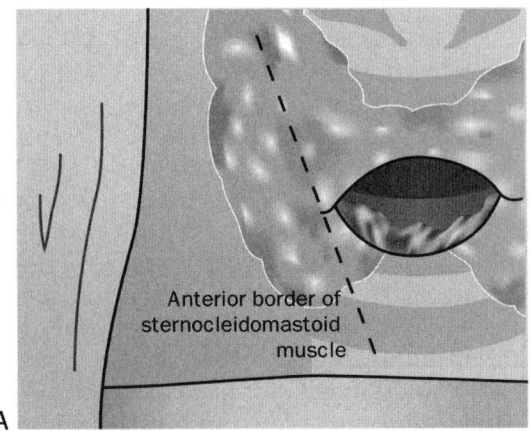

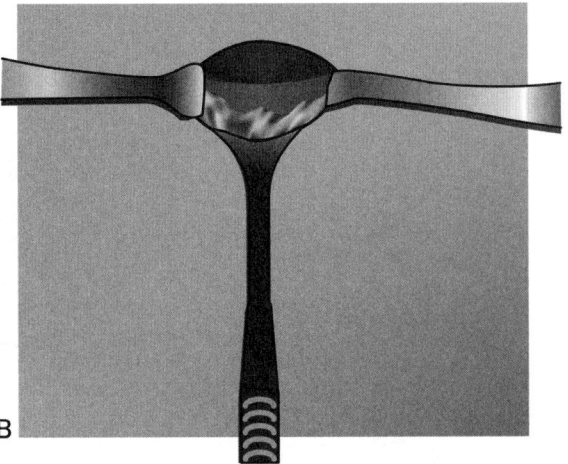

The thyroid gland can be handled in a number of ways. Depending on the location of the isthmus within the surgical wound, the isthmus can be retracted superiorly, inferiorly, or divided and ligated to expose the second and third tracheal rings, where the tracheal window will be performed (Figure 2.5). The cricoid cartilage serves as an important landmark during this portion of the dissection. Often, traction placed on the cricoid cartilage using a cricoid hook mobilizes the laryngotracheal complex into more favorable, superior, and superficial position to allow easier access into the trachea.

The pretracheal fascia is dissected off the proximal trachea using a Kitner sponge. With patients having tracheotomy under local anesthesia, it is important to inject local anesthetic into the pretracheal tissues prior to opening the trachea in order to provide proper analgesia. In addition, a 2% lidocaine solution can be applied transtracheally to obtain topical endoluminal anesthesia. There are multiple incision types for entrance into the trachea. Some surgeons prefer a single horizontal intercartilaginous incision, while others perform an H-type incision or make a tracheal window by removing a centimeter-wide portion of

2.4

Surgical tracheotomy procedure. (A) Exposure of the thyroid isthmus. Note the thyroid isthmus is exposed over the proximal trachea. (B) The thyroid isthmus is cross-clamped and divided.

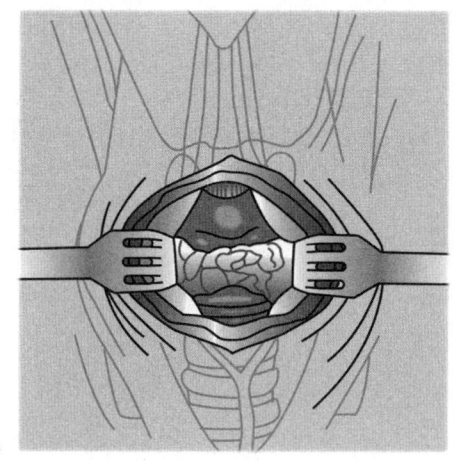
A

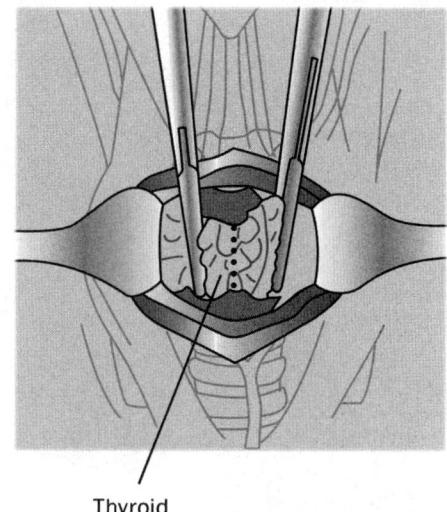
B

Thyroid isthmus

the anterior aspect of the second or third tracheal ring. The type of incision does not seem to affect the development of postoperative tracheal stenosis in either animal models (Natvig & Olving, 1981; Whitley, Castillo, Hassett, Banyas, & Luchette, 1997) or humans. An inferiorly based trap door flap (Bjork flap) can be created by incising the interspace between the second and third tracheal rings as well as the third tracheal ring laterally on both sides, extending inferiorly from the interspace incision. The superior aspect of the flap is then sutured to the inferior aspect of the skin incision with a nonabsorbable suture. This flap facilitates reinsertion of the tracheostomy tube in cases of accidental decannulation, especially in obese patients or those with difficult anatomy. Despite commonly expressed concerns, a study by Malata, Foo, Simpson, and Batchelor (1996) suggests there is no increased rate of either tracheostenosis or tracheocutaneous fistula with use of the Bjork flap. Another option for managing the anterior tracheal wall is the removal of an anterior section of the second or third tracheal rings using a scalpel, Metzenbaum scissors, or tracheal punch.

Once the trachea is entered, a tracheotomy dilator is used to optimize exposure to the tracheal lumen, taking care to prevent excess trauma to the cartilaginous framework of the trachea. Upon visualization of the endotracheal tube within the lumen, the anesthesiologist is asked to withdraw the tube until the posterior tracheal wall is visualized. The tracheostomy tube is then introduced into the lumen of the trachea under direct visualization. In cases of patients with a history of difficult intubation, the endotracheal tube can be withdrawn over a tube exchanger to facilitate reintubation in case tracheostomy tube placement

2.5

Surgical tracheotomy procedure. (A) Removing tracheal ring to form window. (B) Stay sutures are placed superiorly and inferiorly to the stoma.

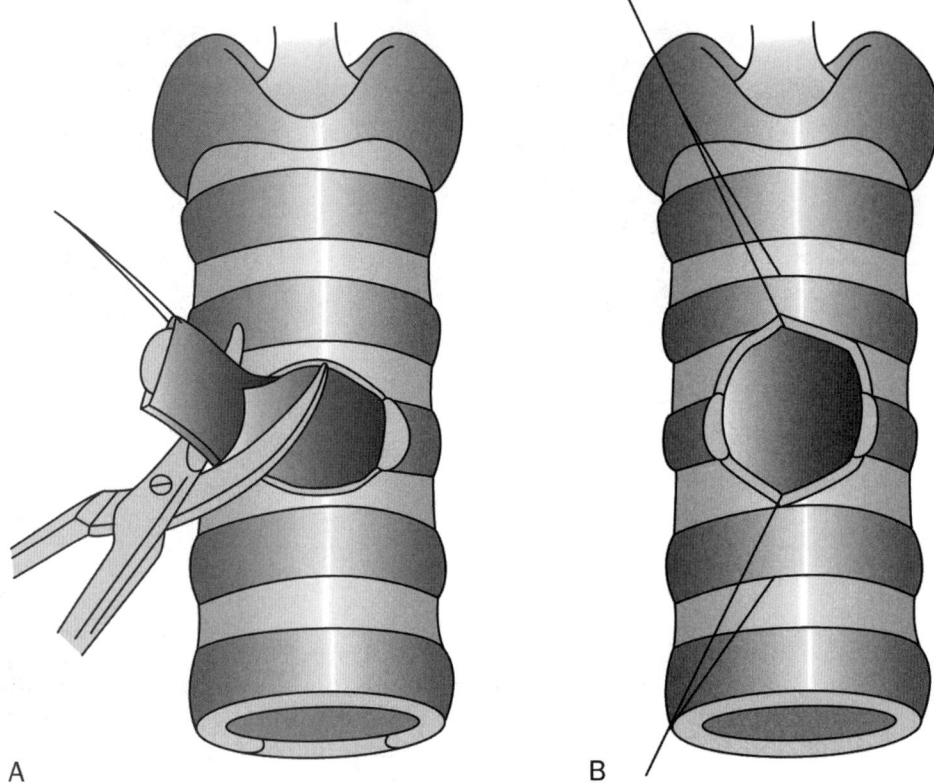

proves difficult. After introduction of the tracheostomy tube, proper placement should be confirmed before the endotracheal tube is removed. This is done by detecting carbon dioxide return from the tracheostomy tube and then suctioning the tracheal contents with a flexible suction catheter. If proper placement of the tracheostomy tube cannot be confirmed via these steps, the endotracheal tube should be reintroduced by the anesthesiologist. Once successfully placed, the tracheostomy tube should be secured into place with nonabsorbable sutures placed through the flanges of the tube (Figure 2.6) as well as tracheostomy ties placed around the patient's neck.

Percutaneous Dilatational Tracheotomy (PDT)

In 1953, Seldinger (1953) introduced the technique of percutaneous guide wire needle placement in arterial catheterization. Soon the guide wire technique, now known as the Seldinger technique, was adapted to various procedures,

2.6

Neck flange sutured in place.

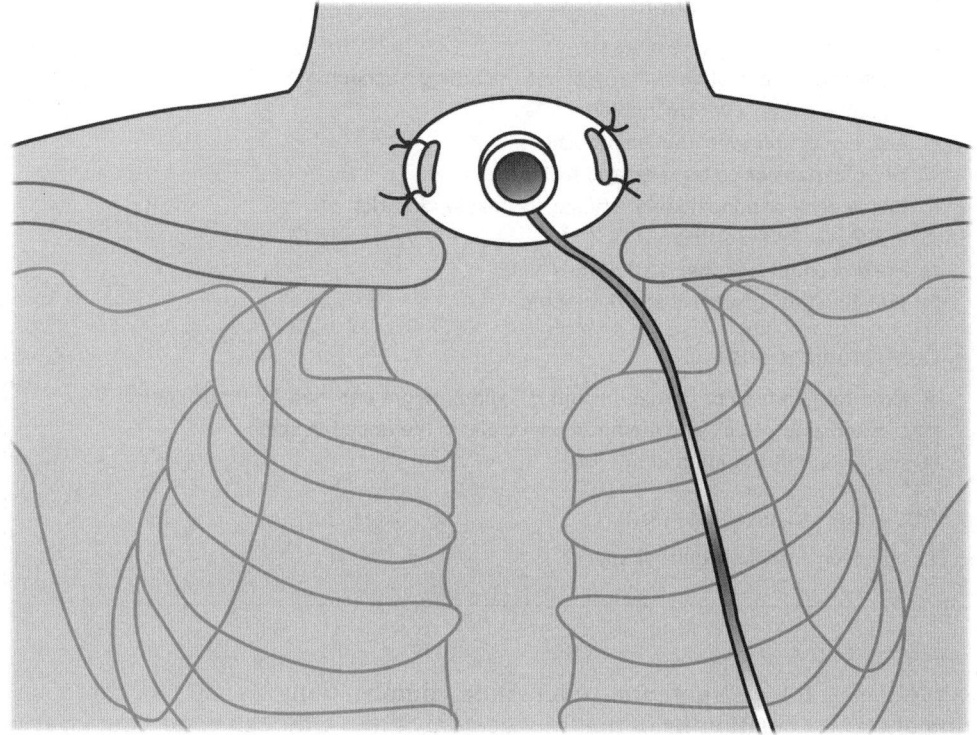

including percutaneous tracheotomy. The first modern percutaneous dilatational tracheotomy (PDT) was reported by Shelden, Pudenz, Freshwater, and Crue (1955) in 1955, but the complication rate was very high due to the laceration of adjacent structures by the trocar. In 1969, Toy and Weinstein (1969) developed a tapered straight dilator with a recessed cutting blade for performing percutaneous tracheotomy over a guiding catheter. The technique of PDT using serial dilators over a guide wire was first described in 1985 by Ciaglia, Firshing, and Synlec (1985). In 1989, Schachner and colleagues developed a dilating tracheotomy forceps over a guide wire. In 1990, Griggs, Worthley, Gilligan, Thomas, and Myburg developed another guide wire dilating forceps specifically for percutaneous tracheotomy. Shortly thereafter, convenient kits to create a full-sized percutaneous tracheotomy became readily available.

PDT involves the placement of a tracheostomy tube without direct visualization of the trachea. The general consensus is that PDT should only be performed on intubated patients. It is considered to be a minimally invasive procedure that can be performed at the bedside in monitored settings. Bronchoscopic guidance is considered the standard of care, and a single surgeon or intensivist aided by a bronchoscopist can easily accomplish the procedure. The main benefit derived from direct bronchoscopic visualization during PDT is close, real-time

2.4 Contraindications to Percutaneous Dilatational Tracheotomy

Relative Contraindications
- Children under 12 years of age
- Anatomic abnormalities of the trachea, including tracheomalacia
- Palpable pulses over tracheotomy site
- Active infection over tracheotomy site
- Thyroid mass or goiter over tracheotomy site
- Obese neck or nonpalpable laryngotracheal landmarks
- PEEP greater than 15 cm H_2O
- Platelet count less than 40,000/mm^3
- Bleeding time greater than 10 minutes

Contraindications
- Prothrombin time or partial thromboplastin time greater than 1.5 times control
- Limited ability to extend the neck, especially in the unstable spine
- History of difficult intubation

Absolute Contraindication
- Need for urgent surgical airway

surveillance for any potential immediate complications, as well as confirmation of proper positioning of the tracheostomy tube. Although some controversy regarding PDT may still linger, numerous large series have been reported with comparable rates of complications.

The criteria for PDT are more stringent than for surgical tracheotomy (Couch & Bhatti, 2002; see Table 2.4). The laryngotracheal framework should be easily palpable through the skin. It is critically important that the patient's neck easily extends and that the patient can be easily reintubated in case of accidental decannulation. Obese patients, children, and those with abnormal coagulation are not candidates for this procedure. Clinicians performing PDT should be well trained in the technique, prepared to convert to an open surgical tracheotomy if needed, and ready to manage any immediate complications.

For this procedure, the patient is positioned and draped as for standard, open tracheotomy. A skin incision is made and the pretracheal tissue cleared with minimal blunt dissection. The endotracheal tube is withdrawn until the cuff is just at the level of the glottis. The endoscopist can place the tip of the bronchoscope such that the light from its tip is visible through the surgical wound, thus highlighting the target area. The operator then enters the tracheal lumen below the second tracheal ring with a needle introducer (Figure 2.7A–B). A guide wire is then inserted through the needle (Figure 2.8A–B). The track extending from the skin to the tracheal lumen is then serially dilated over a guide wire (Figure 2.9A–B). A tracheostomy tube is then introduced under direct bronchoscopic view over the dilator (Figure 2.10A–B). Proper placement is

2.7

Percutaneous tracheotomy procedure. (A) Insertion of needle between second and third tracheal rings. (B) Bronchoscopic view of needle insertion into trachea. (Bronchoscopic image provided courtesy of Alberto de Hoyos, MD.)

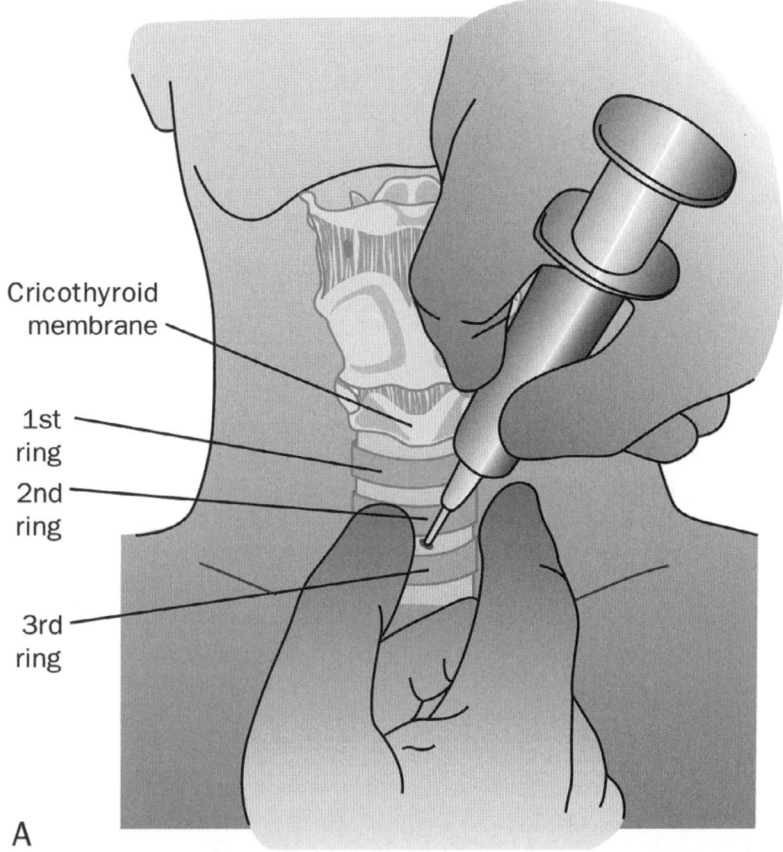

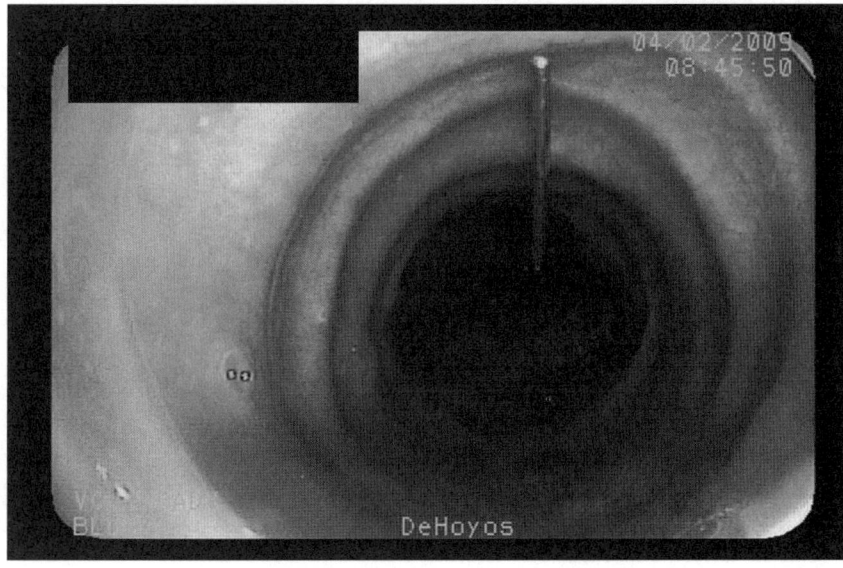

2.8

(A) Guide wire is placed through needle introducer. (B) Bronchoscopic view of guide wire through needle. (Bronchoscopic image provided courtesy of Alberto de Hoyos, MD.)

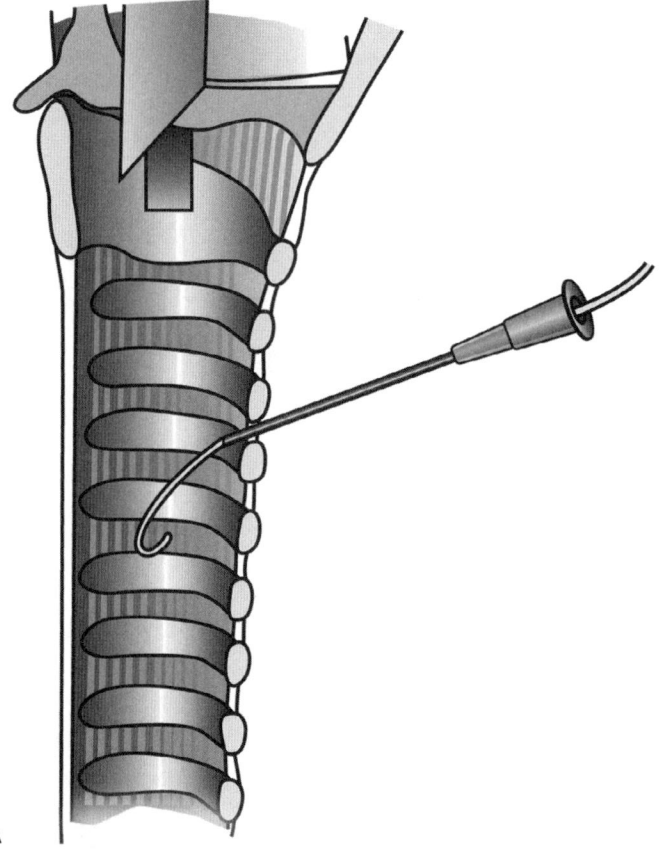

A

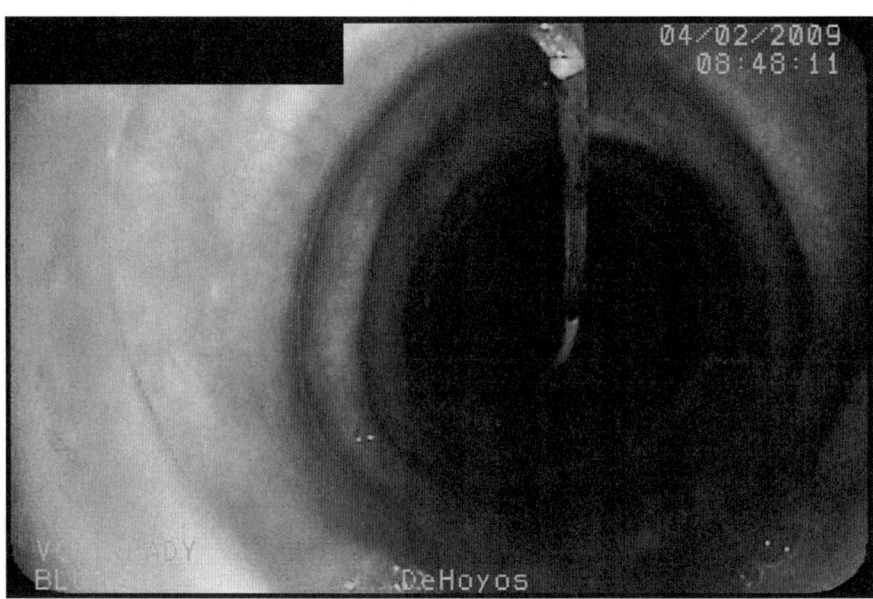

B

2.9

(A) Insertion of dilator over guide wire. (B) Bronchoscopic view of dilator over guide wire. (Bronchoscopic image provided courtesy of Alberto de Hoyos, MD.)

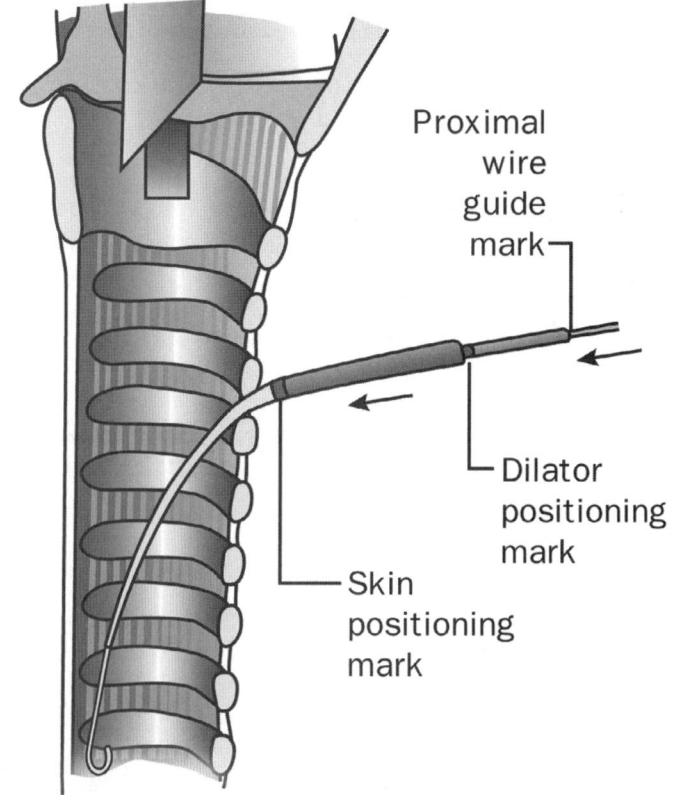

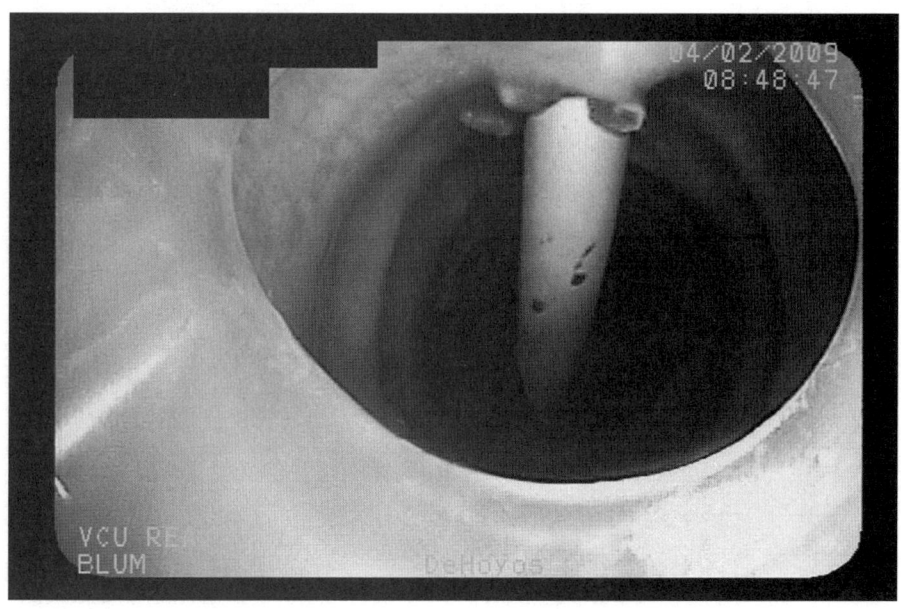

2.10

(A) Insertion of tracheostomy tube over dilator. (B) Bronchoscopic view of tracheostomy placed over dilator. (Bronchoscopic image provided courtesy of Alberto de Hoyos, MD.)

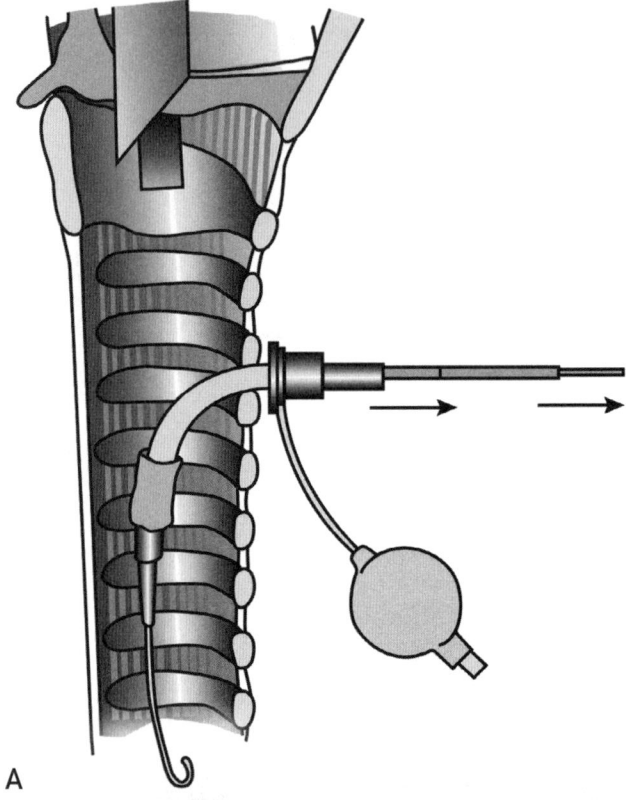

A

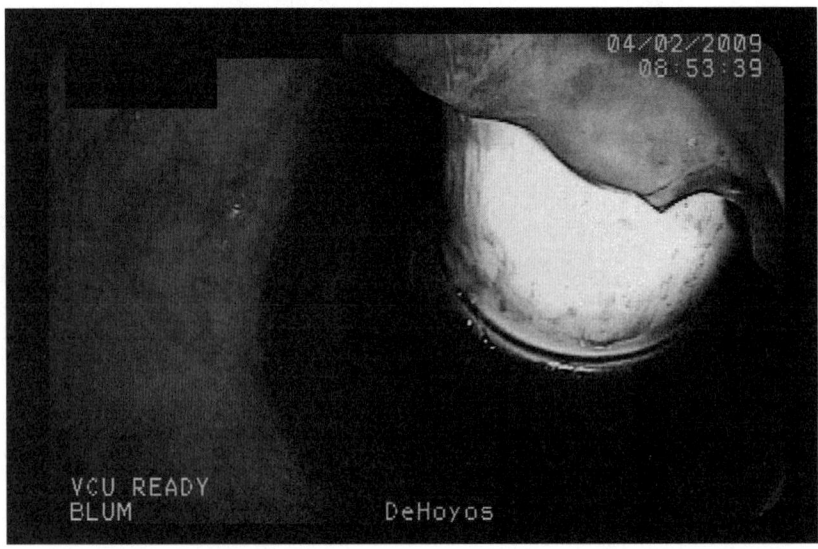

B

then confirmed by viewing the tracheobronchial tree through the tracheostomy tube, and the tube is secured into place with sutures and ties.

Pediatric Tracheotomy

As in adult tracheotomy, identifiable landmarks—including hyoid bone, thyroid notch, cricoid cartilage, thyroid isthmus, and sternal notch—are identified, and a skin incision is marked accordingly. It should be noted that these laryngotracheal landmarks are located relatively superiorly within the neck in the pediatric age group. Dissection then proceeds as in adults. Particular attention should be paid to avoid straying laterally due to the presence of the pulmonary apices within the cervical compartment in the younger age groups, which increases the risk of pleural puncture and resultant pneumothorax.

At the level of the trachea, the incision is generally made vertically through two or three tracheal rings, usually within the second to fifth tracheal rings. As in adults, an incision too close to the cricoid should be avoided, as it is associated with higher rates of subglottic stenosis.

Nylon traction sutures are placed in the trachea on either side of the incision line before the incision is made. These sutures serve to place traction on the tracheal rings during cannulation of the airway and are crucial in locating the tracheal window in cases of accidental tracheal displacement in the early postoperative period (Parnes & Myers, 1976). The vertical transtracheal incision should be long enough to easily allow passage of the tracheostomy tube in order to prevent undue damage to the integrity of the cartilage framework. Too small an incision or a horizontal intercartilaginous incision may lead to the collapse of the suprastomal tracheal ring as the curved tube exerts backward pressure on the ring above the incision.

After the tracheostomy tube is placed, it is secured in a similar fashion to adults. The traction sutures are tied loosely and taped to the skin of the anterior chest wall. Tape labels are used to clearly identify the right and left traction sutures so they are not reversed when used to recannulate the trachea, which would have the counterproductive effect of approximating the edges of the tracheal window.

The position of the tracheostomy tube with respect to the carina and tracheal wall can be determined via either passing a pediatric flexible endoscope through the tube or obtaining a postoperative chest radiograph. The tip of the tracheostomy tube should be 5 to 20 mm from the carina. The tube should not be so short that the lumen faces posteriorly or is at risk for exiting the tracheal window and entering a false pretracheal passage. Certain patients, such as obese children or those with metabolic storage diseases, may have excessively long tracts between the skin and trachea, requiring custom tracheotomy tubes with extra long proximal, extratracheal portions.

Postoperative Care

Postoperative care of the tracheostomy patient is considerably facilitated if there has been preoperative teaching, which helps both children and adults adapt to a new way of breathing. Family counseling is also important in order to optimize postoperative patient support for those able to be discharged. Highly skilled nursing care is crucial for success in this area.

In the initial postoperative period, the patient is usually placed in an intensive care setting in order to continuously monitor vital signs. Indeed, subtle changes in the patient's behavior, pulse, blood pressure, or respiratory rate may herald an obstruction of the tracheotomy tube with dried blood or secretions, which requires immediate attention. Tracheal suctioning must be performed as frequently as needed—often more frequently than would be possible outside of an ICU setting. The humidification of inhaled air is important for the mucociliary transport of secretions and to prevent the obstruction of the airway with dried secretions. The inner cannula must be removed frequently for cleaning and to avoid the accumulation of obstructing crusts. The tracheostomy tube is rarely changed before the third postoperative day to allow the tract to mature and to avoid tissue collapse that would seal off the airway. Tube replacement within the first 72 hours postoperatively should be done in the same conditions as the original procedure and requires adequate headlights, suction, cricoid hook, and assistance. Tube replacement is sometimes necessary if the cuff of the tracheotomy tube fails in a patient continuing to need positive-pressure ventilation after the procedure.

Summary

The surgical technique of tracheotomy should be adapted to the situation at hand, especially for patients with complicated neck anatomy, those with previous tracheotomies, or pediatric patients. Attention to detail during the procedure will help avoid the pitfalls and complications that can plague tracheostomy patients during the postoperative period. There continues to be controversy between open and percutaneous dilatational tracheostomy, but both have long track records, and application of one versus the other depends on the established practice patterns of individual clinicians.

Irrespective of the quality of intervention at the time of the procedure, long-term success and the prevention of complications depends on meticulous care during the postoperative period.

Key Points

- Open surgical tracheotomy can be performed in the operating room or the ICU, with bedside tracheotomies having the advantage of decreased patient transport risk, operating room cost, and schedule burden.
- Percutaneous dilatational tracheostomy has become an important alternative approach and is best performed under bronchoscopic guidance to identify immediate complications and confirm tube placement.
- After the procedure, patients require continuous monitoring of vital signs and are usually placed in an ICU.

Acknowledgment

Bronchoscopic images of percutaneous dilatational tracheotomy were provided by Alberto de Hoyos, MD.

References

American Academy of Ofolaryngology-Head and Neck Surgery (2009). Clinical Indicators Compendium: Tracheostomy. Retrieved November 2, 2009 from www.entnet.org/practice/clinicalIndicators.cfm

Bishop, M. J. (1989). The timing of tracheotomy: An evolving consensus. *Chest, 96,* 712.

Blot, F., Similowski, T., Trouillet, J. L., Chardon, P., Korach, J. M., Costa, M. A., et al. (2008). Early tracheotomy versus prolonged endotracheal intubation in unselected severely ill ICU patients. *Intensive Care Medicine, 34,* 1779–1787.

Brown, B. R. (1996). Anesthesia for ear, nose, throat, and maxillofacial procedures. In C. Prys-Roberts & B. R. Brown (Eds.), *International practice of anaesthesia* (pp. 2–9). Oxford, England: Butterworth-Heinemann.

Ciaglia, P., Firshing, R., & Synlec, C. (1985). Elective percutaneous dilational tracheostomy: A new simple bedside procedure. *Chest, 87,* 715–719.

Colice, G. L., Stukel, T. A., & Dain, B. (1989). Laryngeal complications of prolonged intubation. *Chest, 89,* 877.

Couch, M. E., & Bhatti, N. (2002). The current status of percutaneous tracheotomy. *Advances in Surgery, 36,* 275–296.

Esteban, A., Anzueto, A., Alia, I., Gordo, F., Apeztequia, C., Palizas, F., et al. (2000). How is mechanical ventilation employed in the intensive care unit? An international review. *American Journal of Respiratory Critical Care Medicine, 161*(5), 1450–1458.

Frost, E. A. (1976). Tracing the tracheostomy. *Annals of Otology, Rhinology, and Laryngology, 85*(5, Pt.1), 618–624.

Griffiths, J., Barber, V. S., Morgan, L., & Young, J. D. (2005). Systematic review and meta-analysis of studies of the timing of tracheotomy in adult patients undergoing artificial ventilation. *British Medical Journal, 330,* 1243.

Griggs, W. M., Worthley, L.I.G., Gilligan, J. E., Thomas, P. D., & Myburg, J. A. (1990). A simple percutaneous tracheotomy technique. *Surgery, Gynecology, and Obstetrics, 170,* 543–546.

Grillo, H. C. (2003). Development of tracheal surgery: A historical review. Part 1: Techniques of tracheal surgery. *Annals of Thoracic Surgery, 75,* 610–619.

Heffner, J. E. (1993). Timing of tracheotomy in mechanically ventilated patients. *American Review of Respiratory Disease, 147,* 768.

Malata, C. M., Foo, I. T., Simpson, K. H., & Batchelor, A. G. (1996). An audit of Bjork flap tracheostomies in head and neck plastic surgery. *British Journal of Oral and Maxillofacial Surgery, 34*(1), 42–46.

Natvig, K., & Olving, J. H. (1981). Tracheal changes in relation to different tracheostomy techniques (An experimental study on rabbits). *Journal of Laryngology and Otology, 95*(1), 61–68.

Nekhendzy, V., Guta, C., & Champeau, M. W. (2009). Tracheotomy/tracheostomy and cricothyroidotomy: Anesthetic considerations. In R. A. Jaffe & S. I. Samuels (Eds.), *Anesthesiologist's manual of surgical procedures* (pp. 187–189). Philadelphia: Lippincott Williams & Wilkins.

Parnes, S. M., & Myers, E. N. (1976). Traction sutures in a tracheostomy using a ligature passer. *Transactions. Section on Otolaryngology. American Academy of Opthalmology and Otolaryngology, 82*(4), ORL 479–485.

Plummer, A. L., & Gracey, D. R. (1989). Consensus conference on artificial airways in patients requiring mechanical ventilation. *Chest, 96,* 178–180.

Rumbak, M. J., Newton, M., Truncale, T., Schwartz, S. W., Adams, J. W., & Hazard, P. B. (2004). A prospective, randomized study comparing early percutaneous dilational tracheotomy to prolonged translaryngeal intubation (delayed tracheotomy) in critically ill medical patients. *Critical Care Medicine, 32*(8), 1689–1694.

Scales, D. C., Thiruchelvam, D., Kiss, A., & Redelmeier, D. A. (2008). The effect of tracheostomy timing during critical illness on long-term survival. *Critical Care Medicine, 36,* 2547–2557.

Schachner, A., Ovil, Y., Sidi, J., Rogev, M., Heilbronn, Y., & Levy, M. J. (1989). Percutaneous tracheotomy: A new method. *Critical Care Medicine, 17,* 1052–1056.

Seldinger, S. T. (1953). Catheter replacement of the needle in percutaneous arteriography. *Acta Radiologica, 39,* 368–376.

Shelden, C. H., Pudenz, R. H., Freshwater, D. B., & Crue, B. L. (1955). New method for tracheotomy. *Journal of Neurosurgery, 12,* 428–431.

Stone, D. J., & Bogdonoff, D. L. (1992). Airway considerations in the management of patients requiring long-term endotracheal intubation. *Anesthesia and Analgesia, 74*(2), 276–287.

Toy, F. J., & Weinstein, J. D. (1969). A percutaneous tracheotomy device. *Surgery, 65,* 384–389.

Weber, S. M., Hargunani, C. A., & Wax, M. K. (2006). DuraPrep and the risk of fire during tracheostomy. *Head and Neck, 28*(7), 649–652.

Whitley, R., Castillo, N., Hassett, J. M., Banyas, J., & Luchette, F. A. (1997). Early tracheostomal healing in rabbits with use of various tracheal incisions. *Wound Repair and Regeneration, 5*(4), 323–328.

3

Types of Tracheostomy Tubes and Related Appliances

Linda L. Morris

Each tracheostomy tube has a variety of features, and there are many different tracheostomy tubes to choose from. There are several manufacturers, and all offer different features, materials, lengths, inner and outer diameters, and so forth. Some have a single cannula, while others have dual cannulas—that is, both inner and outer cannulas. Some have low-pressure cuffs, and a few have high-pressure cuffs. Still others are cuffless. The choices are abundant.

Early tracheostomy tubes were composed of metal, either silver or stainless steel. Most modern tracheostomy tubes are composed of medical-grade plastics such as polyvinyl chloride, polyurethane, silicone, or a combination. Although metal tubes are still in use today, softer materials are much more widespread. Plastic tubes have the advantages of being cheaper, lighter, easier to modify for special needs, and, depending on the material, more pliable. These softer materials have allowed for cuffs at the distal end of the tube. Metal tracheostomy tubes have the advantage of thinner walls, but they usually cannot be connected to a ventilator because they do not have cuffs (Dhand & Johnson, 2006; St. John & Malen, 2004).

Tracheostomies

It is important for the clinician to be aware of the many tube choices available. Because of this variety and the specific features of each tracheostomy tube, most hospitals choose one line of tracheostomies for primary use by all clinicians, supplemented with others as the need arises. This is done primarily for safety reasons so that clinical staff can become familiar with the primary features of one particular line of tubes.

An effort will be made here to discuss the major characteristics of most of the tracheostomies currently on the market in the United States; however, it is important to consider that some of these tubes have limited use and information is sparse. First, we will discuss the major parts of the tracheostomy.

Parts of a Tracheostomy Tube

Most tracheostomy tubes are composed of only a few standard parts, as shown in Figure 3.1. For clarity, it is important to be familiar with the names of the major parts of a tracheostomy tube. The shaft of the tracheostomy tube fits,

3.1

Parts of a tracheostomy tube.

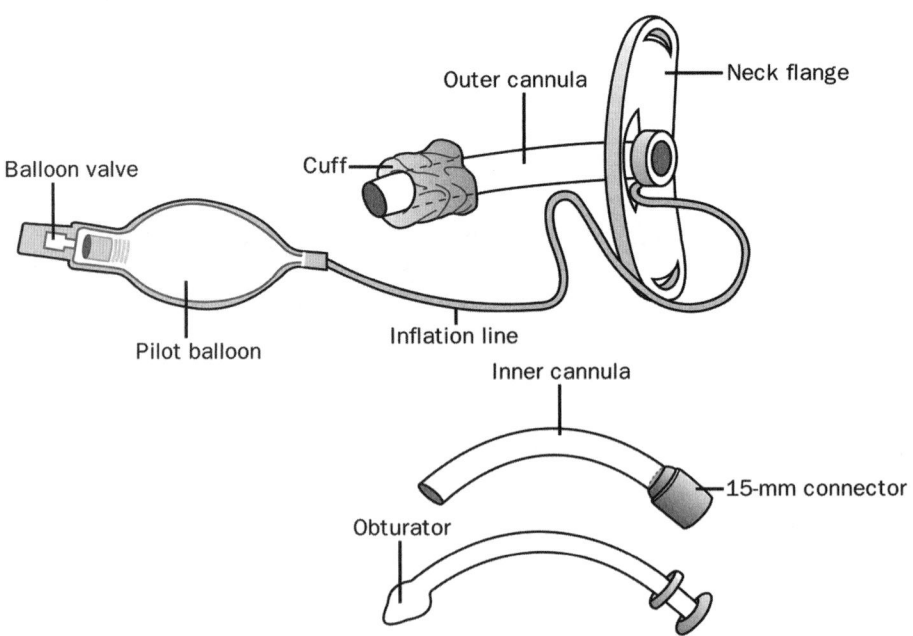

usually entirely, within the trachea. It may be constructed of plastic, silicone, or metal, and may be rigid or flexible. The outer diameter of the tracheostomy tube refers to the widest diameter of the tube itself, excluding the cuff. This diameter varies based on the materials used and the presence of an inner cannula. The outer cannula of each line of tracheostomies varies in terms of materials, length, diameter, angle of curvature, and presence of a cuff.

The curvature of the shaft can be angled differently from one type of tube to another. Figure 3.2 shows the varied curvature of tracheostomy tubes. Some tubes have a 90-degree angle, or an angle like the arc of a circle, and others have a narrower angle.

The neck plate, or neck flange, fits directly against the neck and allows the tracheostomy tube to be anchored to the neck. The outer cannula may or may not have a cuff. There may or may not be an inner cannula. Decisions about when and why to place a cuffed versus an uncuffed tracheostomy will be discussed in chapter 4. If a cuff is present, it is connected to the pilot balloon by means of an inflation line. The inflation port, or inflation valve, at the distal end of the pilot balloon allows for the attachment of a syringe to inflate the cuff. Nothing other than a syringe should be connected to the inflation port.

Sizing of a Tracheostomy Tube

The size of the tracheostomy tube usually refers to the inner diameter of the inner cannula. In other words, the inner diameter reflects the narrowest diameter of a particular tracheostomy tube. However, there are two sizing systems for tracheostomies: the Jackson sizing system and the International Standards Organization (ISO) sizing system. The Jackson sizing system was initially used

3.2

Curvature of shafts on different tracheostomy tubes. Note the relatively narrow angle of the tube on the left (Shiley SCT), compared to the wide angle of the tube on the right (Arcadia Air Cuff).

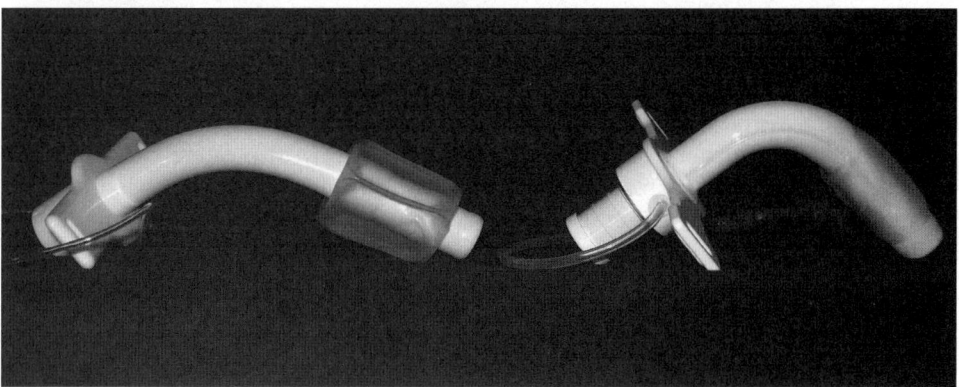

with metal tracheostomy tubes and is still used with the Jackson and Shiley brands. It is important to note that the two largest tracheostomy manufacturers in the United States (Portex and Shiley) use different sizing systems. The Shiley tracheostomies and all of the metal tracheostomy tubes use the Jackson sizing system, while the Portex, Bivona, TRACOE, and Arcadia tracheostomy tubes are sized using the ISO system. The ISO sizing system refers to the inner diameter of the outer cannula; however, the Jackson sizing system does not directly refer to the inner diameter (Dhand & Johnson, 2006; St. John & Malen, 2004). For example, the inner diameter of a size 6 Portex cuffed tracheostomy tube is 6.0 mm; however, the inner diameter of a comparably sized Shiley 6 cuffed tracheostomy tube is 6.4 mm.

St. John and Malen (2004) point out that one must consider the inner diameter of the tracheostomy both with and without the inner cannula in place. Some manufacturers state these two different inner diameters because it may make a difference when fitting a tracheostomy. When the inner cannula is in place, it can decrease the diameter of the tube by up to 2 mm. These 1 or 2 mm can sometimes make a surprising difference in a patient's ability to breathe comfortably.

The Inner Cannula

The inner cannula, when present, nests within the outer cannula and is secured to it. The primary purpose of the inner cannula is to clear secretions through cleaning or replacement at regular intervals. The standard inner cannula is used most often in the hospital setting because it frequently provides a 15-mm adapter—the standard connection for a manual resuscitation bag, ventilator tubing, and other respiratory and airway appliances. Cosmetic inner cannulas lack this adapter and give a low-profile appearance to the tracheostomy. Therefore, cosmetic or low-profile inner cannulas should probably not be used in the hospital to avoid confusion in case of an emergency. Outside of the hospital, the cosmetic inner cannula may be used when a low-profile appearance is desired.

It is important to ensure that the inner cannula, when present, is locked in place at all times. Different manufacturers provide different locking mechanisms for their tracheostomy tubes, and they are not interchangeable from one manufacturer to another, from one model to another, or from one size to another. Failure to lock the inner cannula can result in inadvertent dislodgement, as it may be easily coughed out.

The Obturator

The sole purpose of the obturator, sometimes called a pilot, is to assist with the insertion of the tracheostomy tube. Typically, it is necessary to remove the inner cannula in order for the obturator to fit within the outer cannula. The blunted tip of the obturator cushions the distal tip of the tube as it is inserted, avoiding potential tissue damage as it is advanced into the trachea. Immediately following placement, the obturator should be removed and replaced with the inner cannula (when present). The obturator should then be placed in full view, allowing rapid visualization and access in the event of an emergency, such as inadvertent decannulation.

The Neck Flange or Neck Plate

The purpose of the neck flange is to stabilize the tracheostomy tube, seating it against the neck and preventing it from migrating inward. The neck flange contains an opening at its lateral ends so it can be secured to the neck, typically by means of cloth tape, a soft collar, or sometimes a chain. The neck flange can be fixed to the shaft of the tube, or it can be adjustable and adaptable to a variety of needs.

The neck flange can be rigid or flexible. If rigid, it may tilt on the horizontal plane, the vertical plane, or both. This tilting mechanism is designed to provide comfort as well as adjust for patient movement; however, it can also be a source of inward traction against the stoma.

The neck flange is an important source of clinical information. The specifications of each tube are usually imprinted or embossed on it. One can usually find the manufacturer's name, the model name or code, the inner diameter, the outer diameter, and sometimes the length.

The Pilot Balloon and the Inflation Line

The inflation line is used to inflate or deflate the cuff. At the distal end of the inflation line is the cuff. At the proximal end of the inflation line are the pilot balloon and the inflation valve. The shape of the pilot balloon indicates whether or not there is air within the cuff. A completely flat pilot balloon indicates there is no air in the cuff, and an inflated pilot balloon indicates there is some air in the cuff. Many experienced clinicians believe they can accurately estimate cuff pressure by palpating the pilot balloon; however, one study showed that cuff pressure was accurately estimated by palpation only 61% of the time (Faris et al., 2007).

The Cuff

One of the primary purposes of the cuff is to seal the airway, especially with positive-pressure ventilation. When the cuff is inflated, there is no admixture of room air with inspired gases, and the patient breathes entirely through the tracheostomy tube. Deflation of the cuff allows for the admixture of room air as part of the inspired tidal volume.

Cuffs have evolved over time. Early tracheostomy tubes were made of metal, and early cuffs were detachable and often made of rubber. These rubber cuffs created high pressures against the trachea and resulted in numerous complications, including airway obstruction from detached cuffs. Over the years, these high-pressure cuffs have been almost totally replaced by high-volume, low-pressure cuffs (Quigley, 1988).

3.3

Shape of cuffs on different tracheostomy tubes. From left to right: Bivona TTS (low volume, high pressure), Shiley SCT (barrel shaped, low pressure, high volume), Bivona Fome-Cuf (low pressure, high volume), Portex Blue Line (teardrop shaped, low pressure, high volume).

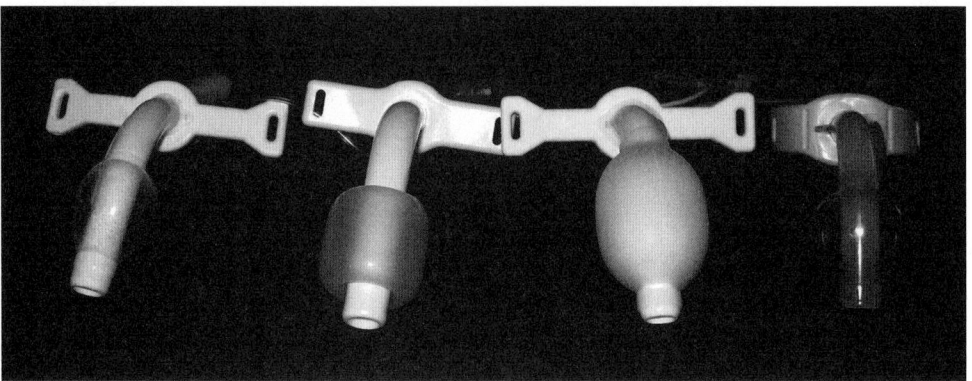

Cuffs come in different shapes, sizes, and types, some of which are illustrated in Figure 3.3. There are barrel-shaped cuffs, teardrop-shaped cuffs, and foam-type cuffs. There are cuffs that are filled with air and others that are filled with fluid. There are still some high-pressure cuffs, but today, most are low pressure. Each of these cuffs has different characteristics.

The barrel-shaped cuff is designed to diffuse pressure along a wider surface area. Rather than creating specific pressure points with a circular balloon, the barrel-shaped cuff minimizes pressure points.

The teardrop-shaped cuff was designed to minimize the pistoning effect—the up-and-down movement of the cuff with positive-pressure breaths. Pistoning will be discussed in chapter 5.

The foam-type cuff tracheostomy tube has an extra-large cuff that naturally expands to fit the shape of the trachea. It was designed to overcome problems with continued leaks around the cuff, while minimizing pressure-related problems.

A deflated cuff that lies tight to the shaft of the tracheostomy tube allows laminar airflow around it, lessening resistance. This is in contrast to the cuffs of most tracheostomy tubes, which have some bulk when deflated. Decisions regarding the most appropriate type of cuff are discussed in chapter 4.

The inflated cuff is used to protect the airway when the patient is unable to do so. It also creates a seal in the airway when delivering positive-pressure ventilation. Inflation of the cuff can help prevent secretions, fluid, or food from entering the lungs, but its success depends on many factors and is not guaranteed. It is important to realize that inflation of the cuff does not prevent aspiration. For a patient who cannot protect his airway, aspiration precautions must be maintained even though the cuff is inflated. This includes elevation of the head of the bed, checking residuals for the patient with enteral feedings, optimizing cuff pressure, and so forth.

Capillary perfusion pressure is considered to be between 20–30 cm H_2O (conversion factor to kPa: 1 cm water = 0.098 kPa; Bernhard, Yost, Joynes, Cothalis, & Turndorf, 1985; Duguet et al., 2007). The challenge is to maintain a cuff pressure high enough to ensure an adequate seal to provide optimal delivery of positive-pressure breaths and prevent the seepage of secretions around the cuff yet low enough to minimize pressure against the trachea.

Another purpose of the cuff is to seat the tube squarely in the center of the trachea and protect it from creating erosion against the trachea. Lateralization of the tube can result from herniation of the cuff and/or additional pressure against the trachea. Lateralization can also lessen optimal delivery of positive pressure, which can result in increased airway pressures.

General Types of Tracheostomy Tubes

Tracheostomy tubes can be classified into four major groups: dual-cannula, cuffed; dual-cannula, uncuffed; single-cannula, cuffed; and single-cannula, uncuffed. However, there are certain types of tracheostomy tubes that, while they fit into one of these general categories, have other unique features that have certain implications and require further discussion. These unique tubes include metal tracheostomy tubes, fenestrated tubes, and extra-length tubes. The following is a discussion of the wide variety of tracheostomy tubes available today, with some explanation of their strengths, weaknesses, and indications for use.

Standard Dual-Cannula Cuffed Tracheostomy Tubes

The standard dual-cannula cuffed tracheostomy tube is often the first choice for a patient who requires positive-pressure ventilation or otherwise cannot protect his or her airway. The inner cannula provides added protection for patients with copious secretions, as it can be easily removed and cleaned or replaced. It is locked in place to the outer cannula, and the method of securing the inner cannula varies by model. The features of different types of dual-cannula tracheostomy tubes are described in the following.

Shiley LPC (Low-Pressure Cuff)

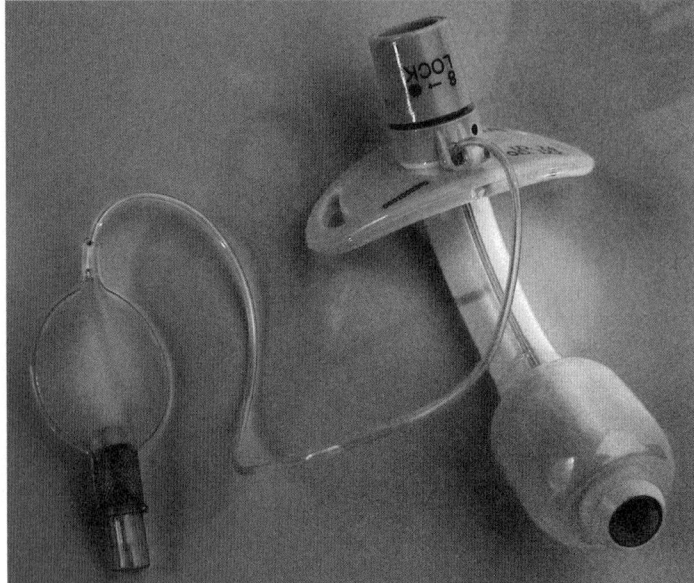

Structure: Cuffed, dual-cannula, arc of circle curvature
Material: Rigid polyvinyl chloride
Manufacturer: Covidien
Unique Features: Nondisposable inner cannula, rigid neck flange that tilts on horizontal plane
Use: Patients who require a cuffed tube for positive-pressure ventilation, airway protection, or when secretions are a concern

Shiley LPC tracheostomy tube (Covidien).

The Shiley LPC dual-cannula tracheostomy tube is made of a rigid polyvinyl chloride. The neck flange has a horizontal swivel mechanism that can accommodate some patient movement. The inner cannula locks in place with a twist-lock mechanism. When the blue dot on the outer cannula aligns with the blue dot on the inner cannula, it is locked in place. Unless the blue dots are aligned, the inner cannula can be easily dislodged or coughed out.

The 15-mm connector is built into the inner cannula of all Shiley dual-cannula tracheostomy tubes; therefore, an inner cannula must be with the patient at all times because respiratory and anesthesia equipment can only be attached when the inner cannula is in place. On the neck flange is printed the size, type, and internal and outer diameter of the tube. The lateral edges of the neck flange have openings of a somewhat softer material so it is easier to attach tracheostomy ties.

Shiley DCT (Disposable Inner Cannula)

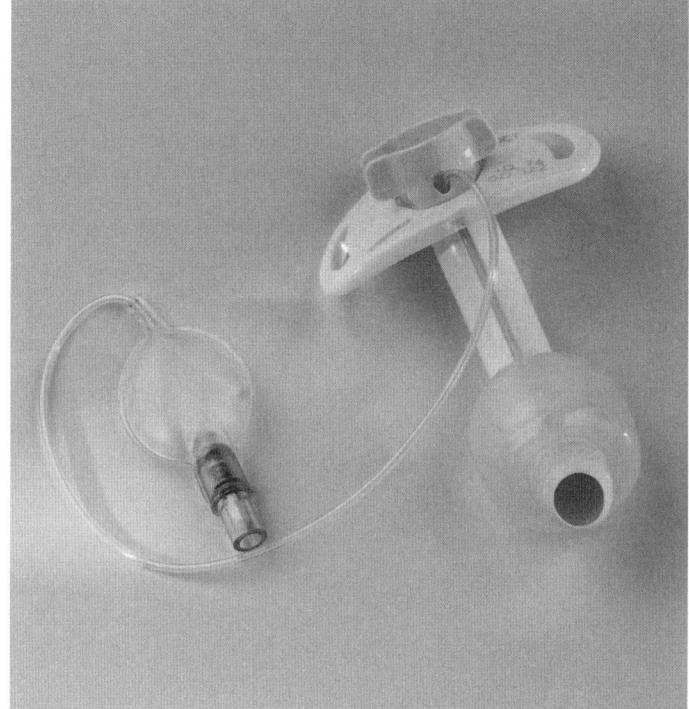

Structure: Cuffed, dual-cannula, arc of circle curvature
Material: Rigid polyvinyl chloride
Manufacturer: Covidien
Unique Features: Disposable inner cannula, rigid neck flange that tilts on horizontal plane
Use: Patients who require a cuffed tube for positive-pressure ventilation, airway protection, or when secretions are a concern

Shiley DCT tracheostomy tube (without inner cannula) (Covidien).

Covidien makes two standard-sized dual-cannula cuffed tracheostomy tubes. The Shiley LPC provides a nondisposable rigid inner cannula, and the Shiley DCT provides a somewhat softer, disposable inner cannula. The outer cannulas of the Shiley LPC and DCT tracheostomies are almost identical and are constructed of rigid polyvinyl chloride. The primary difference between these two tubes is their locking mechanisms and that the inner cannulas are not interchangeable. With the Shiley DCT, "wings" on each side are pinched together and provide a clipping mechanism (not unlike a telephone jack) when the inner cannula is locked in place. This is in contrast to the twist-lock mechanism of the LPC. The inner cannula of the Shiley DCT is constructed of a softer and more flexible material than the inner cannula of the LPC, and it is intended for limited-time use.

Another difference between the Shiley LPC and DCT tubes is the neck flange. The neck flange of the LPC is rounded and semiflexible; however, the neck flange of the DCT can be rectangular and rigid. For both the Shiley LPC and DCT, the inflation line lies on the shaft of the outer cannula. With all Shiley dual-cannula tracheostomy tubes, the attachment of a manual resuscitation bag or ventilator is possible only when the inner cannula is locked in place.

Shiley PERC (Percutaneous)

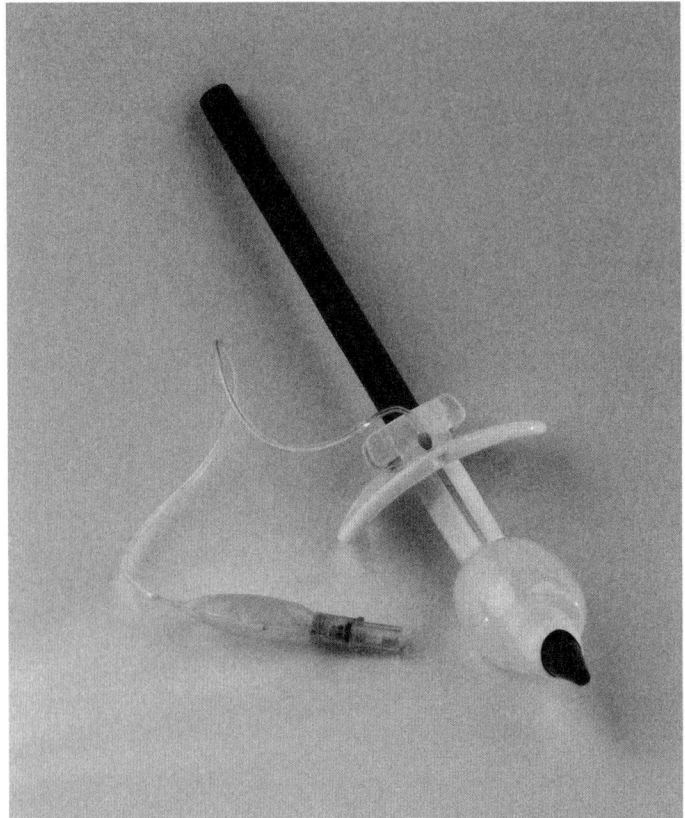

Structure: Cuffed, dual-cannula, arc of circle curvature
Material: Rigid polyvinyl chloride
Manufacturer: Covidien
Unique Features: Tapered distal tip and inverted cuff shoulder allow ease of insertion when loaded on dilator
Use: For use with percutaneous procedure

Shiley PERC tracheostomy tube loaded on Blue Rhino dilator (Covidien).

The Shiley percutaneous tracheostomy tube, PERC, is included in a kit manufactured by Cook Medical in their line of percutaneous tracheostomy introducer sets and trays. The tube itself is very similar to the Shiley DCT tube; however, the distal tip is tapered and the cuff has an inverted shoulder to facilitate its placement with an introducer. With the PERC, the introducer is also a dilator. Using the modified Ciaglia technique, the PERC is advanced into place while it is loaded on the dilator—called the Blue Rhino or the newer, fluid-filled Blue Dolphin.

Portex Per-fit

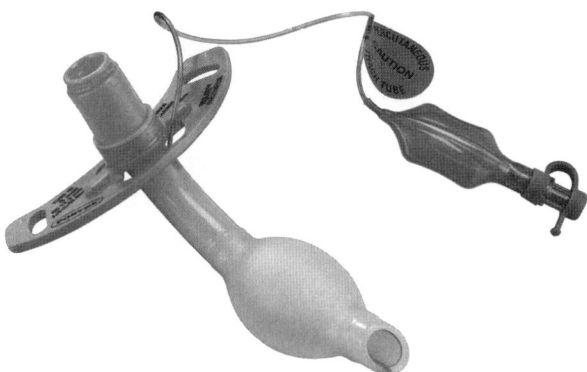

Structure: Cuffed, dual-cannula
Material: Flexible polyvinyl chloride
Manufacturer: Smiths Medical
Unique Features: Tapered distal tip allows ease of insertion over dilator
Use: For use with percutaneous procedure

Portex Per-fit tracheostomy tube. Note tapered distal tip of percutaneous tube for easier insertion over dilator. Photo courtesy of Smiths Medical.

The Portex version of the percutaneous tracheostomy is called the Portex Per-fit. The tube itself is made of flexible polyvinyl chloride with a tapered distal tip and low-profile cuff. The percutaneous tracheostomy kit has a series of dilators for use with the Ciaglia technique. (The percutaneous technique of tracheostomy placement is discussed in chapter 2.) The tapered distal tips of both the Shiley PERC and the Portex Per-fit are designed for an easier fit over a dilator, facilitating easier insertion.

Portex DIC

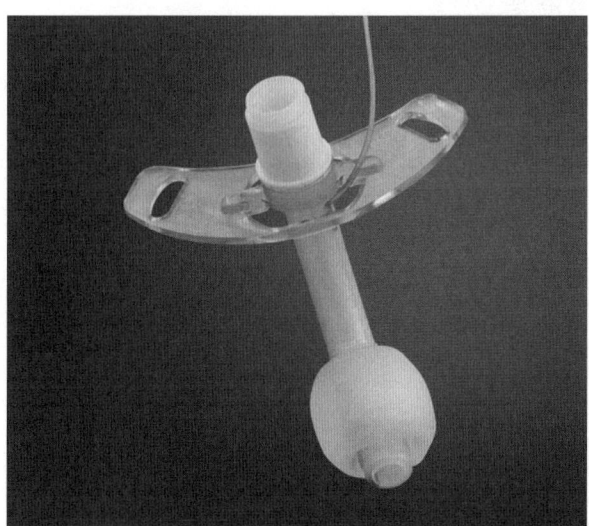

Structure: Cuffed, dual-cannula, arched curve
Material: Rigid polyvinyl chloride
Manufacturer: Smiths Medical
Unique Features: Color-coded inner cannula to identify size; the 15-mm connector is fused with the outer cannula so a manual resuscitation bag can be used without the inner cannula in place
Use: Patients who require a cuffed tube for positive-pressure ventilation, airway protection, or when secretions are a concern

Portex DIC cuffed tracheostomy tube. Photo courtesy of Smiths Medical.

3.1 Color-Coding Guide for Portex DIC Tracheostomies

Color of 15-mm Connector	Size (Inner Diameter)
Orange	6
Green	7
White	8
Blue	9
Yellow	10

Portex also makes two dual-cannula cuffed tracheostomy tubes. Made of polyethylene, the Portex DIC cuffed tracheostomy tube provides a rigid structure to the tube. The 15-mm adapter of the Portex DIC is color coded based on size. Table 3.1 shows the colors related to size.

The neck flange of the Portex tracheostomy tube is soft and pliable and may offer more comfort than a rigid neck flange. The inner cannula of the Portex DIC is removed by lifting up on the ring and pulling it out or pushing it in until it snaps in place. In contrast to the Shiley LPC or DCT, patients with a Portex DIC or Portex Flex DIC tracheostomy can be ventilated with or without the inner cannula in place.

Portex Flex DIC

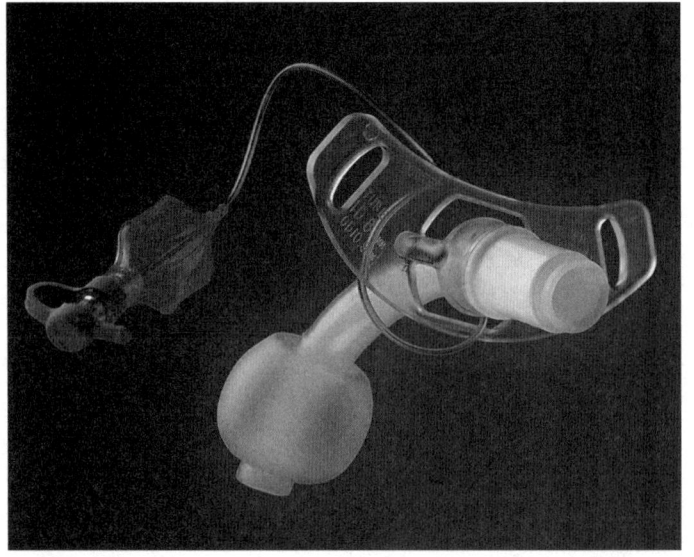

Structure: Cuffed, dual-cannula, arched curve
Material: Flexible polyvinyl chloride with silicone coating
Manufacturer: Smiths Medical
Unique Features: Color-coded inner cannula to identify size
Use: Patients who require a cuffed tube for positive-pressure ventilation, airway protection, or when secretions are a concern

Portex Flex DIC cuffed tracheostomy tube. Photo courtesy of Smiths Medical.

The Portex Flex DIC cuffed tracheostomy tube is made of a softer thermosensitive polyvinyl chloride with a silicone coating. Because of the difference in material, the outer diameters are different than the standard Portex DIC; however, the color-coding system for the inner cannula is the same. The Portex DIC and Flex DIC tubes have an arched curve to the shaft, similar to the Shiley LPC and DIC. The Portex DIC and Flex DIC both have a barrel-shaped cuff.

TRACOE Twist Series

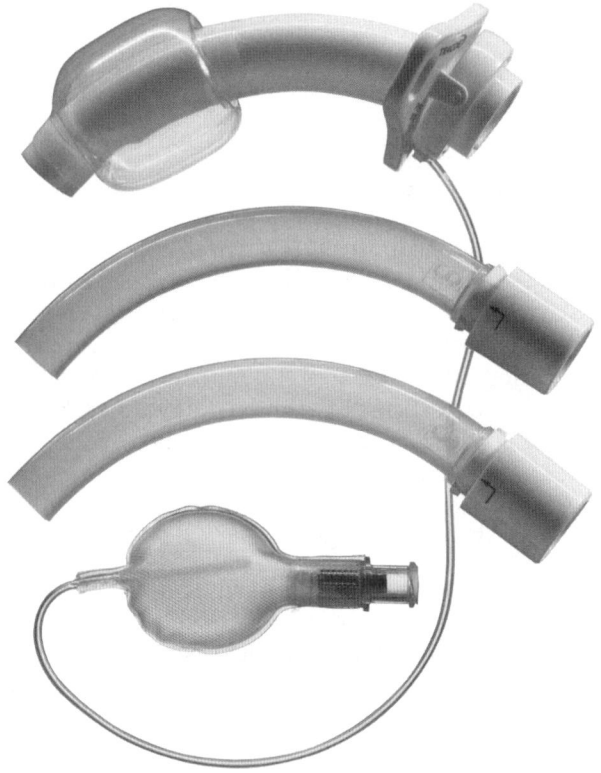

Structure: Cuffed, dual-cannula
Material: Flexible thermoelastic polyurethane
Manufacturer: Boston Medical Products
Unique Features: Neck flange that rotates on two planes
Use: Patients who require a cuffed tube for positive-pressure ventilation, airway protection, or when secretions are a concern

TRACOE Twist cuffed tracheostomy tube. Photo courtesy of Boston Medical Products. All rights reserved.

The TRACOE Twist series of tracheostomy tubes is similar to the Shiley LPC in that it has a cuff and consists of an inner cannula nested into an outer cannula with a twist-lock mechanism. However, it is made of a more flexible material—polyurethane—that becomes more pliable at body temperature. Another difference is that the neck flange moves on two planes, both vertically and horizontally, accommodating more patient movement.

The TRACOE Twist line of tubes comes in a wide variety of features. There are dual-cannula cuffed tubes, dual-cannula cuffless tubes, cuffed tubes with suction lines, cuffless tubes with suction lines, fenestrated cuffed tubes, fenestrated cuffless tubes, cuffed tubes with oxygen supply lines, and cuffed tubes with air supply lines. All these tracheostomy tubes have the same dimensions of inner diameter, outer diameter, and length.

Portex Lo-Profile Cuffed

Structure: Cuffed, dual-cannula
Material: Polyvinyl chloride
Manufacturer: Smiths Medical
Unique Features: Clear neck flange and 15-mm connector; low-profile, semireusable inner cannula
Use: For the patient who requires a cuffed tube but desires a less conspicuous appearance

The Portex Lo-Profile series of tracheostomy tubes are designed "for the active patient." It has a clear neck flange and a clear, low-profile inner cannula. It is also packaged with a standard inner cannula with a clear, 15-mm connector. It comes in cuffed and cuffless versions. The inner cannula is semireusable, meaning it can be cleaned and reused up to 21 times. As opposed to the Portex Blue Line series, DIC series, and Flex DIC series of tracheostomy tubes, the inflation line and pilot balloon of the Portex Lo-Profile tubes are clear.

Dual-Cannula Cuffless Tracheostomy Tubes

Cuffless dual-cannula tracheostomy tubes should be used only in those patients who can protect their airway and are best used for those who also have thick or large quantities of secretions. In this circumstance, the inner cannula can be removed and cleaned or replaced to prevent obstruction of the tube. This type of tube is ideally suited to the patient who can protect his airway, who does not require positive-pressure ventilation, and who wishes to speak; however, secretions may be an issue.

The Portex versions of dual-cannula cuffless tracheostomy tubes are the Portex DIC uncuffed and the Portex Flex DIC uncuffed tubes. Both tubes have color-coded inner cannulas.

Chapter 3 Types of Tracheostomy Tubes and Related Appliances

Portex DIC Uncuffed

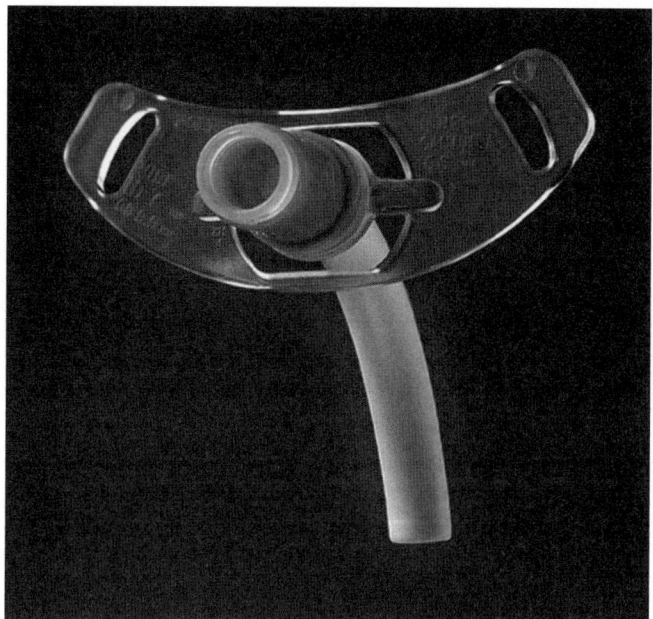

Structure: Dual-cannula, cuffless, curved arch to the shaft
Material: Rigid polyvinyl chloride
Manufacturer: Smiths Medical
Unique Features: Disposable and color-coded inner cannula
Use: For the patient who can protect his airway, yet secretions may be a concern; when capped, phonation can occur

Portex DIC uncuffed tracheostomy tube. Photo courtesy of Smiths Medical.

The Portex DIC uncuffed tracheostomy tube is identical to the Portex DIC except that it is cuffless. The inner cannula is color coded based on size (see Table 3.1). It includes a locking ring that secures the inner cannula to the outer cannula. The disposable inner cannula is removed and replaced on a regular basis—usually every 8 hours—to prevent the accumulation of secretions. The disposable inner cannula is often preferred by nurses because it saves cleaning time (see chapter 7).

Portex Flex DIC Uncuffed

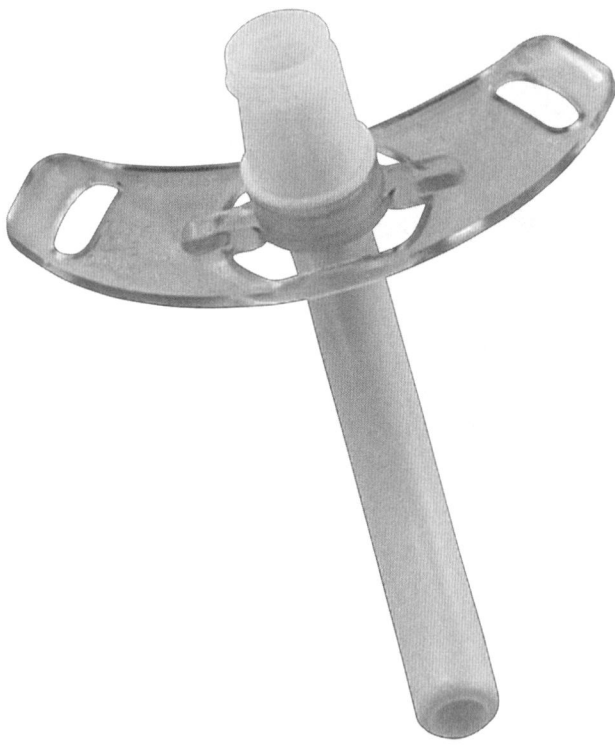

Structure: Dual-cannula, cuffless, arched curve to the shaft
Material: Flexible thermosensitive polyvinyl chloride with silicone coating
Manufacturer: Smiths Medical
Unique Features: Color-coded inner cannula to identify size
Use: For the patient who can protect his airway, yet secretions may be a concern; when capped, phonation can occur

Portex Flex DIC uncuffed tracheostomy tube. Photo courtesy of Smiths Medical.

The materials for these uncuffed tubes are the same as the cuffed versions. The Portex Flex DIC tracheostomy tube is made of a softer thermosensitive polyvinyl chloride with a silicone coating, and the Portex DIC is made of a rigid polyvinyl chloride. The color-coding system for the inner cannula is also the same (see Table 3.1). The Portex DIC and Portex Flex DIC tracheostomy tubes have an arched curve to the shaft, similar to the Shiley LPC and DCT.

Chapter 3 Types of Tracheostomy Tubes and Related Appliances

Shiley CFS

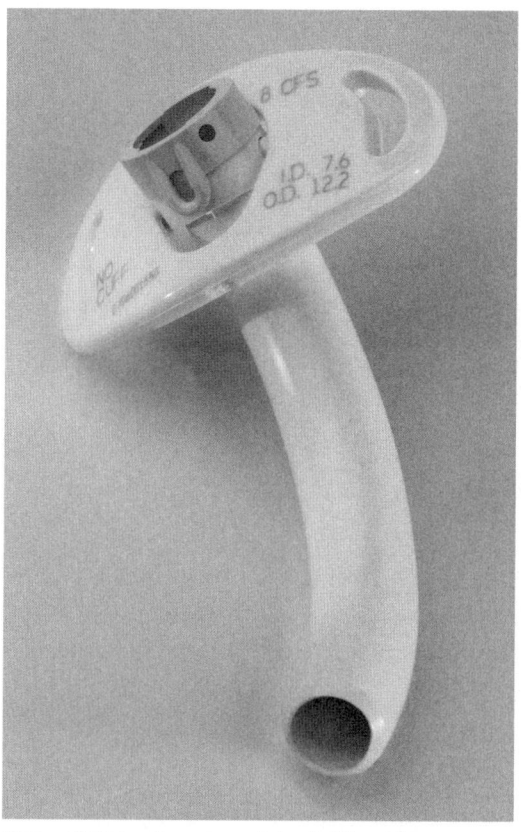

Structure: Dual-cannula, cuffless, arched curve to the shaft
Material: Rigid polyvinyl chloride
Manufacturer: Covidien
Unique Features: Cosmetic inner cannula and capped inner cannula are included in kit
Use: For the patient who can protect his airway, yet secretions may be a concern; when capped, phonation can occur

Shiley CFS tracheostomy tube (without inner cannula) (Covidien).

The Shiley CFS is identical to the LPC except that it is cuffless. It is constructed of rigid polyvinyl chloride. The CFS is packaged with a standard inner cannula, a capped inner cannula, a cosmetic inner cannula, and an obturator.

The cosmetic inner cannula may be used to provide a low-profile appearance; however, its use should be restricted in the hospital because it does not provide a 15-mm connector, so it is impossible to connect to a manual resuscitation bag or ventilator. The capped inner cannula is used to provide a low-profile appearance when a cap is in place. The outer aspect of the capped inner cannula is red for clear visibility.

58 Tracheostomies

Shiley DCFS

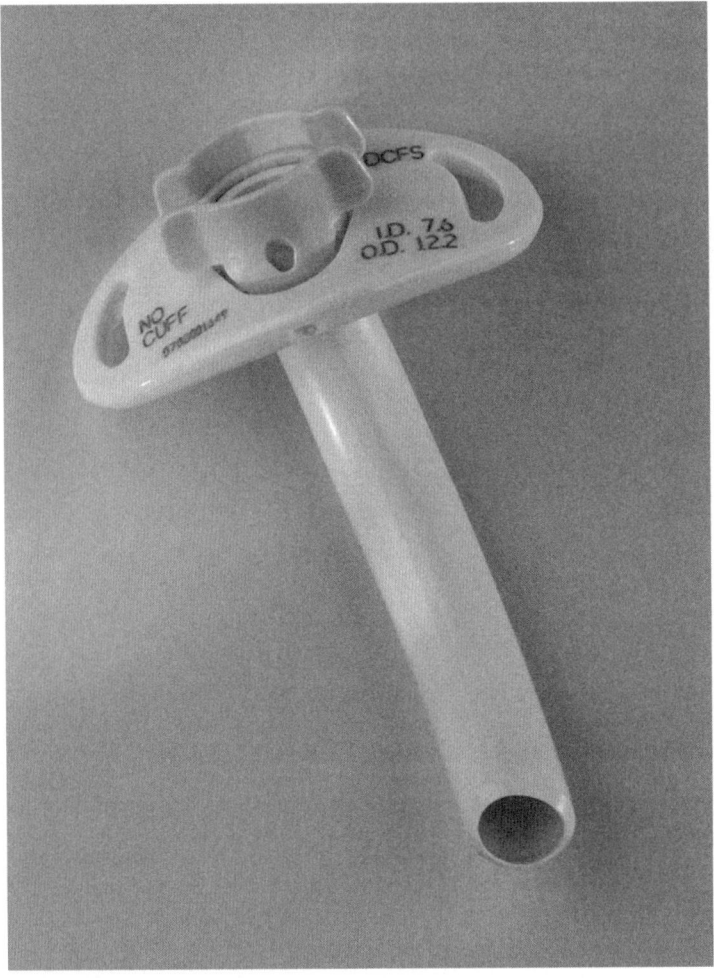

Structure: Dual-cannula, cuffless
Material: Rigid polyvinyl chloride
Manufacturer: Covidien
Unique Features: Disposable inner cannula
Use: For the patient who can protect his airway, yet secretions may be a concern; when capped, phonation can occur

Shiley DCFS tracheostomy tube (without inner cannula) (Covidien).

The Shiley DCFS tracheostomy tube is identical to the Shiley DCT tube except that it is cuffless. Like the DCT, the inner cannula is disposable and locks in place with a clipping mechanism.

TRACOE Twist Cuffless

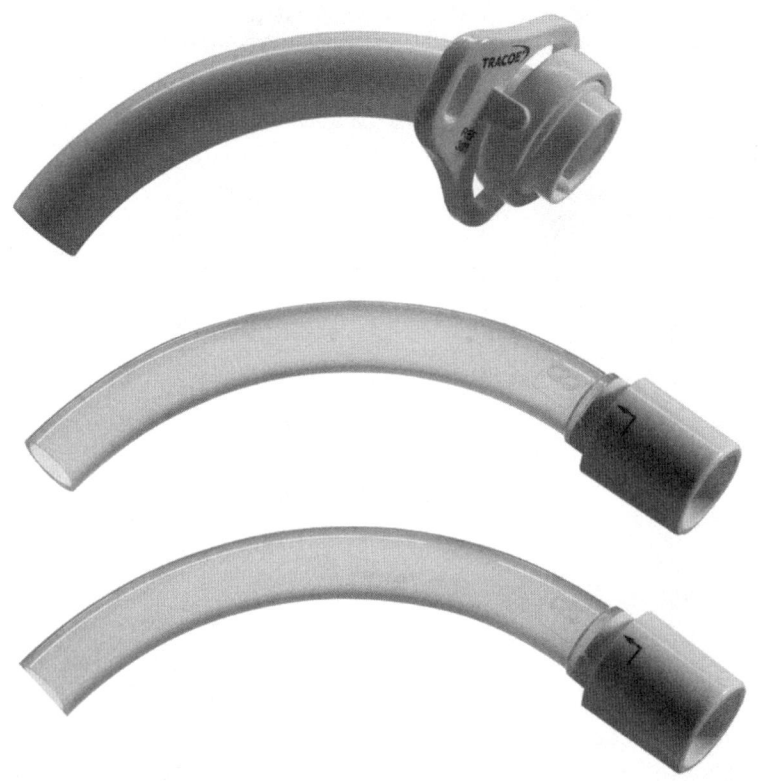

Structure: Dual-cannula, cuffless
Material: Flexible thermoelastic polyurethane
Manufacturer: Boston Medical Products
Unique Features: Packaged with two inner cannulas
Use: For the patient who can protect his airway, yet secretions may be a concern; when capped, phonation can occur

TRACOE Twist cuffless tracheostomy tube. Photo courtesy of Boston Medical Products. All rights reserved.

The TRACOE Twist cuffless tracheostomy tubes are made of medical-grade polyurethane and are identical to the TRACOE Twist cuffed tubes, without the cuff. It is packaged with two individual inner cannulas with 15-mm connectors.

TRACOE Comfort

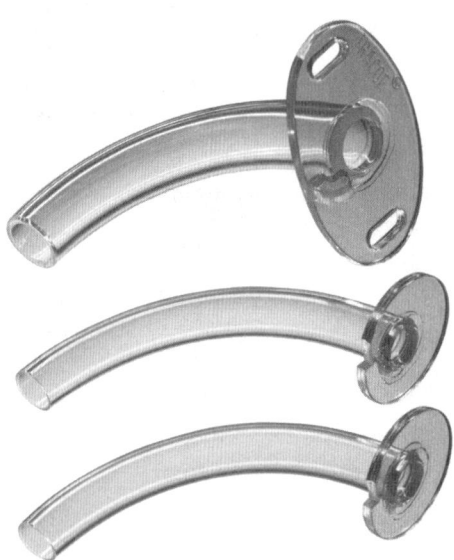

Structure: Uncuffed, single- or dual-cannula
Material: Flexible polyvinyl chloride
Manufacturer: Boston Medical Products
Unique Features: Clear
Use: When positive-pressure ventilation is not required and secretions are not a concern

TRACOE Comfort dual-cannula tracheostomy tube (with additional inner cannula). Photo courtesy of Boston Medical Products. All rights reserved.

The TRACOE Comfort line of tracheostomies is made of a very soft, flexible, clear, and lightweight medical polymer. They are always cuffless and come with or without an inner cannula. Most of the models are low profile in nature and do not have 15-mm adapters; however, one of the models (103.A) comes with a 15-mm adapter on the inner cannula so positive pressure can be used. Model 104 comes with a swivel speaking valve. Model 103 comes with a silver speaking valve and can also be ordered with an oxygen supply port. The manufacturer recommends that paraffin oil be used with the dual-cannula tracheostomy tubes. It should be used at least every other day to lubricate the inner cannula and ensure it is easy to insert and remove.

Portex Lo-Profile Uncuffed

Structure: Dual-cannula, cuffless
Material: Polyvinyl chloride
Manufacturer: Smiths Medical
Unique Features: Clear neck flange and 15-mm connector; clear, low-profile, semireusable inner cannula
Use: For the patient who desires a less conspicuous appearance

Chapter 3   Types of Tracheostomy Tubes and Related Appliances

The Portex Lo-Profile tracheostomy tubes also come in cuffless versions. For specific information about this tube, refer to the earlier section describing the Portex Lo-Profile cuffed tracheostomy tube.

Single-Cannula Cuffed Tracheostomy Tubes

Single-cannula cuffed tracheostomy tubes are used for patients who require a cuffed tube for airway protection or positive-pressure ventilation but for whom secretions are not a major concern. Because there is no inner cannula, single-cannula tracheostomy tubes have a narrower outer diameter than comparably sized dual-cannula tubes.

Shiley SCT

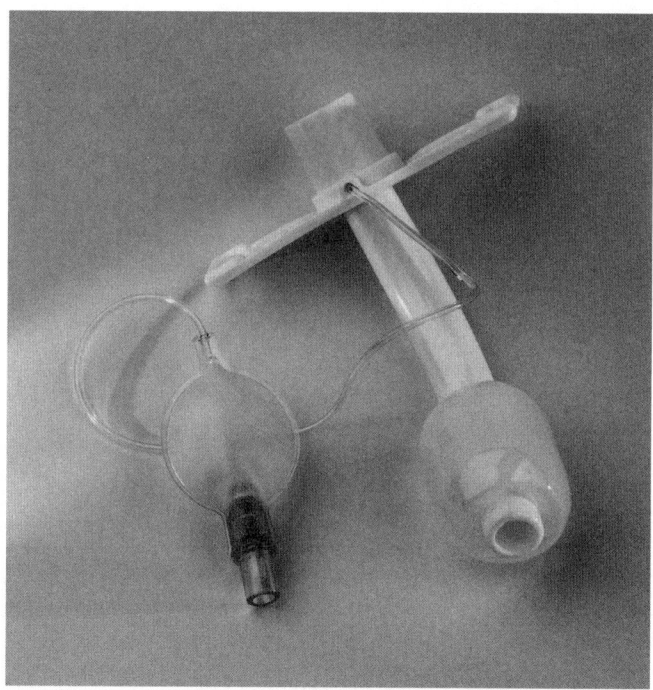

Structure: Cuffed, single-cannula
Material: Flexible polyvinyl chloride
Manufacturer: Covidien
Unique Features: Longer shaft than comparably sized tube
Use: For the patient who requires a cuff, yet for whom secretions are not a concern; can also be used when a longer tube is desired

Shiley SCT tracheostomy tube (Covidien).

The Shiley SCT is constructed of polyvinyl chloride but is more flexible than standard Shiley tubes. It is the only Shiley tracheostomy tube without an inner cannula, and as such the outer diameter is narrower than a comparable dual-cannula tracheostomy tube. It is also distinctly longer than a comparably sized Shiley DCT or LPC. As opposed to the standard Shiley tubes, the SCT uses the ISO sizing system. The manufacturer recommends that no solution other than saline be used to clean any part of the tube.

Tracheostomies

Portex Blue Line

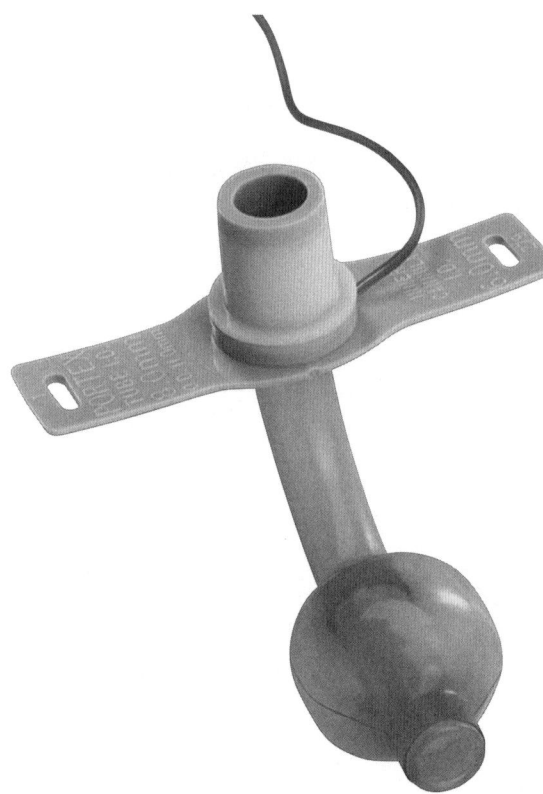

Structure: Cuffed, single-cannula, 90-degree curvature to the shaft
Material: Siliconized polyvinyl chloride
Manufacturer: Smiths Medical
Unique Features: The Blue Line tube is identifiable by its blue neck flange, inflation line, and pilot balloon
Use: For the patient who requires a cuff, yet for whom secretions are not a concern; however, a separate inner cannula can be used when necessary

Portex Blue Line cuffed tracheostomy tube. Photo courtesy of Smiths Medical.

The Portex Blue Line series of tracheostomy tubes is primarily single-cannula tubes; however, they do have a corrugated inner cannula that can be used when needed (ordered separately). When used, the inner cannula decreases the diameter of the airway by 2 mm. The Blue Line cuffed tracheostomy tube is recognizable by its soft, flexible blue neck flange and shaft as well as its blue pilot balloon and inflation line. The Blue Line tracheostomy tubes have a 90% curvature to the shaft, and the inflation line is buried within the outer cannula. The Blue Line tracheostomy tube has a teardrop shaped cuff, which is thought to allow better placement of the tube within the airway.

Chapter 3 Types of Tracheostomy Tubes and Related Appliances

Portex Blue Line Ultra

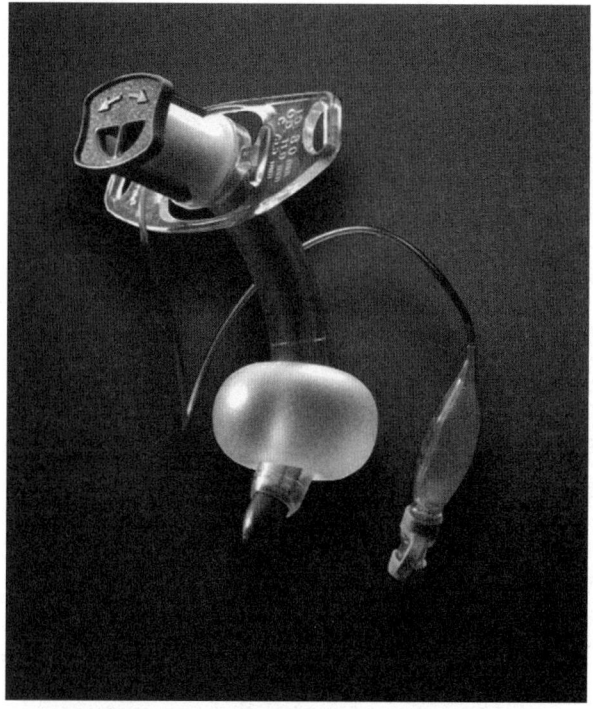

Portex Blue Line Ultra cuffed tracheostomy tube. Photo courtesy of Smiths Medical.

Structure: Cuffed, single-cannula
Material: Siliconized polyvinyl chloride
Manufacturer: Smiths Medical
Unique Features: Presence of a central channel to accommodate guide wire; larger curvature than standard Blue Line tube
Use: For the patient who requires a cuff, yet for whom secretions are not a concern

The Portex Blue Line Ultra series of tracheostomy tubes is very similar to the standard Portex Blue Line tubes but with a larger curvature. This feature theoretically allows the cuff to be more centrally placed within the airway. The inner cannula of the Blue Line Ultra decreases the diameter of the airway by 1 mm, as opposed to 2 mm for the other Portex tracheostomy tubes.

There is also a type of Blue Line Ultra tracheostomy tube that provides an extra port for subglottic suctioning of secretions that accumulate above the cuff (Suctionaid). One of the most unique features of the Blue Line Ultra is the presence of a central channel through the obturator that can accommodate a guide wire for insertion.

Bivona Mid-Range Aire-Cuf

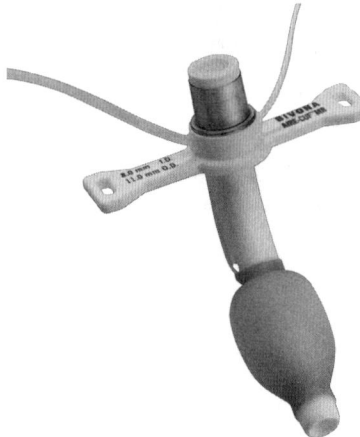

Structure: Cuffed, single-cannula
Material: Silicone
Manufacturer: Smiths Medical
Unique Features: 360-degree swivel adapter; soft, "low-trauma" tip
Use: For the patient who requires a cuff, yet for whom secretions are not a concern

Bivona Mid-Range Aire-Cuf tracheostomy tube. Photo courtesy of Smiths Medical.

The Bivona Mid-Range Aire-Cuf tracheostomy tube has a flexible neck flange, a white inflation line, and a blue pilot balloon.

All of the Bivona tracheostomy tubes, regardless of the line, are constructed entirely of silicone and are more flexible. The theoretical advantage to silicone is that secretions are less likely to adhere to the material; however, no studies have been done to verify this claim. All Bivona tracheostomy tubes are single-cannula tubes and have 360-degree swivel adapters to accommodate some patient movement. Bivona tracheostomy tubes also come with a disconnect wedge, which is helpful because the 15-mm swivel connector can sometimes get wedged into the adaptor of a manual resuscitation bag or ventilator tubing. The forceful removal of any device from a Bivona tracheostomy tube can result in permanent damage to the tube, so the use of the disconnect wedge is advised whenever removing any device from this tube.

There have been two important manufacturing changes to adult Bivona tracheostomy tubes. First, the swivel mechanism has been replaced with a single-molded piece as the 15-mm connector. Second, the solid obturators have been redesigned to be hollow. This redesign supports the introduction of a guide wire as a tube exchanger (personal communication Mark Lareau, Smiths Medical, November 2008).

Arcadia Silicone Air Cuff

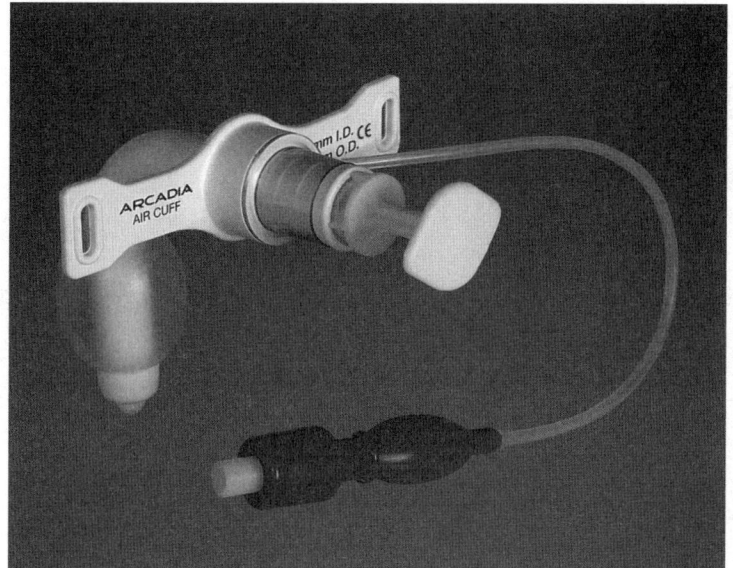

Structure: Cuffed, single-cannula, wide arch curvature
Material: Flexible silicone
Manufacturer: Arcadia Medical Corporation
Unique Features: 360-degree swivel adapter; angled design allows tube to be centered within the airway
Use: For the patient who requires a cuff, yet for whom secretions are not a concern

Arcadia Air Cuff tracheostomy tube. Latex free. Arcadia Medical Corporation, www.arcadiamedical.com.

The Arcadia line of tracheostomies is new to the United States as of January 2009. The line is constructed of silicone and consists of single-cannula tracheostomy tubes. The neck flange has a 15-mm swivel connector, and a disconnect wedge is included to facilitate the removal of respiratory equipment.

The curvature of many of the Arcadia tracheostomy tubes is unique in that they have a more horizontal orientation to the proximal portion of the shaft while the distal portion has a more vertical orientation, giving a 90-degree angle to the tube.

Bivona Fome-Cuf

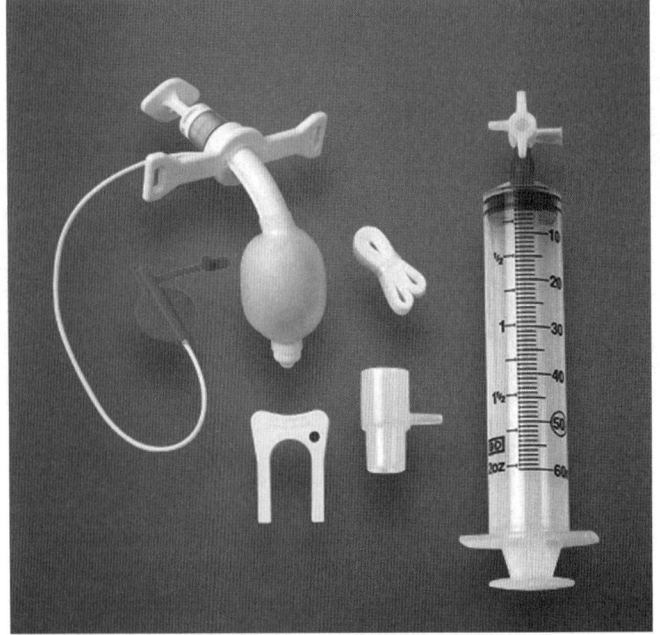

Structure: Cuffed, single-cannula
Material: Silicone
Manufacturer: Smiths Medical
Unique Features: Foam-filled cuff that expands automatically to fit tracheal diameter
Use: For the patient who has repeated cuff leaks and does not desire to speak

Bivona Fome-Cuf tracheostomy tube. Photo courtesy of Smiths Medical.

The Bivona Fome-Cuf tracheostomy tube is constructed entirely of silicone. The Fome-Cuf tube is unique in that it provides a large, self-inflating cuff that adjusts itself to the patient's trachea. Once in place, the pilot balloon should remain open to air at all times, and no additional air should be injected into this cuff. This tracheostomy tube is inserted by first deflating the cuff completely. Because of the extra-large cuff, this is often best done with the large syringe and three-way stopcock that come in the tracheostomy kit. The deflated cuff is particularly bulky; however, when inflated it is usually able to provide a complete seal within the airway.

The Fome-Cuf tracheostomy tube is often chosen when positive-pressure ventilation is required, yet because of this a good seal is difficult because of a continued leak around the outside of the tracheostomy tube. Over time, moisture may collect within the cuff especially when using the ventilator adapter, so routine cuff deflation is recommended every 8 hours. It is recommended that this tracheostomy tube be routinely changed at least every month to minimize the collection of moisture and debris and prevent solidification within the cuff.

If the ventilator tubing should become difficult to remove from the 15-mm connector of the tube, the Fome-Cuf tube has a disconnect wedge that can be used as a lever to simplify removal. Forceful attempts to remove the tubing can result in damage to the tracheostomy tube itself. The manufacturer's recommendations state that these tracheostomy tubes should not be used with lasers or electrosurgical devices.

Arcadia Foam Cuff

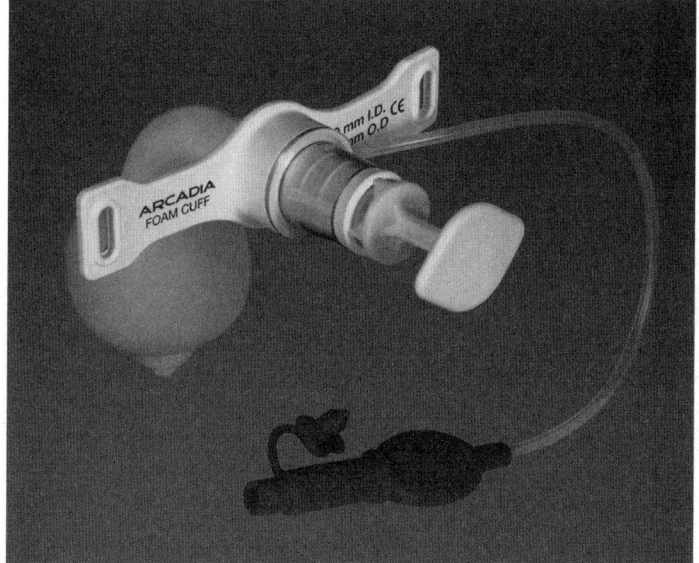

Structure: Cuffed, single-cannula
Material: Flexible silicone
Manufacturer: Arcadia Medical Corporation
Unique Features: Foam-filled cuff that expands automatically to fit tracheal diameter
Use: For the patient who has repeated cuff leaks and does not desire to speak

Arcadia Foam Cuff tracheostomy tube. Latex free. Arcadia Medical Corporation, www.arcadiamedical.com.

The Arcadia Foam Cuff tube is made of silicone with an auto-expandable cuff. The neck flange has a 15-mm swivel connector. The Arcadia tubes also have disconnect wedges to simplify the removal of any respiratory equipment.

Bivona TTS (Tight-to-Shaft)

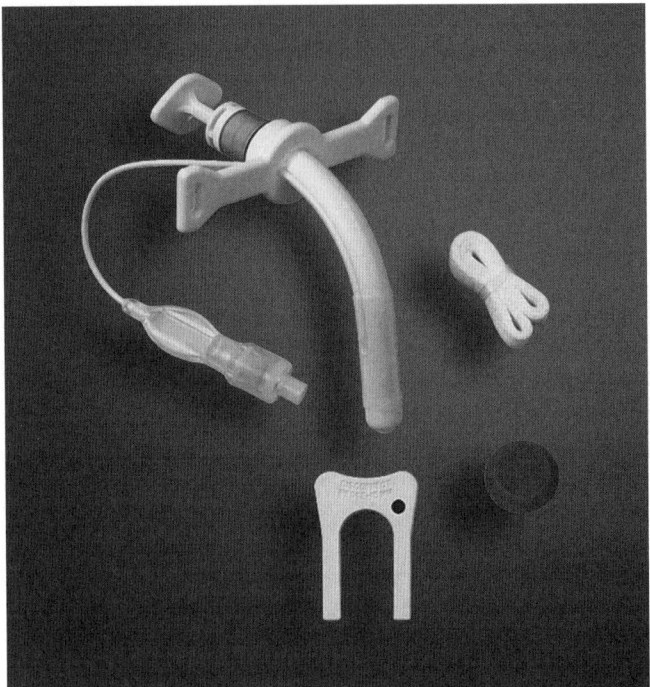

Bivona TTS tracheostomy tube. Note deflated cuff that lies snugly against the shaft of the tube. Photo courtesy of Smiths Medical.

Structure: Cuffed, single-cannula
Material: Silicone
Manufacturer: Smiths Medical
Unique Features: When this high-pressure cuff is deflated, it lies tight to the shaft, minimizing resistance when breathing around the tube (when prolonged cuff inflation in desired, it should be inflated with sterile water); other than the Arcadia CTS tube, the TTS tracheostomy tube is the only cuffed tube that may be safely capped when deflated
Use: Ideal for the patient who requires intermittent positive-pressure ventilation yet who also desires to speak

The Bivona Tight-to-Shaft, or TTS, tracheostomy tube is constructed of silicone material and provides some flexibility. It is a single-cannula tracheostomy tube whose most notable feature is its cuff, which, when deflated, lies tight to the shaft of the tube—hence its name. The TTS is ideally suited for the patient who may require intermittent cuff inflation (perhaps for nocturnal ventilation) yet who wishes to speak at intervals when the cuff is deflated. The TTS design provides laminar flow around the outside of the tube, so it can be capped to allow phonation. (The details of phonation will be discussed in chapter 6.) It is important to note that the cuff of the TTS is a high-pressure cuff, so precautions must be taken to minimize pressure against the tracheal wall. This is best done with the minimal leak technique.

The cuff of the TTS tracheostomy tube is inflated with sterile water (not saline) in order to minimize gas permeability across the cuff that might otherwise result when air is used for cuff inflation. This gas permeability is manifested as cuff deflation over time. The TTS tracheostomy tube is packaged with a disconnection wedge to be used in case the ventilator tubing becomes difficult to remove from the 15-mm connector. If force is used, the TTS tracheostomy tube can become damaged.

Arcadia Silicone CTS Cuff (Close-to-Shaft)

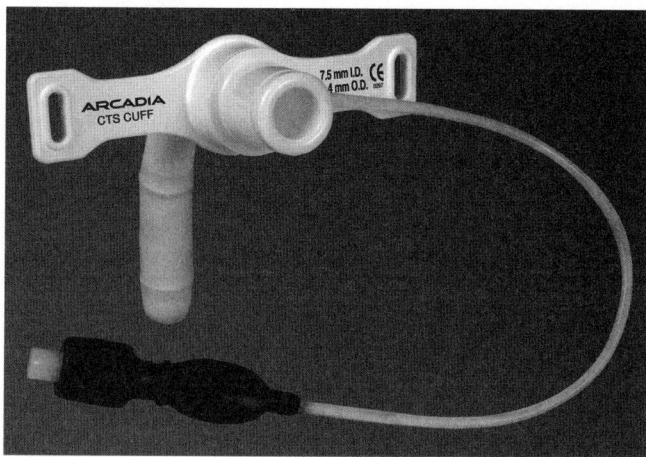

Arcadia Silicone CTS Cuff tracheostomy tube. Note deflated cuff lying snugly against the shaft of the tube. Arcadia Medical Corporation, www.arcadiamedical.com.

Structure: Cuffed, single-cannula, curved shaft
Material: Silicone
Manufacturer: Arcadia Medical Corporation
Unique Features: When the high-pressure cuff is deflated, it lies close to the shaft, minimizing resistance when breathing around the tube (when prolonged cuff inflation is desired, it should be inflated with sterile water); the CTS tracheostomy tube is one of only two cuffed tracheostomy tubes that may be safely capped when deflated (the other is the Bivona TTS)
Use: Ideal for the patient who requires intermittent positive-pressure ventilation yet who also desires to speak

The Arcadia Silicone CTS Cuff tracheostomy tube has a radiopaque silicone shaft with a curved design to make insertion and removal easier. It has a silicone cuff that lies flat against the shaft when deflated. Like the Bivona TTS, it is a single-cannula tracheostomy tube with a high-pressure cuff, and its cuff should be inflated with sterile water.

Single-Cannula Cuffless Tracheostomy Tubes

Single-cannula cuffless tracheostomy tubes are used when exclusive breathing through the tube is not necessary (or not desired) and secretions are not a concern.

Bivona Uncuffed

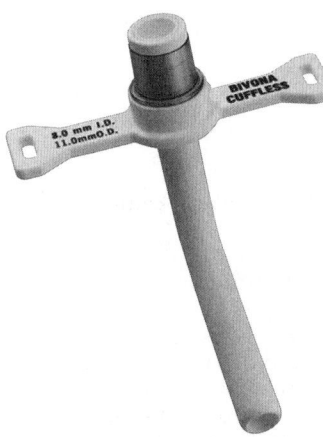

Structure: Cuffless, single-cannula
Material: Silicone
Manufacturer: Smiths Medical
Unique Features: Swivel mechanism of 15-mm adapter
Use: When positive-pressure ventilation is not required and secretions are not a concern

Bivona uncuffed tracheostomy tube. Photo courtesy of Smiths Medical.

The Bivona uncuffed tracheostomy tube is a single-cannula tube and is composed of silicone. The neck flange is flexible, and the 15-mm connector has a swivel mechanism that accomodates some patient movement.

Air-Lon Tracheostomy Tube and Inhalation Set

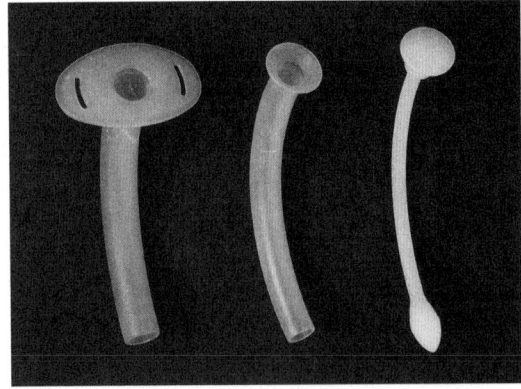

Air-Lon™ tracheostomy tube. Premier Medical Products Company.

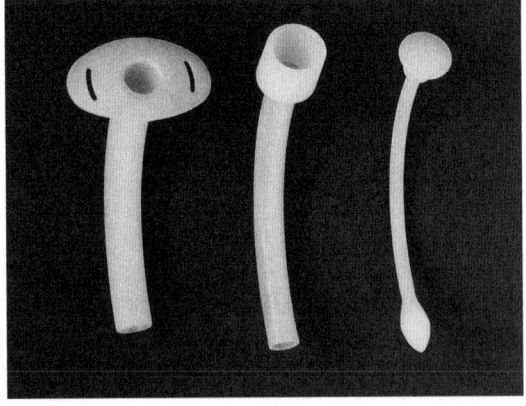

Air-Lon™ inhalation set. Premier Medical Products Company.

Structure: Uncuffed, single-cannula; 90-degree curvature to the shaft
Material: Nylon
Manufacturer: Premier Medical Products
Unique Features: Low-profile inner cannula
Use: When positive-pressure ventilation is not required and secretions are not a concern

The Air-Lon™ tracheostomy tube is cuffless and made of nylon. The outer cannula has a 90-degree arc. It comes with an obturator and low-profile inner cannula. If positive-pressure ventilation is desired, the Air-Lon™ Inhalation Set can be used.

TRACOE Comfort

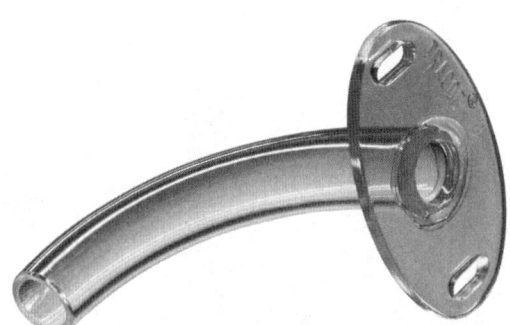

Structure: Uncuffed, single- or dual-cannula
Material: Flexible polyvinyl chloride
Manufacturer: Boston Medical Products
Unique Features: Clear, flexible material; low-profile appearance
Use: When positive-pressure ventilation is not required and secretions are not a concern

TRACOE Comfort single-cannula tracheostomy tube. Photo courtesy of Boston Medical Products. All rights reserved.

The TRACOE Comfort line of tracheostomy tubes is made of a very soft, flexible, clear, and lightweight medical polymer. They are always cuffless and come with or without an inner cannula. The TRACOE Comfort single cannula (Model 101) is a single-cannula tube that is low profile in nature. Paraffin oil should be used to lubricate the inner cannula within the outer cannula.

Portex Blue Line Uncuffed

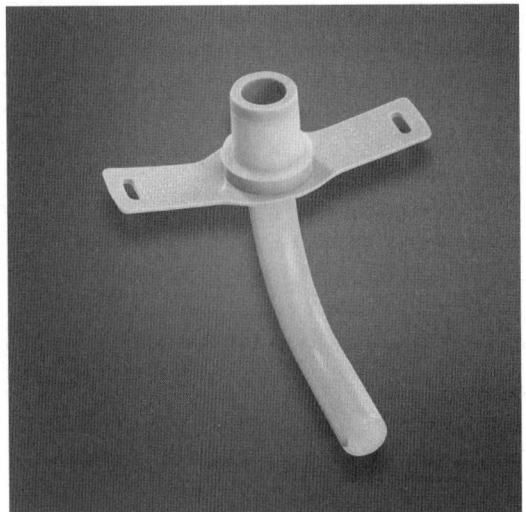

Structure: Cuffed, single-cannula, 90-degree curvature to the shaft
Material: Siliconized polyvinyl chloride
Manufacturer: Smiths Medical
Unique Features: The Blue Line tube is identifiable by its blue neck flange, inflation line, and pilot balloon
Use: For the patient who does not require a cuff and for whom secretions are not a concern (however, a separate inner cannula can be used when necessary)

Portex Blue Line uncuffed tracheostomy tube. Photo courtesy of Smiths Medical.

The Portex Blue Line series of tracheostomy tubes are primarily single-cannula tubes; however, they do have a corrugated inner cannula that can be used when needed (ordered separately). When used, the inner cannula decreases the diameter of the airway by 2 mm. The Blue Line tracheostomy tube is recognizable by its soft, flexible blue neck flange and shaft. The Blue Line tracheostomy tubes have a 90% curvature to the shaft.

Portex Blue Line Ultra Uncuffed

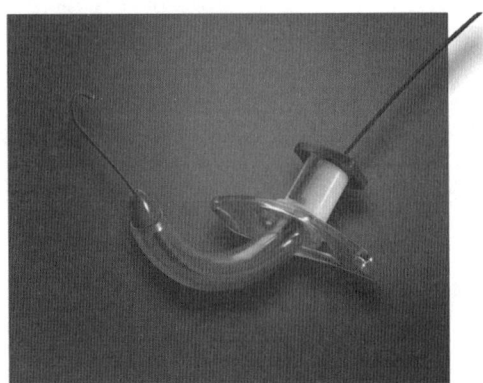

Structure: Uncuffed, single-cannula
Material: Siliconized polyvinyl chloride
Manufacturer: Smiths Medical
Unique Features: Presence of a central channel to accommodate guide wire; larger curvature than standard Blue Line tube
Use: For the patient who does not require a cuff and for whom secretions are not a concern

Portex Blue Line Ultra uncuffed tracheostomy tube over guide wire. Photo courtesy of Smiths Medical.

The Portex Blue Line Ultra series of tracheostomy tubes are very similar to the standard Portex Blue Line tubes but have a larger curvature. This feature theoretically allows the cuff to be more centrally placed within the airway. The inner cannula of the Blue Line Ultra decreases the diameter of the airway by 1 mm, as opposed to 2 mm for the other Portex tubes. One of the most unique features of the Blue Line Ultra is a central channel through the obturator, which can accommodate a guide wire for insertion.

Moore

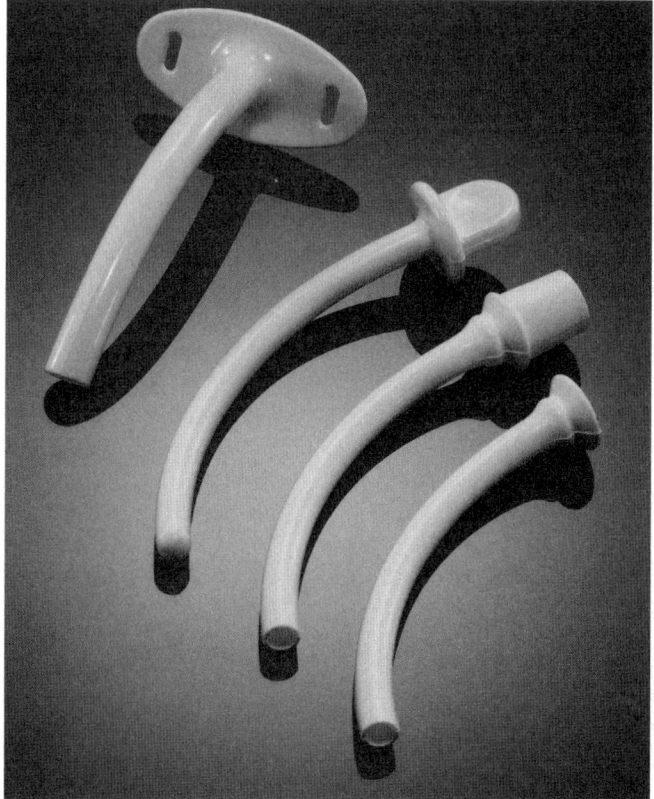

Structure: Uncuffed, single- or dual-cannula
Material: Silicone
Manufacturer: Boston Medical Products
Unique Features: Soft and flexible, conforms to shape of individual neck and trachea
Use: When positive-pressure ventilation is not required and comfort is desired

Moore tracheostomy tube (pictured with two inner cannulas and obturator). Courtesy of Boston Medical Products. All rights reserved.

The Moore tracheostomy tube is a flexible, single- or dual-cannula cuffless tube made of silicone. It comes in two sizes (6 and 8), and both have a standard length of 115 mm. The manufacturer reports that the extra-long length can be trimmed to fit. The outer cannula comes with a standard inner cannula, a low-profile inner cannula, and an obturator. The inner cannula can be soaked in warm soapy water for 10 minutes to loosen any crusts. If necessary, the inside of the inner cannula can be cleaned with a soft-bristle bottle brush.

Arcadia Silicone Cuffless

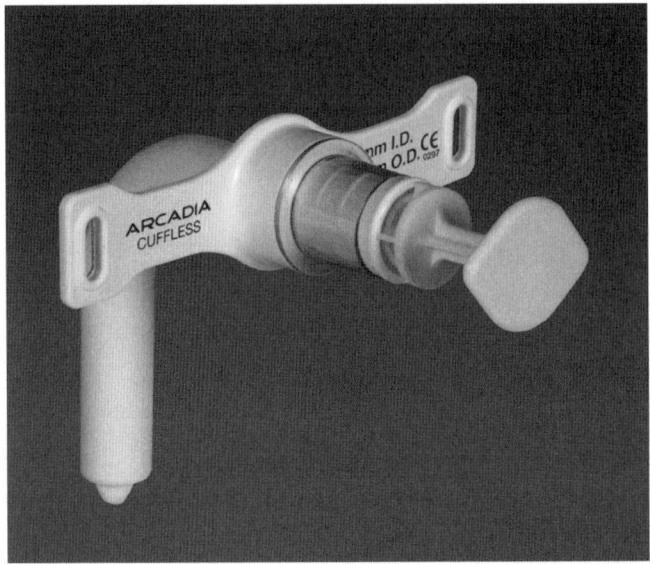

Structure: Uncuffed, single-cannula
Material: Flexible silicone
Manufacturer: Arcadia Medical Corporation
Unique Features: Soft contoured neck flange minimizes stomal irritation
Use: When positive-pressure ventilation is not required and when secretions are not a concern

Arcadia Silicone Cuffless tracheostomy tube (with obturator in place). Arcadia Medical Corporation, www.arcadiamedical.com.

The Arcadia Silicone Cuffless tracheostomy tube has a 90-degree angle to the shaft for better placement within the airway. The neck flange has a 15-mm swivel connector.

Bivona Sleep Apnea

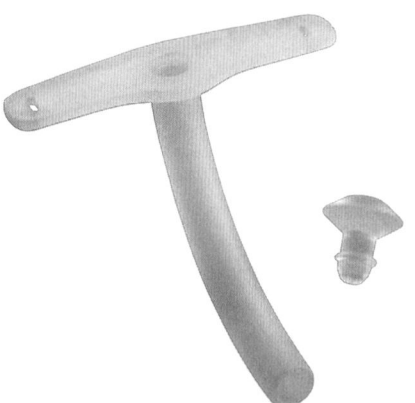

Structure: Uncuffed, single-cannula
Material: Flexible silicone
Manufacturer: Smiths Medical
Unique Features: Low-profile appearance; comes with two plugs
Use: When positive-pressure ventilation is not required and when secretions are not a concern

Bivona Sleep Apnea tracheostomy tube (with plug). Photo courtesy of Smiths Medical.

The Bivona Sleep Apnea tubes are always cuffless and have a low profile. They are made of flexible silicone. Because of their low-profile nature, they are not recommended for patients who require ventilatory support or airway access for suctioning and pulmonary hygiene. Its low-profile design makes it easily capped and concealed during waking hours. The Bivona Sleep Apnea tracheostomy tube also comes in a version with an inner cannula with a 15-mm connector, which is called an "inhalation set."

Special Use Tracheostomy Tubes

There are several specialty tracheostomy tubes available for specific needs. These include talking tracheostomy tubes, extra-long tubes, fenestrated tubes, double-cuffed tubes, and custom-designed tubes.

Talking Tracheostomy Tubes

A few tracheostomy tubes available are called "talking trachs." These tracheostomy tubes are typically cuffed tubes with an additional lumen that terminates above the cuff and allows air to reach the vocal cords. When the tube is in the proper position and the proximal connector is attached to oxygen or an air-regulated gas source, air flows into the line. The patient or assistant must occlude the thumb port of this air supply line to direct the gas flow upward through the vocal cords. Gas flow usually starts at 4–6 liters per minute and can be adjusted upward until optimal voice quality is attained; however, a maximum of 10–15 liters per minute is recommended.

Another method of phonation with the talking tracheostomy tube is connecting the gas line to a suction source. When the thumb port is occluded, air is drawn in through the nose and mouth and passes through the vocal cords from the opposite direction. The product literature for the Portex Blue Line Trach Talk recommends setting the initial negative pressure on the suction system to 80 mm Hg and adjusting to voice quality with a maximum of 180 mm Hg.

This suction port can also be used as a suction line to remove secretions produced above the cuff, rather than for phonation. By occluding the thumb port, these secretions are easily removed. The disadvantage, however, is that the suction line may become clogged with secretions and can be a source of infection. Because of this, its use as a suction line should be limited to a select group of patients.

Portex Blue Line Trach Talk

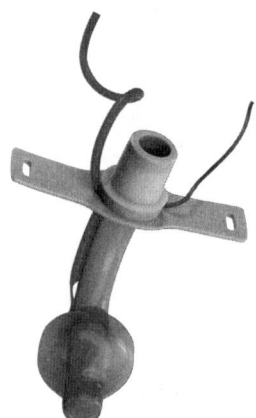

Structure: Cuffed, single-cannula
Material: Siliconized polyvinyl chloride
Manufacturer: Smiths Medical
Unique Features: Air supply line (green) with port that terminates above the cuff
Use: For the ventilator-dependent patient who desires to speak

Portex Blue Line Trach Talk tracheostomy tube. Photo courtesy of Smiths Medical.

The Portex Blue Line Trach Talk is similar to a Blue Line tracheostomy tube but has an additional lumen for gas flow. The distal port of the green gas line terminates just above the cuff of the tube.

TRACOE Twist With Air Supply Line

Structure: Cuffed, dual-cannula
Material: Flexible thermoelastic polyurethane
Manufacturer: Boston Medical Products
Unique Features: Air supply line with port that terminates above the cuff
Use: For the ventilator-dependent patient who desires to speak

The TRACOE Twist cuffed tracheostomy tube with air supply line is another version of the talking tracheostomy tube. It has all of the features of the TRACOE twist tubes previously disucssed.

Bivona Fome-Cuf With Talk Attachment

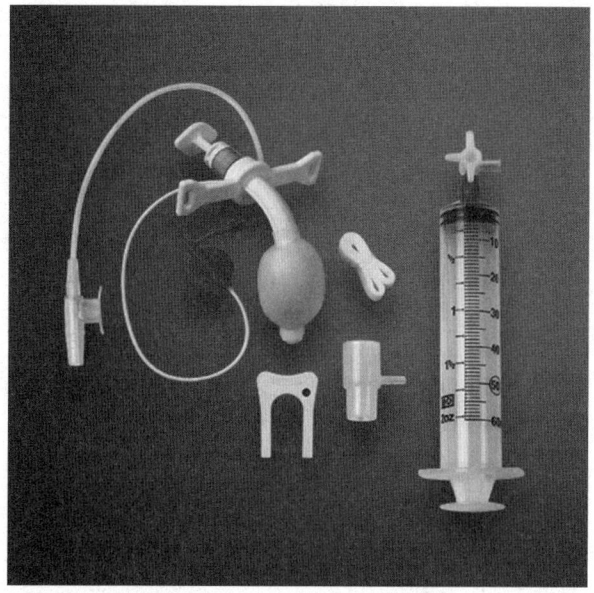

Structure: Cuffed, single-cannula
Material: Silicone
Manufacturer: Smiths Medical
Unique Features: Air supply line with port that terminates above the cuff
Use: For the ventilator-dependent patient who desires to speak

Bivona Fome-Cuf tracheostomy tube with talk attachment (pictured with decannulation wedge, cotton twill ties, ventilator adapter, and large syringe with stopcock). Photo courtesy of Smiths Medical.

The Bivona Fome-Cuf with talk attachment is the only tube that allows a patient with a Fome-Cuf tracheostomy to talk. Otherwise, the bulkiness of this cuff, as well as its default-inflated position, does not allow any air to pass around the cuff.

Extra-Long Tracheostomy Tubes

There are several circumstances in which an extra-long tracheostomy tube is beneficial. Extra-long tubes can be useful in cases of tracheomalacia, unusual anatomy, or morbid obesity. In the case of tracheomalacia, an extra-long tube will place the cuff in a more distal position within the trachea, which can allow the damaged area to heal. There are different types of extra-long tracheostomy tubes, and they all have different features.

Bivona Hyperflex

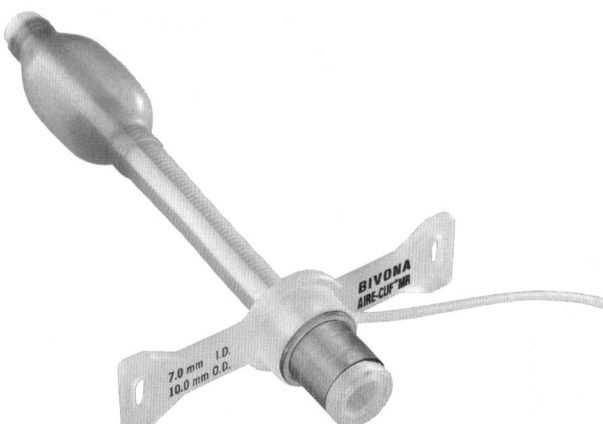

Structure: Cuffed, single-cannula, no curvature to the shaft
Material: Flexible silicone; wire reinforced
Manufacturer: Smiths Medical
Unique Features: Adjustable neck flange to accommodate variable length, shaft has no predetermined shape and can conform to a wide variety of anatomical variations, while wire reinforcement allows it to maintain its diameter without kinking regardless of its position
Use: For the patient who requires an extra-long tracheostomy tube; ideal for the patient with unusual anatomy such as an extra-long or extra-wide neck

Bivona Hyperflex tracheostomy tube with fixed-neck flange. Note wire-reinforced shaft. Photo courtesy of Smiths Medical.

The Bivona Hyperflex tracheostomy tube is a single-cannula, extra-long tracheostomy with a silicone shaft reinforced with wire, allowing it to retain its shape no matter its position. Because it is armored with wire, it is not compatible with magnetic resonance imaging (MRI). If the patient requires an MRI, this tube must be changed out.

The Bivona Hyperflex was designed to provide extra length to accommodate patients with thick bull necks, anatomical airway anomalies, or other conditions such as tracheomalacia. The neck flange is manufactured with an adjustable or fixed neck. The adjustable-neck flange is designed as a temporary measure to accommodate individual needs. It is secured in place with a wrap-and-snap connection in which a band of silicone wraps around the shaft of the tube and hooks to itself. Even when locked in place, this adjustable-neck flange can move when traction is exerted on it, especially in a patient with a large amount of secretions. The manufacturer cautions that it is meant for temporary use until the proper length tube can be obtained. It should be replaced with a tracheostomy tube with a fixed-neck flange. The fixed-neck flange of the Hyperflex is flexible but fused to the shaft of the tube. The adjustable-neck flange model comes in two varieties of cuff: Aire-Cuf and TTS. The fixed-neck flange model used to be a custom order; however, it currently comes in standard lengths with three standard cuff varieties: Aire-Cuf, uncuffed, and TTS.

Arcadia Air Cuff Adjustable-Neck Flange

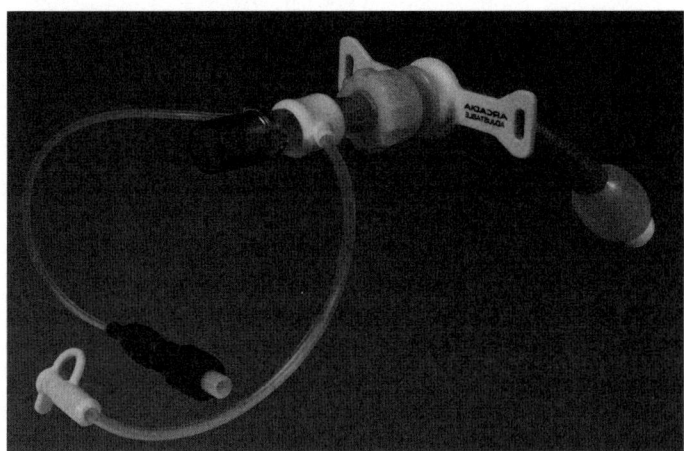

Arcadia Air Cuff Adjustable-Neck Flange tracheostomy tube. Note subglottic suction port in addition to inflation line. Arcadia Medical Corporation, www.arcadiamedical.com.

Structure: Cuffed, single-cannula, no curvature to the shaft
Material: Flexible silicone; wire reinforced
Manufacturer: Arcadia Medical Corporation
Unique Features: Adjustable-neck flange to accommodate variable length, shaft has no predetermined shape and can conform to a wide variety of anatomical variations, while wire reinforcement allows it to maintain its diameter without kinking regardless of its position (an access port located above the cuff can be connected to suction to prevent aspiration or to direct airflow above the cuff to allow for phonation)
Use: Designed to accommodate patients with unusual anatomy, airway complications, and trauma

The Arcadia adjustable-neck flange tracheostomy tube is a single-cannula, extra-long tube with a silicone shaft reinforced with wire, allowing it to retain its shape no matter its position. Because it is armored with wire, it is not compatible with MRI. If a patient requires an MRI, this tube must be changed out. This tube also has a port above the cuff that may be used to remove secretions. In addition to this subglottic suction channel, one of the most unique features of the Arcadia adjustable-neck flange tracheostomy tube is its locking mechanism. The shaft passes through a twist-lock mechanism that locks it into place. When locked, this mechanism will not move, unlike the Bivona Hyperflex adjustable-neck flange, which may move especially when exposed to secretions. The manufacturer, however, cautions that the Arcadia adjustable-neck flange tube should also be replaced with a fixed-neck flange tube.

Shiley TracheoSoft XLT

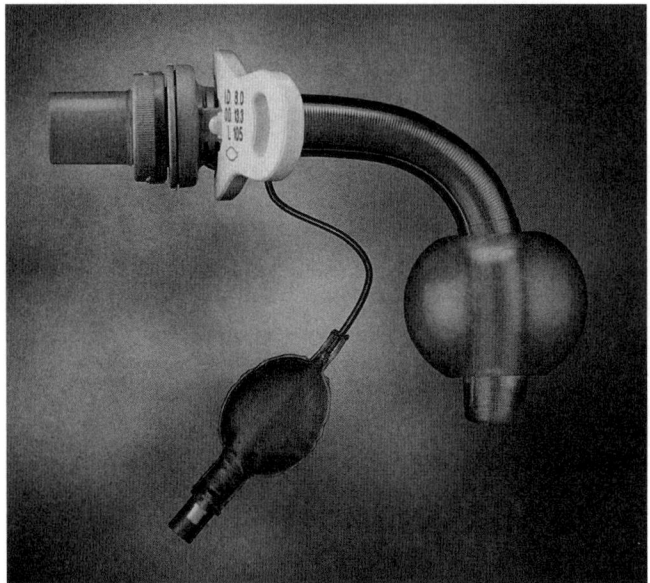

Structure: Cuffed, dual-cannula
Material: Semisoft polyvinyl chloride
Manufacturer: Covidien
Unique Features: Extra-long, dual-cannula tracheostomy tube comes in either extra distal or extra proximal length
Use: For the patient with a thick or extra-long neck and for whom thick secretions are a concern

Shiley TracheoSoft XLT tracheostomy tube. Note extended horizontal length (Covidien).

The Shiley TracheoSoft XLT tracheostomy tube is an extra-long tube constructed of semisoft polyvinyl chloride. It has a disposable inner cannula and comes in an extra distal as well as extra horizontal length. It was taken off the market in 2004 because of design issues but has since been redesigned and reintroduced. Its most valuable feature is that it is currently the only extra-length tracheostomy tube with an inner cannula. Because of its inner cannula and extra length, it is ideal for the patient with an extra-large or extra-long neck who also has a large amount of secretions.

TRACOE Vario

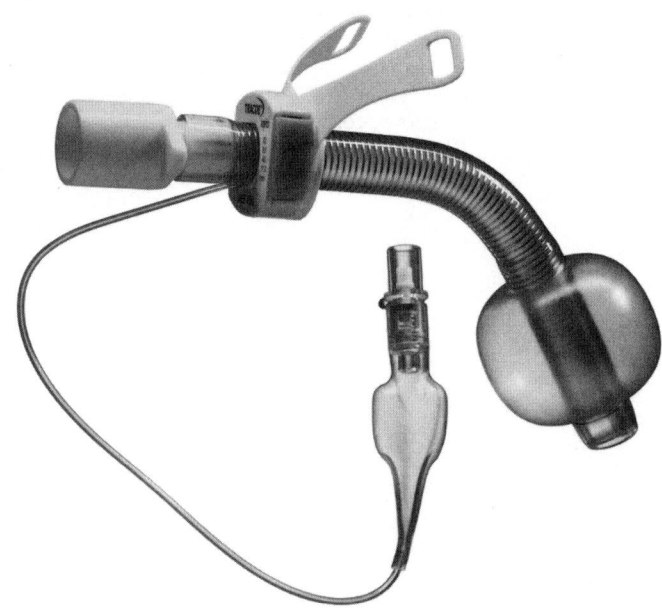

Structure: Cuffed or uncuffed; single-cannula
Material: Spiral reinforced polyvinyl chloride or clear polyvinyl chloride
Manufacturer: Boston Medical Products
Unique Features: Extra length and adjustable wings on the neck flange; models include cuffed, cuffless, wire-reinforced, and one model with a suction port above the cuff
Use: For the patient with unique anatomical needs

TRACOE Vario tracheostomy tube. Photo courtesy of Boston Medical Products. All rights reserved.

The TRACOE Vario tracheostomy tubes are extra-long, single-cannula tubes with adjustable-neck flanges. Two of the TRACOE Vario models are wire reinforced (models 450 and 455), and an MRI is contraindicated with these tubes in place. The TRACOE Vario tubes have a wide angle to the shaft and come in cuffed (models 450, 460, and 470) and cuffless (models 455 and 465) versions. In addition, one of the models also has a suction attachment port above the cuff for the patient with copious subglottic secretions (model 470). The wings of the neck flange can be placed in different positions.

TRACOE Comfort Extra Long

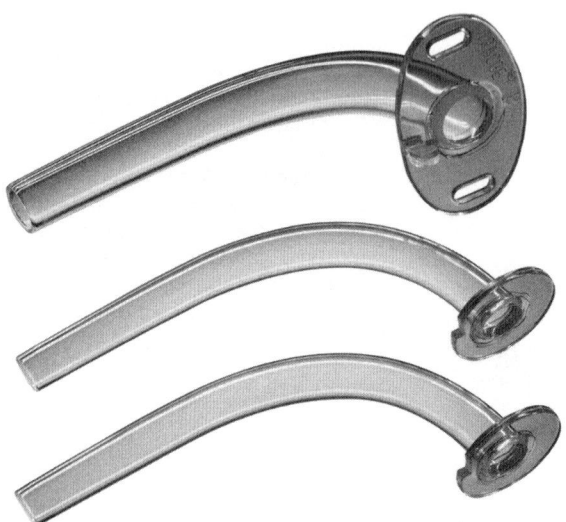

Structure: Uncuffed, single- or dual-cannula, fenestrated or nonfenestrated
Material: Flexible polyvinyl chloride
Manufacturer: Boston Medical Products
Unique Features: Clear, flexible material; extra length; low profile
Use: When positive-pressure ventilation is not required and secretions are not a concern

TRACOE Comfort extra-long tracheostomy tube. Photo courtesy of Boston Medical Products. All rights reserved.

The TRACOE Comfort line of extra-length tracheostomy tubes is made of a very soft, flexible, clear, and lightweight medical polymer. They are always cuffless and come with or without an inner cannula. Most of the models are low profile in nature and do not have a 15-mm adapter; however, one of the models (205) comes with a 15-mm adapter on the inner cannula so positive pressure can be used. Model 204 comes with a swivel speaking valve. Model 203 comes with a silver speaking valve and can also be ordered with an oxygen supply port. The manufacturer recommends that paraffin oil be used with the dual-cannula tracheostomy tubes at least every other day to lubricate the inner cannula and ensure it is easy to insert and remove.

Portex Blue Line Extra Horizontal Length

Structure: Cuffed, single-cannula
Material: Siliconized polyvinyl chloride
Manufacturer: Smiths Medical
Unique Features: Extra horizontal length
Use: For the patient with a thick neck

The Portex Blue Line Extra Horizontal Length tracheostomy tube is made of siliconized polyvinyl chloride. The proximal length is elongated to accommodate large or thick necks. This tracheostomy tube is no longer available (personal communication, Mark Larue, Portex sales representative, November 2008).

Tracheostomy Tubes With Additional Suction Channel

A few tracheostomy tubes on the market have specifically designed suction channels. The accumulation of secretions above the cuff has been implicated in the development of ventilator-associated pneumonia. The Portex Blue Line Ultra Suctionaid tube has been developed to meet that need. In addition, the TRACOE Twist and Vario tubes both have specifically designed suction ports. Any talking tracheostomy tubes or those with an additional air supply line have also been used successfully for intermittent or continuous suctioning above the cuff. The major problem with a suction channel of any kind is that it tends to get clogged with secretions. However, simply flushing the line with water or saline (with the cuff inflated) usually remedies the problem.

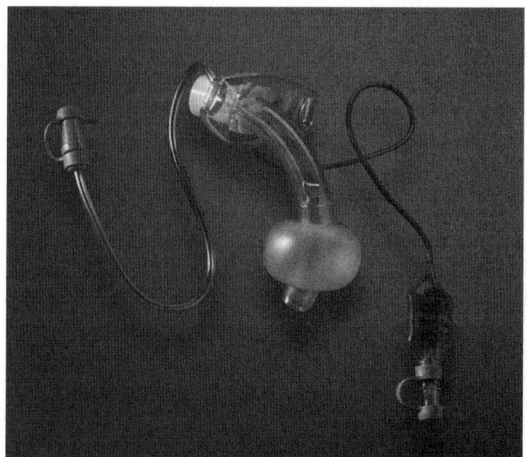

Portex Blue Line Ultra Suctionaid tracheostomy tube. Note subglottic suction port in addition to inflation line. Photo courtesy of Smiths Medical.

Metal Tracheostomy Tubes

Metal tracheostomy tubes are always uncuffed. There are several types of metal tracheostomy tubes, but the Jackson tracheostomy is the oldest and probably best known. Metal tracheostomy tubes can be constructed of stainless steel or silver. They are heavier than plastic tubes and can reflect ambient temperature. The primary differences among these metal tubes are the design of the neck flange, the length, and the angle of tube curvature. A metal tracheostomy tube can last a lifetime, but it does require regular cleaning, as do tubes made of plastic and other softer materials. For this reason, a metal tracheostomy tube may be preferred in patients who pay out of pocket or those who will be returning to a country where plastic tubes are difficult to obtain.

Some medical centers frequently use metal tracheostomy tubes; in other centers, they are rarely seen. Metal tracheostomy tubes are sometimes preferred when it is known the tube will be permanent, such as in head or neck cancer or trauma.

Metal tracheostomy tubes cannot be customized as easily as plastic tubes. For this reason, they often come in a variety of lengths. Many metal tubes are completely interchangeable within a size and style. One of the biggest advantages of metal tracheostomy tubes is that the walls of the tube are thinner. A unique advantage of silver tubes is that they are reported to have bactericidal properties.

One manufacturer recommends that metal tracheostomy tubes be cleaned daily. Chemical cleaners such as hydrogen peroxide, enzyme cleaners, or sodium hydroxide should not be used with metal tubes because they can cause damage. More detailed instructions for cleaning metal tracheostomy tubes can be found in chapter 7.

Jackson

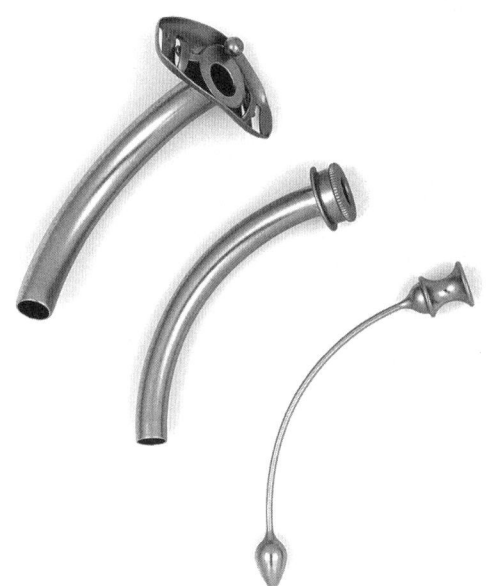

Jackson tracheostomy tube. Note low-profile inner cannula. Pilling product image provided courtesy of Teleflex Medical.

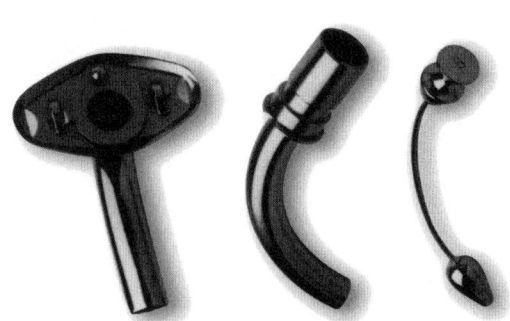

Jackson Improved tracheostomy tube with 15-mm adapter. Premier Medical Products.

Structure: Uncuffed, dual-cannula
Material: Stainless steel or sterling silver
Manufacturers: Pilling (Teleflex Medical), Premier Medical Products
Unique Features: Parts are completely adaptable within a size and style
Use: For the patient who prefers a metal tracheostomy

The Jackson tracheostomy tube was the original metal tube. The original Jackson tracheostomy tubes came in stainless steel, but there is also a model in sterling silver. This sterling silver model has a rotating lock to hold the low-profile inner cannula in place, and this swivel-locking ring is also found on the Jackson Improved models. The original Jackson tracheostomy tubes have a swivel lock to hold the inner cannula in place and as such are low profile, but they can be fitted with 15-mm adapters for use with positive-pressure ventilation. There are currently two manufacturers of the Jackson tracheostomy tube: Pilling (Teleflex Medical) and Premier Medical Products. At Premier, the 15-mm adapter is permanently attached to the Improved pattern tube. The neck flange may have different shapes depending on the size of the tube. With Premier tubes, sizes 00 to 8 have a small rectangular shape, while sizes 9 and 10 have a larger oval neck flange (personal communication, Toni Banet, Premier Medical Products, May 2009).

Holinger

Structure: Uncuffed, dual-cannula
Material: Sterling silver
Manufacturer: Pilling
Unique Features: Tube is attached to the neck flange at a 65-degree, acute downward angle; sterling silver has bactericidal effect
Use: For patients who prefer a metal tracheostomy tube

Holinger tracheostomy tubes are sterling silver with a rectangular neck flange. Sizes vary from 000 to 8. The Holinger tube is attached to the neck flange at an acute downward angle of 65 degrees, rather than the usual alignment of 90 degrees. Holinger tracheostomy tubes are low-profile tubes, with an inner cannula but without a 15-mm connector.

Tracheostomies

Tucker

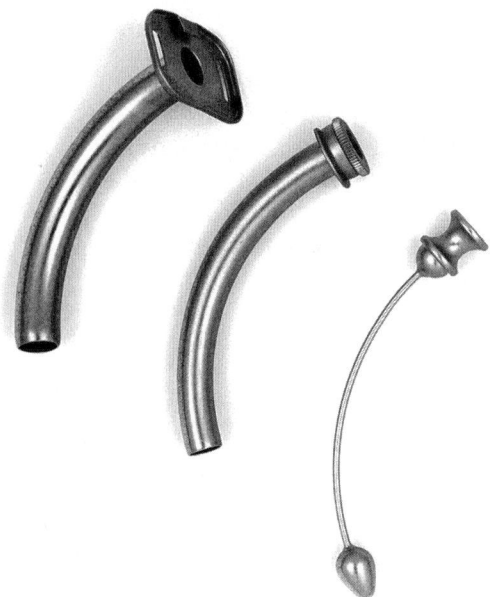

Structure: Uncuffed, dual-cannula
Material: Sterling silver
Manufacturer: Pilling
Unique Features: Valved inner cannula allows speech without digital occlusion; sterling silver has bactericidal effect
Use: For the patient who prefers a metal tracheostomy tube

Tucker tracheostomy tubes.

Tucker tracheostomy tubes are made of sterling silver and may or may not have a Tucker valve along the shaft of the inner cannula. The Tucker valve bulges outward during inspiration, allowing the patient to speak without finger occlusion of the tube. This internal valve is quite different than other types of speaking valves, which are connected to the outside of the tube. The Tucker valve is for use with sterling silver tubes only. See chapter 6 for further discussion of phonation.

Mayo Clinic

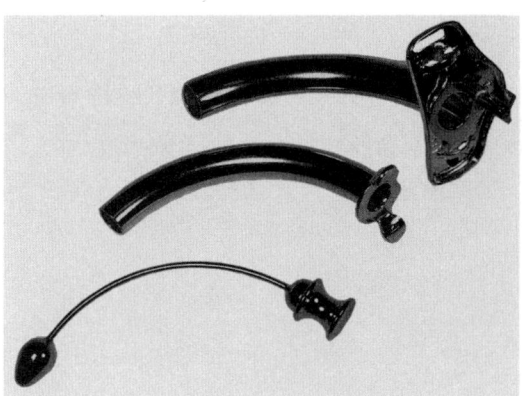

Structure: Uncuffed, dual-cannula
Material: Stainless steel
Manufacturer: Pilling
Unique Features: Holinger-style neck flange on Jackson stainless steel shaft
Use: For the patient who prefers a metal tracheostomy tube

Mayo Clinic tracheostomy tube. Pilling product image provided courtesy of Teleflex Medical.

The Mayo Clinic tube is a metal tracheostomy tube with a Holinger-style neck flange (rectangular) on a Jackson stainless steel shaft.

Martin

Structure: Uncuffed, dual-cannula
Material: Sterling silver
Manufacturer: Pilling
Unique Features: Additional inner cannula with proximal extension of 2.5 cm
Use: For the patient who prefers a metal tracheostomy tube; extended inner cannula projects out of bulky dressings

The Martin tracheostomy tube is sterling silver and has a low-profile inner cannula as well as an additional inner cannula with a 2.5-cm proximal extension that can project beyond bulky dressings. It has a standard Jackson curve and so is interchangeable with Jackson tracheostomy tubes. The Martin tracheostomy tube is no longer manufactured (Patti Pandya, personal communication, Teleflex Medical, November 4, 2009).

Luer

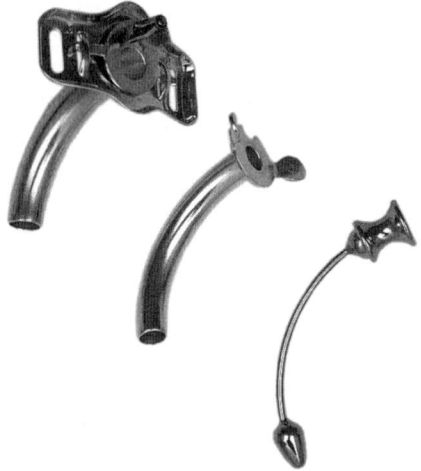

Structure: Uncuffed, dual-cannula
Material: Sterling silver
Manufacturer: Pilling
Unique Features: Shorter and more acute curve than Jackson tracheostomy tube
Use: For the patient who prefers a metal tracheostomy tube

Luer tracheostomy tube. Pilling product image provided courtesy of Teleflex Medical.

The Luer tracheostomy tube is made of sterling silver and is shorter in length than the comparable Jackson tube. It has a more acute curve than the Jackson tracheostomy tubes, but it has the original Jackson-style neck flange. These are low-profile tubes without 15-mm connectors.

Laryngectomy Tubes

Laryngectomy tubes are always cuffless because laryngectomy patients are neck breathers. The laryngectomy tube is typically shorter than the comparable tracheostomy tube and the angle of curvature is narrower. It can have either a single outer cannula or a dual cannula. Like tracheostomy tubes, laryngectomy tubes can be rigid or flexible. Because laryngectomy is a permanent stoma, the tube itself is often not required beyond a few months after initial placement.

Chapter 3   Types of Tracheostomy Tubes and Related Appliances

Shiley LGT

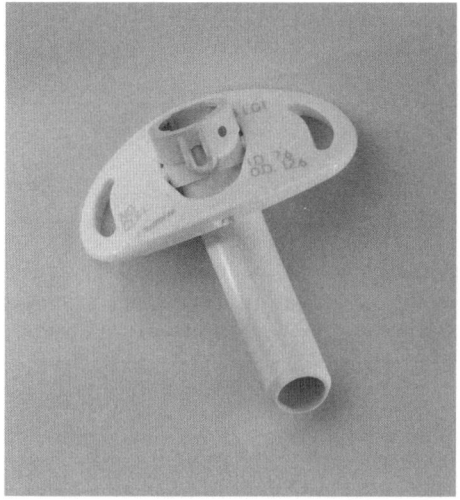

Structure: Uncuffed, dual-cannula, short, narrow curvature
Material: Rigid polyvinyl chloride
Manufacturer: Covidien
Unique Features: Shorter length and narrower curvature than standard tracheostomy tube
Use: For the laryngectomy patient in whom secretions are a concern

Shiley LGT laryngectomy tube (without inner cannula) (Covidien).

The Shiley LGT tracheostomy tube is a rigid tube made of polyvinyl chloride. It has an inner cannula that nests within the outer cannula and, like the Shiley CFS and LPC, is attached by means of a twist lock. It also comes with a low-profile, cosmetic inner cannula.

Portex DIC Laryngectomy

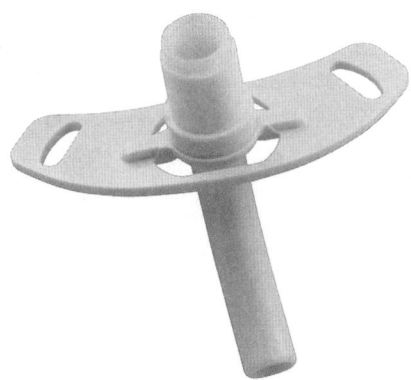

Structure: Uncuffed, single-cannula, short, narrow curvature
Material: Silicone
Manufacturer: Smiths Medical
Unique Features: Shorter length and narrower curvature than standard tracheostomy tube
Use: For the laryngectomy patient in whom secretions may be a concern

Portex DIC laryngectomy tube. Photo courtesy of Smiths Medical.

The Portex DIC laryngectomy tube is a flexible silicone tube with an inner cannula.

TRACOE Twist Laryngectomy

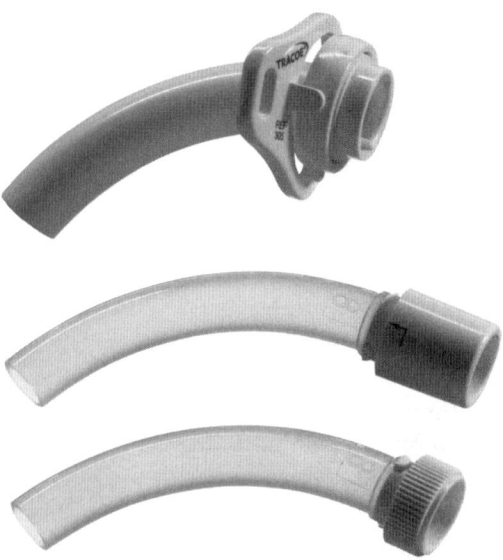

Structure: Uncuffed, dual-cannula, short, narrow curvature
Material: Flexible thermoelastic polyurethane
Manufacturer: Boston Medical Products
Unique Features: Shorter length and narrower curvature than standard tracheostomy tube
Use: For the laryngectomy patient in whom secretions may be a concern

TRACOE Twist laryngectomy tube. Photo courtesy of Boston Medical Products. All rights reserved.

The TRACOE Twist laryngectomy tube is made of medical-grade polyurethane, similar to the TRACOE Twist tracheostomy tubes. It has a standard inner cannula with a 15-mm connector and a low-profile inner cannula.

TRACOE Comfort Laryngectomy

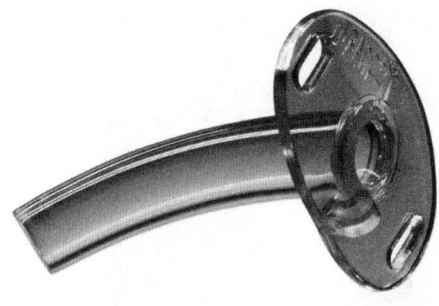
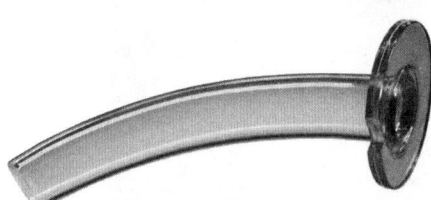

Structure: Uncuffed, dual-cannula, short, narrow curvature
Material: Flexible polyvinyl chloride
Manufacturer: Boston Medical Products
Unique Features: Clear, flexible material; comes with one or two inner cannulas
Use: To maintain patency of the stoma following laryngectomy

TRACOE Comfort laryngectomy tube.
Photo courtesy of Boston Medical Products.
All rights reserved.

The TRACOE Comfort laryngectomy tube is clear and flexible with an inner cannula that can be removed for cleaning.

Singer Laryngectomy

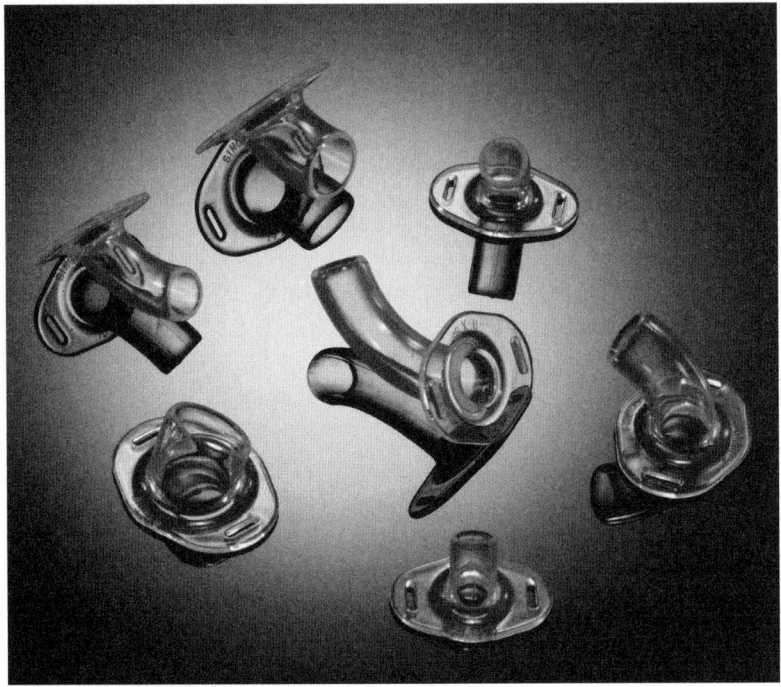

Singer laryngectomy tube. Photo courtesy of Boston Medical Products. All rights reserved.

Structure: Uncuffed, single-cannula, short, narrow curvature
Material: Silicone
Manufacturer: Boston Medical Products
Unique Features: Clear and very flexible material
Use: To maintain patency of the stoma following laryngectomy

The Singer laryngectomy tube is clear, flexible, and made of silicone. It has a low-profile appearance and comes in 28 sizes. The flange is designed to cover a wide surface area to keep tracheostomy ties away from the healing stoma. The Singer tube should be rinsed under running water to clean. If crusts or mucus plugs are seen, it should be soaked in hot, soapy water for at least 10 minutes and cleaned with a nonabrasive brush. The manufacturer recommends it be soaked overnight in a 3% hydrogen peroxide solution and then rinsed and air dried.

Provox LaryTube

Structure: Uncuffed, single-cannula, short, narrow curvature
Material: Silicone
Manufacturer: Natus Medical
Unique Features: Fenestrated model is for use with voice prosthesis; can be used with its own heat moisture exchanger (HME) system
Use: For the laryngectomy patient in whom secretions are not a concern

The Provox LaryTube is made of flexible silicone and has a conical gradation from the short neck flange to the shaft. It comes in a standard model, a fenestrated model (for use with a voice prosthesis), and a model with a ring that attaches to an adhesive base plate for wear without ties around the neck. This tube can also be used with its own HME system.

Bivona Laryngectomy

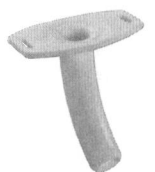

Structure: Uncuffed, single-cannula, short, narrow curvature
Material: Silicone
Manufacturer: Smiths Medical
Unique Features: Wider neck flange; short and long lengths for three different sizes
Use: For the laryngectomy patient in whom secretions are not a concern

Bivona laryngectomy tube. Photo courtesy of Smiths Medical.

The Bivona laryngectomy tube comes in three different sizes (9.5, 11, and 13) in three different lengths (55, 85, and 105 mm).

Fenestrated Tracheostomy Tubes

Fenestrated tracheostomy tubes can be cuffed or uncuffed. The term comes from the French word *la fenêtre,* meaning window. The shaft of the fenestrated tube has an opening on the dorsal aspect that allows for an added boost of air to the vocal cords. The standard placement of the fenestration is at a point on the shaft one-third of its length as measured from the neck flange. Many clinicians do not realize that this fenestration must be measured to fit so that it aligns centrally within the airway. A failure to precisely fit this tracheostomy tube can result in the abutment of the fenestration with the anterior or posterior wall of the trachea, resulting in the growth of granulation tissue within the fenestration. The removal of a tracheostomy tube with a growth of this granulation tissue can be a surgical challenge. Manipulation of a fenestrated tracheostomy tube should be preceded by a thorough assessment of its placement within the airway. Initially, this can be done by shining a light within the opening of the tracheostomy and looking through the tube, with the patient's head in different positions. If a pale pink color is seen, it may be granulation tissue within the fenestration, and a consultation with an otolaryngologist should be done immediately. One can also attempt to gently move the tracheostomy within the stoma to assess for the mobility of the tube itself. The forceful removal of a fenestrated tracheostomy tube with an unrecognized growth of granulation tissue can result in hemorrhage and an airway catastrophe. For these reasons, many centers do not routinely place fenestrated tracheostomies. If a fenestrated tracheostomy remains the best option for the patient, the procedure to fit the tracheostomy tube is discussed in chapter 4.

Shiley Fenestrated FEN, CFN, DFEN, DCFN

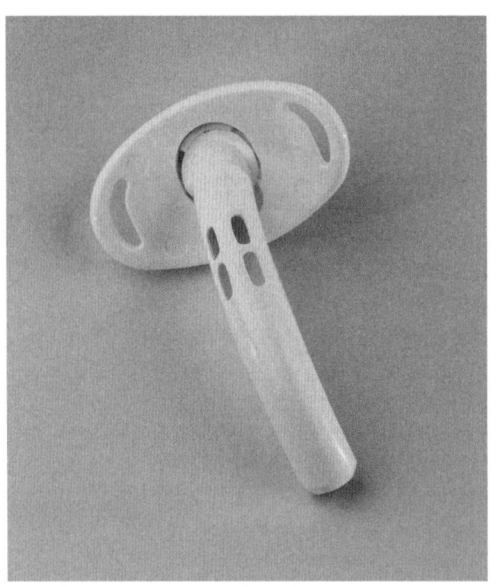

Structure: Cuffed (FEN, DFEN) or uncuffed (CFN, DCFN), dual-cannula
Material: Rigid polyvinyl chloride
Manufacturer: Covidien
Unique Features: FEN and DFEN tubes have one large oval fenestration; CFN and DCFN tubes have narrower fenestrated slits
Use: For the patient who desires to speak

Shiley DCFN tracheostomy tube (Covidien).

Shiley manufactures four types of fenestrated tracheostomy tubes—the FEN, CFN, DFEN, and DCFN—which are all made of rigid polyvinyl chloride. The Shiley FEN and DFEN are cuffed tubes; the CFN and the DCFN are cuffless tubes. Both the FEN and the CFN have a standard, nondisposable inner cannula and a fenestrated, nondisposable inner cannula. The DFEN and the DCFN have only a standard (nonfenestrated) disposable inner cannula. The fenestration of the FEN and the CFN is a large oval aperture on the dorsal aspect of the shaft. The fenestration of the DFEN and the DCFN is a set of linear slits along the dorsal aspect of the tube. Because the DFEN and DCFN have only a standard (nonfenestrated) inner cannula, they can only be used as a fenestrated tube without the inner cannula in place.

Portex DIC Fenestrated

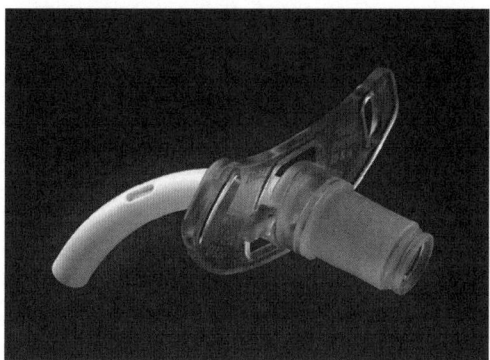

Structure: Cuffed or uncuffed, dual-cannula, fenestrated
Material: Rigid polyvinyl chloride
Manufacturer: Smiths Medical
Unique Features: Color-coded disposable inner cannula
Use: For the patient who wishes to speak but for whom secretions may be a concern

Portex DIC fenestrated uncuffed tracheostomy tube. Photo courtesy of Smiths Medical.

The Portex DIC fenestrated tube has all the features of the other DIC tubes, including a color-coded inner cannula based on size (see Table 3.1). The fenestration is composed of two slits along the shaft of the tube to allow air up to the vocal cords.

Portex Flex DIC Fenestrated

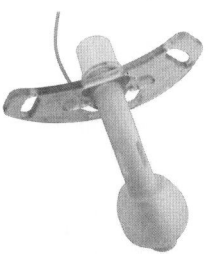

Structure: Cuffed or uncuffed, dual-cannula, fenestrated
Material: Flexible polyvinyl chloride with silicone coating
Manufacturer: Smiths Medical
Unique Features: Color-coded disposable inner cannula
Use: For the patient who wishes to speak but for whom secretions may be a concern

Portex Flex DIC fenestrated cuffed tracheostomy tube. Photo courtesy of Smiths Medical.

The Portex Flex DIC fenestrated tube has all of the features of the other Flex DIC tubes, including a color-coded inner cannula based on size.

Portex Lo-Profile Fenestrated

Structure: Cuffed or uncuffed, dual-cannula, fenestrated
Material: Rigid polyvinyl chloride
Manufacturer: Smiths Medical
Unique Features: Low-profile inner cannula (without 15-mm adapter) and standard inner cannula (with 15-mm adapter)
Use: For the patient who wishes to speak but for whom secretions may be a concern

Portex Blue Line Fenestrated and Portex Blue Line Ultra Fenestrated

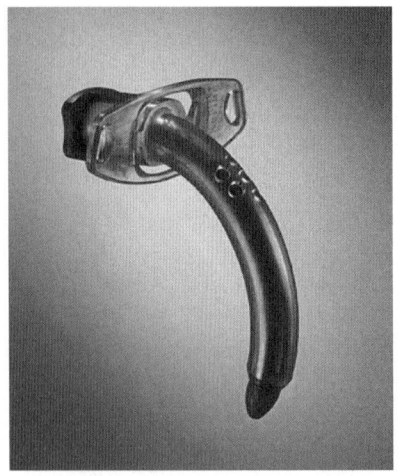

Structure: Cuffed or uncuffed, dual-cannula, fenestrated
Material: Siliconized polyvinyl chloride
Manufacturer: Smiths Medical
Unique Features: Blue neck flange, inflation line, and pilot balloon
Use: For the patient who wishes to speak

Portex Blue Line Ultra fenestrated tracheostomy tube. Photo courtesy of Smiths Medical.

The Portex Blue Line Ultra tracheostomy tubes also come in fenestrated versions. These fenestrated tubes come in cuffed and cuffless models. The fenestration of the Portex fenestrated tube is a series of linear slits along the dorsal aspect of the tube. The pictures the Portex Blue Line Ultra fenestrated tracheostomy tube.

TRACOE Twist Fenestrated

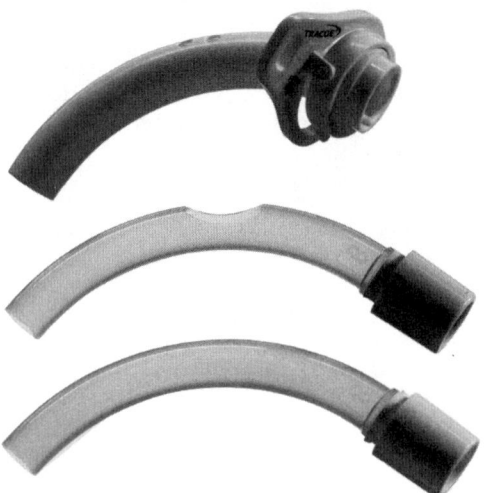

Structure: Cuffed or cuffless, dual-cannula
Material: Flexible thermoelastic polyurethane
Manufacturer: Boston Medical Products
Unique Features: Fenestrations consist of several small circular holes on dorsal aspect of shaft
Use: For the patient who wishes to speak but for whom secretions may be a concern

TRACOE Twist fenestrated tracheostomy tube. Photo courtesy of Boston Medical Products. All rights reserved.

The TRACOE Twist tracheostomy tubes also come in fenestrated versions. These fenestrated tubes come in cuffed and cuffless models. They have all the features of the standard TRACOE Twist tubes, with the addition of an oval-shaped fenestration. Unlike other fenestrated models, the fenestrations on this tube are a series of small circular holes on the dorsal aspect of the outer cannula and a large oval aperture on the inner cannula. Model numbers for the fenestrated versions of the TRACOE Twist tubes are 302 and 304. They are packaged with a standard inner cannula with a 15-mm connector, a fenestrated inner cannula, and an obturator.

TRACOE Comfort Fenestrated

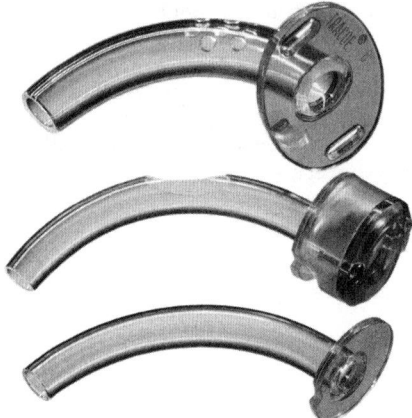

Structure: Uncuffed, dual-cannula
Material: Flexible polyvinyl chloride
Manufacturer: Boston Medical Products
Unique Features: Clear, low profile; fenestrations are a series of round holes; one model comes with a silver speaking valve
Use: For the patient who desires to speak

TRACOE Comfort fenestrated tracheostomy tube. Photo courtesy of Boston Medical Products. All rights reserved.

The TRACOE Comfort line of tracheostomy tubes also includes four models that are fenestrated: 103, 103A, 104, and 104A. This type of fenestration is unique to TRACOE tubes; the inner cannula has one large oval aperture while the outer cannula has a series of round holes on the dorsal aspect of the shaft. Two of the models (103 and 103A) also include a detachable silver speaking valve. Model 104 comes with a swivel speaking valve attached to the inner cannula.

Jackson Fenestrated

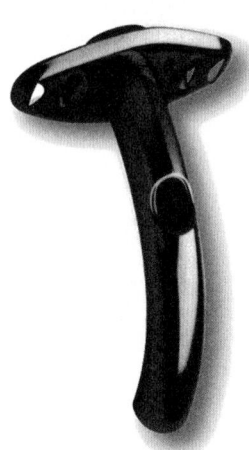

Structure: Uncuffed, dual-cannula
Material: Stainless steel or sterling silver
Manufacturer: Pilling (Teleflex Medical), Premier Medical Products
Unique Features: Large oval fenestration on dorsal aspect of shaft
Use: For the patient who prefers a metal tracheostomy tube and who desires to speak

Jackson fenestrated tracheostomy tube. Premier Medical Products.

The Jackson metal tracheostomy tube also comes in a fenestrated version. Unless otherwise ordered, the fenestration is placed one-third of the distance between the neck flange and the distal tip of the tube.

Double-Cuffed Tracheostomy Tubes

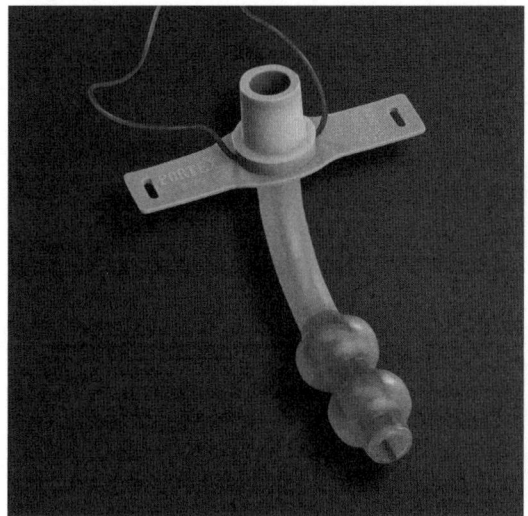

Structure: Double-cuffed, single-cannula
Material: Siliconized polyvinyl chloride
Manufacturer: Smiths Medical
Unique Features: Extra vertical length with two separate cuffs
Use: For the patient with unusual tracheal anatomy, fistulas, stenosis, or tracheomalacia

Portex Blue Line tracheostomy tube with extra vertical length with double cuff. Photo courtesy of Smiths Medical.

In rare circumstances, a double-cuffed tube may be beneficial. The presence of two cuffs can be useful in special circumstances, such as cases of tracheomalacia, fistulas, or stenosis. One cuff can be inflated, allowing delivery of positive-pressure ventilation. When a leak becomes apparent, that cuff can be deflated and the other cuff inflated. This alternate deflation and inflation allows for the reperfusion of the affected area. However, Quigley (1988) reported that this advantage is somewhat controversial and suggested that mucosal injury may extend over a greater surface area. Portex is the only company that currently manufacturers a double-cuffed tube, but this model is reportedly scheduled to be discontinued (personal communication, Mark Larue, Portex sales representative, November 2008). If a double-cuffed tube is desired, it can be custom ordered.

T-Tubes

T-tubes are tracheal stents designed to maintain an open airway for patients with tracheal stenosis or an airway reconstruction. First used in the mid-1960s, T-tubes were used for the repair of tracheal injuries and tracheomalacia (Huang, 2001; Wouters, Byreddy, Gleeson, & Morley, 2008). The long limb is positioned within the trachea, and the short limb projects through the stoma. T-tubes are thought to be superior to silicone stents because they seldom migrate, can be suctioned, and are easily removable. They are well tolerated and have been reported to remain in place for up to 20 years (Wahidi & Ernst, 2003).

Montgomery Safe-T-Tube

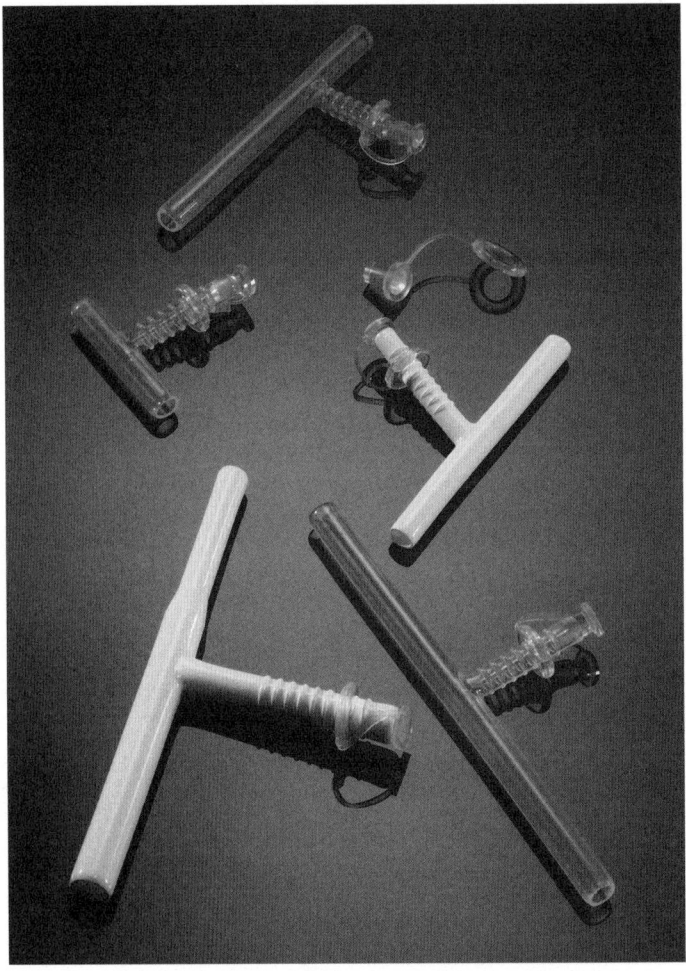

Montgomery Safe-T-Tube. Photo courtesy of Boston Medical Products. All rights reserved.

Structure: T-shaped airway stent
Material: Silicone
Manufacturer: Boston Medical Products
Unique Features: Clear or radiopaque; includes plug/ring set; Hebeler model has internal balloon system to facilitate positive-pressure ventilation
Use: To maintain adequate airway or stent stenotic trachea during reconstruction

The Montgomery Safe-T-Tube comes in adult sizes 4.5–16 mm in external diameter and pediatric sizes 4.5 to 8 mm in external diameter and has tapered ends to minimize trauma to the tracheal tissue (Guha, Mostafa, & Kendall, 2001; Wouters et al., 2008). It is made of silicone and is available in both clear and radiopaque models in five sizes: pediatric, standard, thoracic, extra long, and tapered. In addition, a Hebeler model has an internal balloon to adjust airflow through the upper end of the tube. It can be inflated for intermittent closure of the upper limb in order to create a closed system between the tracheostomy tube and the lungs. When positive-pressure ventilation is no longer required, the balloon can be deflated, opening the upper limb for access to the upper respiratory tract.

Mini-Tracheostomy Tubes

Patients who have weak secretion clearance may benefit from a mini-tracheostomy. Indications for use of the mini-tracheostomy include patients after major thoracic or abdominal surgery at particular risk for pulmonary complications due to advanced age, chronic lung disease, or poor functional status. In this case, the mini-tracheostomy is a percutaneous procedure in the operating room. It can be considered a useful adjunct in the care of patients with sputum retention.

Wright (2003) reported the success rate for the mini-tracheostomy at 96%–100%. The average duration of use is about 1 week, although cannulas are sometimes in place for several months. When the patient has regained an adequate cough and no longer requires suctioning, the mini-tracheostomy can be removed. Swallowing is reported to be normal while the cannula is in place and complications are rare. Contraindications to the procedure include morbid obesity, neck mass, calcified cricothyroid membrane, coagulopathy, and impending respiratory failure.

The Portex Mini-Trach II is a small-bore cannula of 4 mm internal diameter. The kit also includes a scalpel, suction catheter, 15-mm connector, and cotton twill tape.

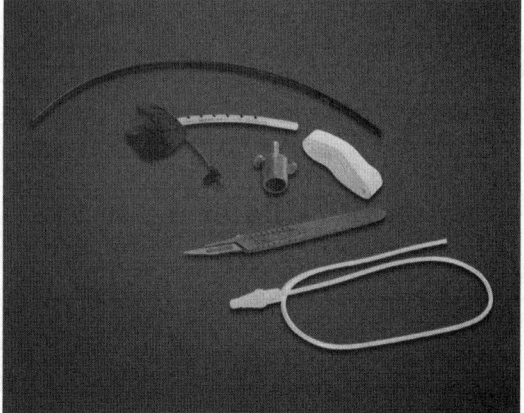

Portex Mini-Trach II Kit. Photo courtesy of Smiths Medical.

Custom-Designed Tracheostomy Tubes

Occasionally, patients have special needs that cannot be met by the standard tracheostomy tubes available. For these patients, it is possible to custom order a tracheostomy tube to meet their needs. A specific length of tracheostomy tube can be ordered, or a specific curvature of the tube can be ordered, often by sending CT scans to the manufacturer. Other options are a TTS cuff on an extra-long shaft or specifying the placement of a fenestration. These custom tracheostomy tubes often come at a premium price. In addition, depending on the manufacturer, custom-designed tubes often take up to 2 weeks, so some advance planning is necessary. Because of the time and expense required to manufacture these custom tubes, it is important that exact measurements be taken and the goals of treatment be clearly discussed between the managing service, the tracheostomy specialist, and the manufacturer.

New Tracheostomy Products

New types of tracheostomy tubes are being introduced with the purpose of overcoming the complications of standard tubes and meeting the specific needs of patients. One of these tubes is discussed here.

Blom Tracheostomy Tube System

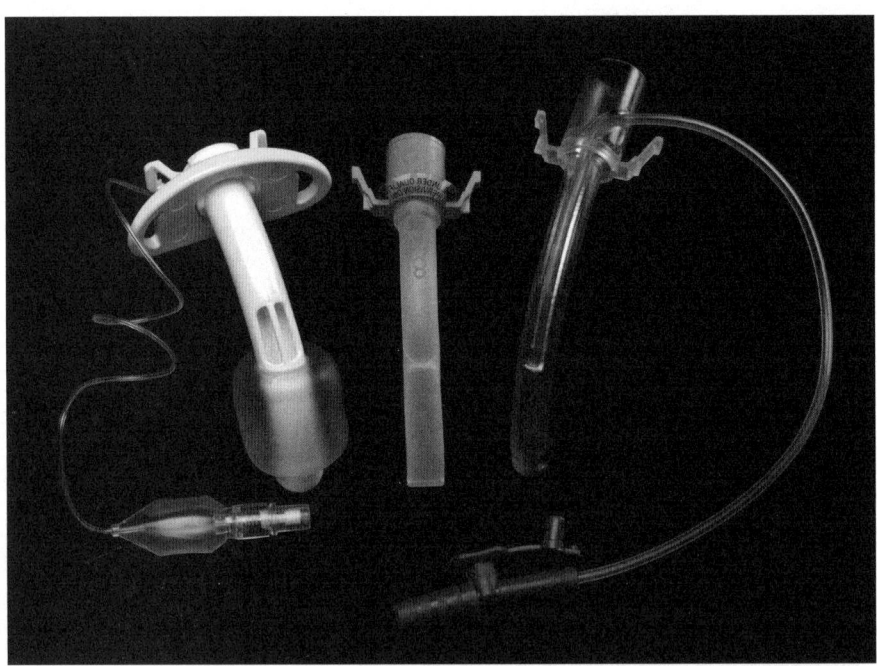

Blom tracheostomy tube system. Reprinted by permission of Pulmodyne (Indianapolis, Indiana).

Structure: Cuffed, dual-cannula, fenestrated
Material: Outer cannula—kostrate and barium; cuff—polyvinyl chloride; neck flange—polycarbonate and polyvinyl chloride; standard cannula—polyurethane and polypropylene; speech cannula—silicone and polypropylene

Manufacturer: Pulmodyne
Unique Features: Speech cannula with two valves (flap valve and bubble valve), exhaled volume reservoir, subglottic suctioning cannula; fenestration is 1 mm above the cuff so the fenestration does not contact the tracheal mucosa when inflated
Use: For the ventilator-dependent patient who wishes to speak

The Blom tracheostomy tube system is new and was designed for the ventilator-dependent patient who desires to speak regardless of cuff inflation. It has a fenestrated shaft; however, the fenestration is only 1 mm above the cuff. When the cuff is fully inflated, the fenestration is reported to avoid contact with the tracheal mucosa. It also has two valves that redirect air. During inspiration, the flap valve opens, and the bubble valve expands into the fenestration and seals it. This allows all the air to be delivered to the patient's lungs and prevents air from escaping into the upper airway. On exhalation, the mechanism is reversed—the flap valve closes and the bubble valve collapses to unblock the fenestration and allow air up through the fenestration to the vocal cords. The actual use and potential of this tracheostomy tube cannot be fully appreciated until the results of clinical trials have been evaluated.

Tracheostomy Accessories and Appliances

There are many appliances and supplies available for the tracheostomy patient. These include speaking valves, tracheostomy buttons, disconnect wedges, HMEs, decannulation plugs, shower protection devices, and more. Some of these supplies and the conditions in which they may be helpful are discussed in this section.

Speaking Valves

Speaking valves are one-way valves used to facilitate phonation. Air enters the tracheostomy on inspiration but is diverted on expiration through the oropharynx. The variety of valves is discussed in detail in chapter 6.

Stoma Maintenance Devices

There are a variety of devices available that maintain stoma patency. Often these devices are employed during the rehabilitation phase or for patients who cannot otherwise be decannulated. Using these devices, patients can proceed through the rigors of rehabilitation; however, the airway can be immediately accessed if problems are encountered.

Tracheostomy Button and Stoma Stent. A tracheostomy button is used as a temporary stent to maintain the patency of the stoma (Figure 3.4). The tracheostomy button must fit within the stoma tract and not into the airway. Spacers are used to ensure a snug fit. In order to properly fit a tracheostomy button, the stoma must be round rather than irregular. Fitting a tracheostomy button is

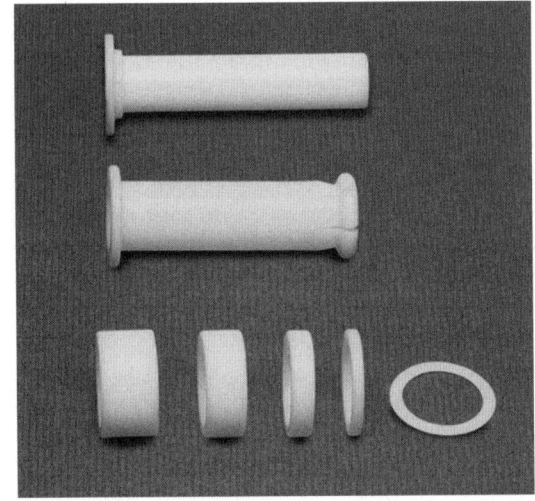

3.4

Olympic tracheostomy button with spacers. Image courtesy of Natus Medical.

discussed in chapter 4. A tracheostomy button provides a low-profile appearance while allowing breathing through the upper airway; however, a ventilator adapter is available when access to the airway is desired (Figure 3.5).

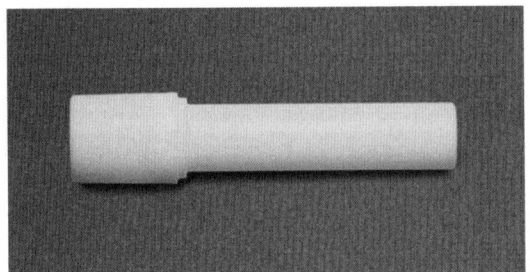

3.5

Ventilator adapter for Olympic tracheostomy button. Image courtesy of Natus Medical.

A stoma stent (Figure 3.6) is similar to a tracheostomy button; however, the cap may be directly attached to the stent itself. Stoma stents have been used in patients with high spinal cord injury to access the airway for mechanical ventilation or bronchial hygiene (Hall & Watt, 2008).

Tracheal Cannula. A tracheal cannula is similar to a tracheostomy button in that it stents open the stoma and does not interfere with airflow. However, the tracheal cannula is meant to allow direct access to the airway. The Montgomery cannula (Figure 3.7) is a corrugated tube that is an open system; however, a tracheostomy button closes off access to the airway. It is easy to suction a patient with a tracheal cannula, but the tracheostomy button does not provide regular access to the airway for suctioning. The Montgomery cannula is made of silicone and is very flexible. A ring washer holds it in place, and it comes with its own detachable plug/ring set to allow phonation. The Montgomery speaking valve was designed for use with the Montgomery cannula and comes in compatible sizes.

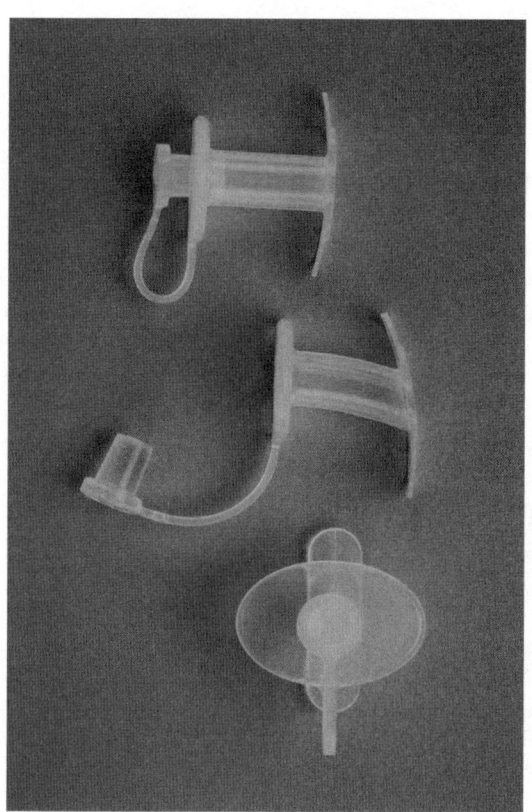

3.6
Hood stoma stent. Hood Labs (Pembroke, Massachusetts).

3.7
Montgomery cannulas. Photo courtesy of Boston Medical Products. All rights reserved.

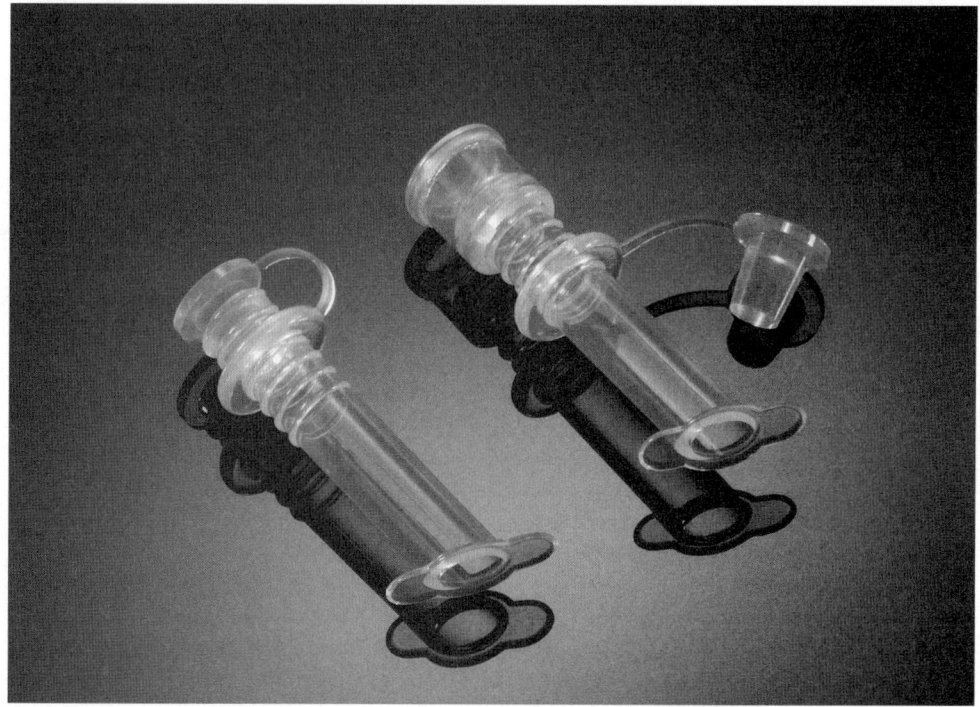

Disconnect Wedges

A disconnect wedge (Figure 3.8) is used when airway equipment (e.g., ventilator tubing or a manual resuscitation bag) is difficult to remove from the 15-mm connector of the tracheostomy tube. Forceful removal should be avoided because the tube can be damaged. The wedge is used as a lever on the 15-mm connecter to disconnect the airway equipment from the tracheostomy tube. Disconnect wedges are packaged with the Bivona and Arcadia lines of tracheostomy tubes.

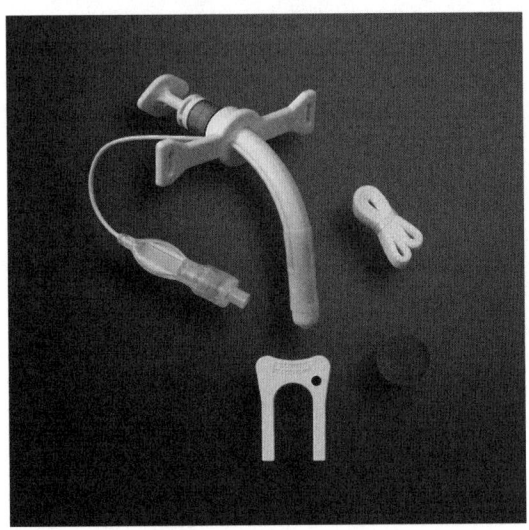

3.8 Bivona TTS tracheostomy tube and disconnect wedge (also pictured are cotton twill ties and red cap). Photo courtesy of Smiths Medical.

Caps and Decannulation Plugs

A tracheostomy cap or plug (Figures 3.9 and 3.10) is used to prevent air from entering the tracheostomy tube, which forces the patient to breathe through his or her mouth and nose, simulating normal breathing. The decannulation plug is differentiated from the cap because it typically is applied by removing the inner

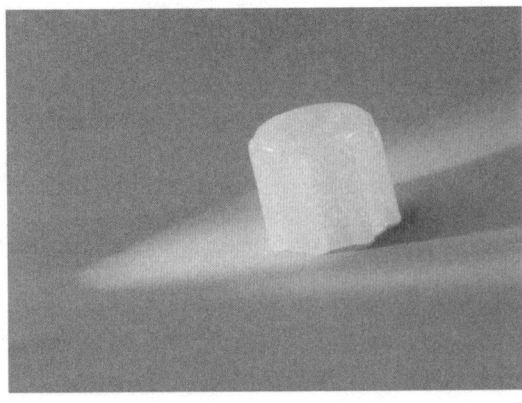

3.9 Shiley CAP (Covidien).

cannula. The advantage of the cap or plug is that it allows the patient to phonate easily without the use of digital occlusion.

Caps. There are three primary types of caps: those applied to the tracheostomy tube, those that replace the inner cannula, and graded plugs. A standard cap is applied externally to the tracheostomy tube to "plug the hole." The Shiley CFS is the only tracheostomy tube with its own capped inner cannula (Figure 3.11). One must first remove the standard inner cannula and replace it with the capped inner cannula. Caps should never be used with standard cuffed tracheostomy tubes, even if the cuff is completely deflated. The proper use of caps is discussed in chapter 6.

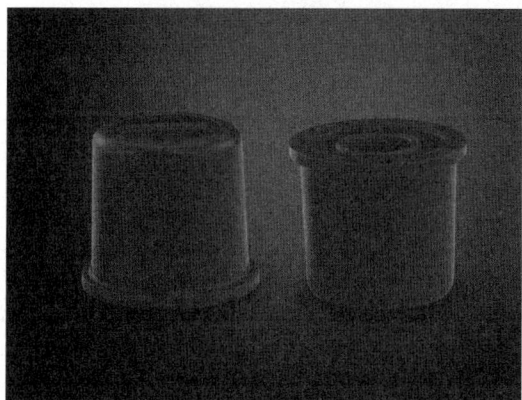

3.10
Bivona red cap.
Photo courtesy of
Smiths Medical.

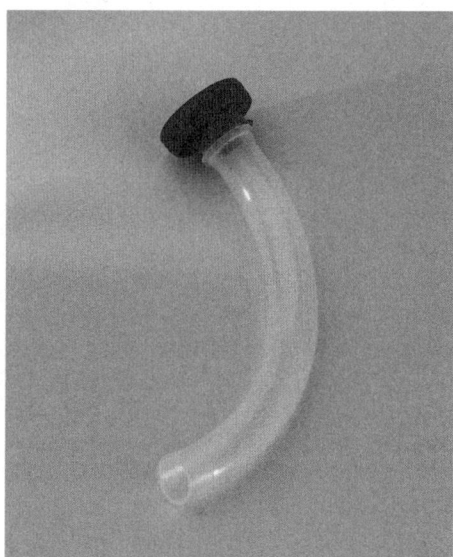

3.11
Shiley CFS capped
inner cannula
(Covidien).

Decannulation Plugs: Shiley DCP, DDCP. Rather than capping a tracheostomy tube, a decannulation plug (Figure 3.12) can be used as a low-profile cap. The use of a decannulation plug often requires the removal of the inner cannula and the attachment of the decannulation plug to the outer cannula. However, TRACOE provides red decannulation plugs for the outer cannulas of the TRACOE Twist tubes (Models 505–04, 505–10) or blue decannulation plugs for the inner cannulas (Models 504–04, 504–10).

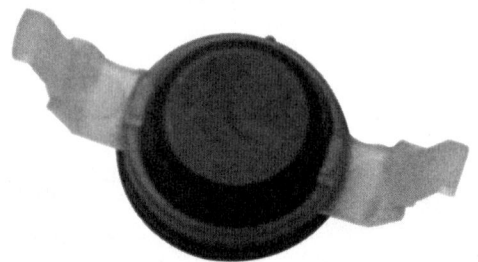

3.12 Blom decannulation plug. Reprinted by permission of Pulmodyne (Indianapolis, Indiana).

Decannulation Corks or Stoppers. A cork or stopper is similar to a cap or decannulation plug; however, it fits within (rather than around) the inner or outer cannula of a tracheostomy tube. Typically, these corks are used for metal tracheostomy tubes and can be ordered to fit based on tube size. They can be ordered in gradations of occlusion in order to facilitate a gradual transition to full upper-airway breathing (Figure 3.13). For example, they can be ordered for one-fourth partial obstruction, one-half partial obstruction, three-fourths partial obstruction, or full obstruction.

3.13

Graduated corks. Corks are graduated to provide partial to full obstruction. From left: 25%, 50%, 75%, and 100% obstruction.

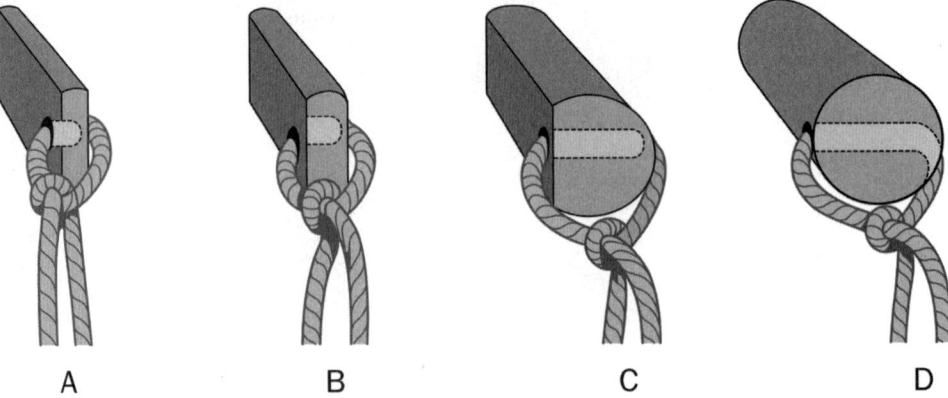

Disposable and Spare Inner Cannulas

There are several types of inner cannulas meant for temporary use.

The Shiley SIC. The inner cannula of a Shiley tracheostomy tube must be in place in order to provide positive-pressure ventilation. Because of this, one must have an extra inner cannula when cleaning the inner cannula of a Shiley tube. The Shiley SIC, or spare inner cannula (Figure 3.14), is identified by its red 15-mm connector and is a temporary inner cannula for use with the Shiley LPC, CFS, FEN, or CFN. It is not intended for long-term use and should be replaced with the permanent inner cannula as soon as tracheostomy care has been completed.

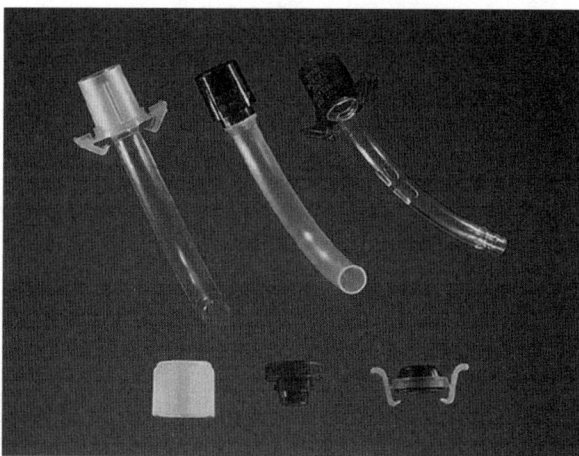

3.14 Clockwise from top left: Shiley disposable inner cannula (DIC), spare inner cannula (SIC), disposable fenestrated inner cannula (DFIC), disposable decannulation plug, decannulation plug, cap (Covidien).

Shiley DIC. The Shiley DCT tracheostomy tube inner cannulas require regular replacement, rather than cleaning. The disposable inner cannula for these tubes is called the DIC.

Portex Per-Fit Inner Cannula. The Portex Per-fit tracheostomy tube has a beveled distal tip for ease of insertion using the Seldinger technique over a dilator. The Per-fit inner cannula has a beveled tip to match the outer cannula. Figure 3.15 shows the angled distal tip, which allows easier placement over a dilator during insertion.

Disposable Inner Cannulas for Portex DIC. Portex DIC tracheostomy tubes also have disposable inner cannulas that are color coded based on size (Figure 3.16).

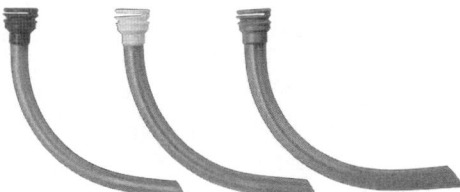

3.15 Portex Per-fit inner cannulas. Photo courtesy of Smiths Medical.

These inner cannulas must be replaced, rather than cleaned, on a regular basis. These inner cannulas are for use with all versions of Portex DIC and Flex DIC tracheostomy tubes.

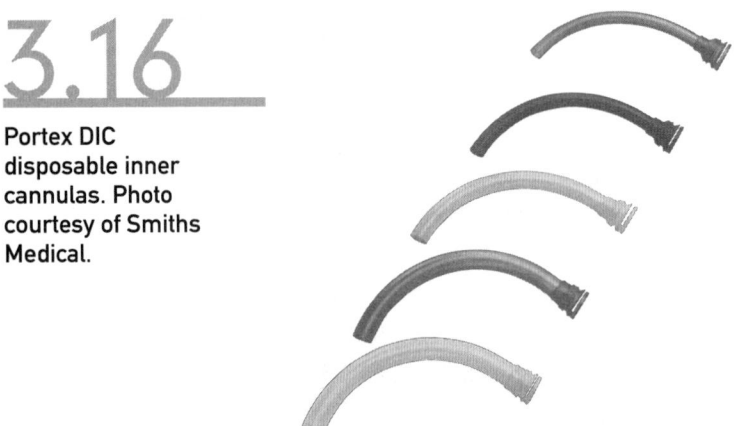

3.16 Portex DIC disposable inner cannulas. Photo courtesy of Smiths Medical.

Antidisconnect Device ("Stronghold," Covidien)

An antidisconnect device helps eliminate accidental disconnection of equipment from the tracheostomy tube (Figure 3.17). It is available in adult and pediatric sizes and is used to secure the tracheostomy tube to the ventilator tubing circuit.

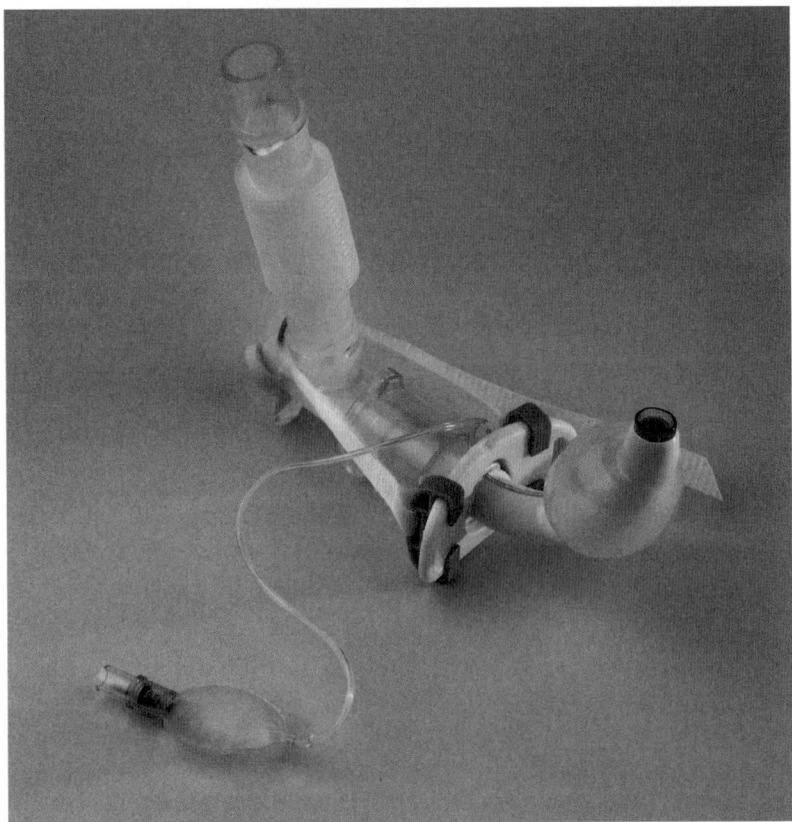

3.17 Shiley Stronghold (Covidien).

Heat Moisture Exchanger

An HME is used to trap the moisture of exhaled gas, allowing the inspiration of added humidity. These devices are especially helpful when patients experience discomfort from dry mucus membranes. These devices can be used in-line with the ventilator circuit or attached separately onto the 15-mm connector of the tracheostomy tube.

Patients who prefer not to use an HME, but who have uncomfortably dry mucous membranes, can use a thin layer of damp gauze draped over the tracheostomy. Saline nasal mist can also be sprayed within the tracheostomy at intervals to moisten mucus membranes.

Ventilator Adapters

A ventilator adapter is available for use with the Bivona Fome-Cuf tracheostomy tube (Figure 3.18). The ventilator adapter provides an additional inflation of air into the cuff with inhalation and a slight deflation of the cuff with exhalation. It is designed to be attached distally from an HME attached directly to the tracheostomy tube. The HME normally collects exhaled moisture from the circuit and delivers it during inhalation. However, this ventilator adapter delivers moisturized air from the ventilator directly to the cuff. For this reason, an auto-control device is connected to the dry side of the ventilator, and the port from the device is connected to the pilot balloon. This will inflate the cuff with dry gas.

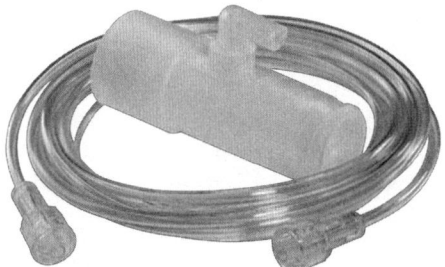

3.18
Bivona auto control device for Fome-Cuf. Photo courtesy of Smiths Medical.

Tracheostomy-Securing Devices

Tracheostomy tubes can be secured to the neck in a variety of ways, including cotton twill tape or softer collars with Velcro closures. Some patients prefer to secure their tracheostomy to their neck with a chain. There is no one recommended device; however, the priority is tube security, especially in the early postoperative period. It is recommended that no more than one finger fit under the securing device. If the securing device is too loose, the patient can easily cough out or otherwise dislodge the tracheostomy tube. If the device is too tight, it can erode into the skin of the neck.

Tracheostomy-Related Supplies

There are a variety of tracheostomy-related supplies and equipment available for the patient's convenience that are primarily for home use.

Tracheostomy Bibs. Patients who have a large amount of secretions may find it helpful to wear a type of bib designed to protect their clothing. Bibs are also available that can filter and warm the environmental air.

Scarves or Ascots. Patients who are concerned about the appearance of their tracheostomy may camouflage it by wearing decorative scarves or ascots. Some of these are available in materials that resist staining and moisture.

Shower Protection Devices. Patients who are concerned water may enter their tracheostomy or laryngectomy tube while showering can use a shower protection device. Otherwise, patients should be taught to avoid facing the water flow.

Tube Spacer. A tube spacer can be used to prevent blocking the aperture when the patient is wearing protective clothing around the stoma.

Grid or Mesh Screens. A mesh screen can be used to filter air in order to prevent inhalation and aspiration of particulate matter or foreign bodies.

Summary

There are many choices of tracheostomy tubes. Each tube has its own characteristics with inherent strengths and precautions. The major categories of tracheostomy tubes include cuffed or cuffless and single- or dual-cannula. Many special-use tracheostomy tubes are also available, such as extra-length or talking tracheostomy tubes. One must have a clear understanding of the primary goals in order to choose the best tube for a particular patient. Chapter 4 discusses the details of the next step—fitting and changing the tracheostomy tube.

Key Points

- Tracheostomy tubes can be classified into four categories: dual-cannula, cuffed tubes; single-cannula, cuffed tubes; dual-cannula, cuffless tubes; and single-cannula, cuffless tubes.
- Tracheostomy tubes are constructed of a variety of materials, including polyvinyl chloride, silicone, nylon, stainless steel, and silver.
- Tracheostomy tubes with inner cannulas should be used in patients who have large amounts of secretions.
- Laryngectomy tubes are always cuffless and are usually shorter than a standard tube.
- Cuffless tracheostomy tubes can be used in patients who can protect their airway.

References

Bernhard, W. N., Yost, L., Joynes, D., Cothalis, S., & Turndorf, H. (1985). Cuff pressures in endotracheal and tracheostomy tubes. Related cuff physical characteristics. *Chest, 87,* 720–725.

Dhand, R., & Johnson, J. C. (2006). Care of the chronic tracheostomy. *Respiratory Care, 51*(9), 984–1001.

Duguet, A., D'Amico, L., Biondi, G., Prodanovic, H., Gonzalez-Bermejo, J., & Similowski, T. (2007). Control of tracheal cuff pressure: A pilot study using a pneumatic device. *Intensive Care Medicine, 33,* 128–132.

Faris, C., Koury, E., Philpott, J., Sharma, S., Tolley, N., & Narula, A. (2007). Estimation of tracheostomy tube cuff pressure by pilot balloon palpation. *Journal of Laryngology and Otology, 121*(9), 869–871.

Guha, Q., Mostafa, S. M., & Kendall, J. B. (2001). The Montgomery T-tube: Anaesthetic problems and solutions. *British Journal of Anaesthesia, 87*(5), 787–790.

Hall, A. M., & Watt, J. W. (2008). The use of tracheal stoma stents in high spinal cord injury: A patient-friendly alternative to long-term tracheostomy tubes. *Spinal Cord, 46*(11), 753–755.

Huang, C. (2001). Use of the silicone T-tube to treat tracheal stenosis or tracheal injury. *Annals of Thoracic and Cardiovascular Surgery, 7*(4), 192–196.

Quigley, R. L. (1988). Tracheostomy—an overview. Management and complications. *British Journal of Clinical Practice, 42*(10), 430–434.

St. John, R. E., & Malen, J. F. (2004). Contemporary issues in adult tracheostomy management. *Critical Care Nursing Clinics of North America, 16*(3), 413–430.

Wahidi, M. M., & Ernst, A. (2003). The Montgomery T-tube tracheal stent. *Clinics in Chest Medicine, 24,* 437–443.

Wouters, K.M.A., Byreddy, R., Gleeson, J., & Morley, A. P. (2008). New approach to anaesthetizing a patient at risk of pulmonary aspiration with a Montgomery T-tube in situ. *British Journal of Anaesthesia, 101,* 354–357.

Wright, C. D. (2003). Minitracheostomy. *Clinics in Chest Medicine, 24*(3), 431–435.

Web Resources

Arcadia Medical Corporation, manufacturer of Arcadia tracheostomy tubes, http://www.arcadiamedical.com

Boston Medical, manufacturer of TRACOE, Montgomery, and Singer tracheostomies and related devices, http://www.trachs.com

Covidien, manufacturer of Shiley tracheostomy tubes, http://www.nellcor.com

Premier Medical Products, manufacturer of Jackson original, Jackson Improved, and Air-Lon™ tracheostomy tubes, http://www.premusa.com

Pulmodyne, manufacturer of the Blom tracheostomy tube, http://www.pulmodyne.com

Smiths Medical, manufacturer of Bivona and Portex tracheostomies and related devices, http://www.smiths-medical.com

Teleflex Medical, Pilling, manufacturer of Jackson, Mayo Clinic, Holister, and Tucker tracheostomy products, http://www.teleflexmedical.com

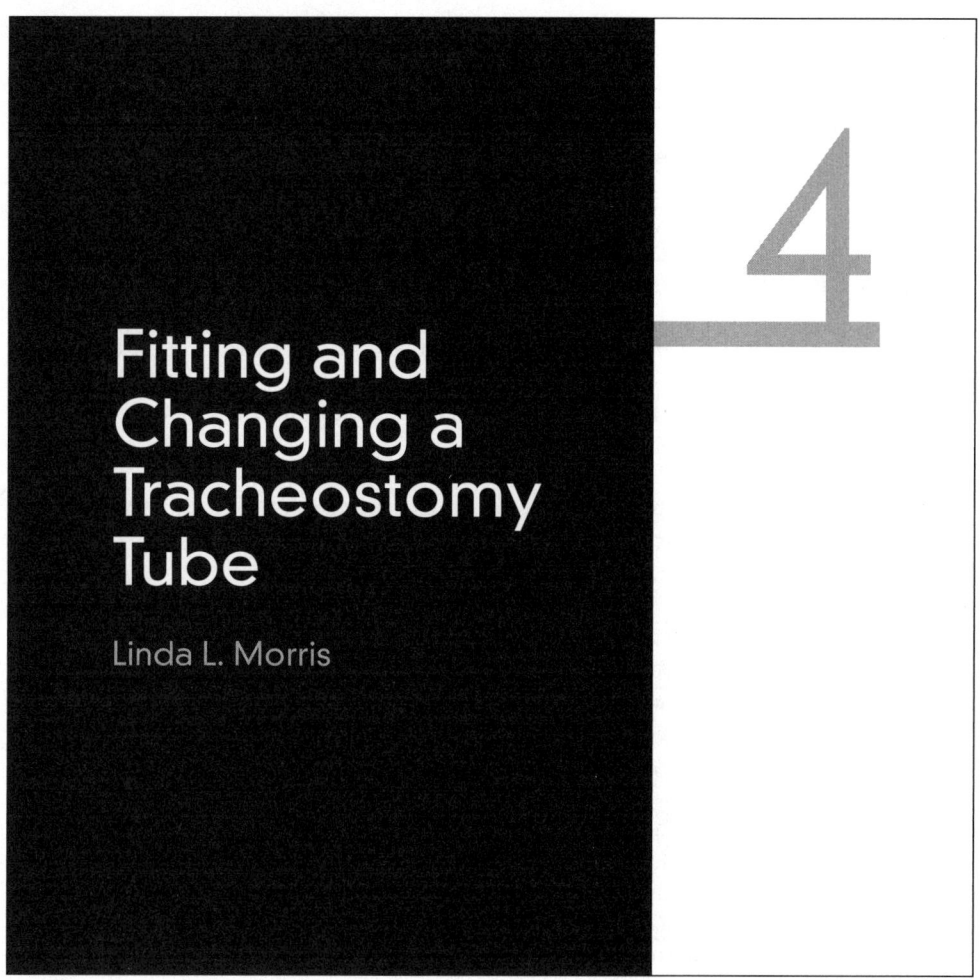

Fitting and Changing a Tracheostomy Tube

Linda L. Morris

Fitting tracheostomy tubes is both a science and an art. One might believe it is a routine and straightforward procedure, but this is hardly the case. There are numerous factors to consider when determining the optimal size and type of tracheostomy tube, particularly the patient's ability to protect his or her airway, the amount and thickness of secretions, if positive-pressure ventilation is required, anatomical considerations, if the patient wishes to speak, airway pressures, the size of the tracheostomy tube versus the size of the airway, and lung mechanics. Each of these factors must be taken into consideration in order to provide for the individual needs of each patient.

Considerations When Fitting a Tracheostomy Tube

Before Fitting a Tracheostomy Tube

There are numerous factors to consider when fitting a patient with a tracheostomy tube. Short-term and long-term goals should be identified and reviewed on a regular basis. Questions include the following:

- Will the patient require mechanical ventilation for the next week, next month, or some other time frame?
- Does the patient desire to speak?
- Is the patient able to manage airway secretions?
- Is the patient ready to be weaned from mechanical ventilation?
- Can the patient be managed with nocturnal positive-pressure ventilation and a tracheostomy collar during the day?
- Is the patient on a path to rehabilitation, or will the patient require long-term care?
- Does the family have the capability to safely manage the patient at home?

There are questions to ask at each point in the patient's hospitalization, discharge planning, rehabilitation, and outpatient settings because the goals often change as the patient progresses through each phase of treatment and recovery.

When fitting a tracheostomy tube, it is necessary to examine the inner diameter, outer diameter, and length of the tracheostomy tube in place; consider individual patient issues; and then determine the primary and secondary goals. If wishing to speak is a secondary goal, enough air must pass around the outside of the tube to easily reach the vocal cords. If a primary goal is to deliver positive-pressure ventilation, then an adequate seal would be the priority. The challenge comes when there are multiple or conflicting goals—for example, a patient who requires positive-pressure ventilation but who also desires to speak. Another challenging example is a patient who requires a longer tracheostomy tube but who also has copious thick secretions. One must constantly balance goals with priorities.

Assessing the Resistance of the Tracheostomy Tube

When fitting the optimal tracheostomy tube, one must first consider size. Poiseuille's Law states that flow is dependent on the radius and length of the tube.

$$P = \dot{V}8Ln/\pi r4$$

In this equation, P is the pressure gradient across the tube, $\dot{V}$ represents gas flow, L represents tube length, n represents gas viscosity, r represents the tube radius, and 8 and π represent constants. In other words, when flow is laminar, resistance is directly proportional to the radius of the tube raised to the fourth power. However, when flow is turbulent, resistance becomes inversely proportional to the radius raised to the fifth power. Because of this, a small decrease in radius will dramatically increase resistance (Beachey, 2007; Epstein, 2005). Compared to endotracheal tubes, a tracheostomy tube makes the elastic and resistive work of breathing easier. The shorter length of the tracheostomy tube, as well as its more rigid structure and placement in the subglottic region, makes it easier to facilitate effective bronchial hygiene (Epstein). By lessening the resistance that secretions create, intrinsic PEEP is reduced, decreasing the elastic work of breathing.

Pierson (2005) clearly outlined the general principles of airflow with regard to artificial airways:

- The larger the inner diameter, the lower the resistance.
- The shorter the tube, the lower the resistance.
- Irregular walls of the tube (such as those produced by secretions) increase resistance.
- The sharper the curve of the tube, the greater the resistance.

All these factors contribute to work of breathing and must be considered when fitting a tracheostomy tube. Major indications for placing a tracheostomy tube include prolonged mechanical ventilation with endotracheal intubation, upper airway obstruction, airway protection, and the facilitation of bronchial hygiene (Shapiro, Harrison, Kacmarek, & Cane, 1985)—the acronym VOPS (ventilation, obstruction, protection, secretions).

In hospitals, it is advisable to fit the tracheostomy patient with a tube with a standard 15-mm connector to enable the use of a mechanical resuscitation bag or ventilator in the event of an emergency. Some low-profile tubes eliminate the 15-mm connector for a more cosmetic appearance. However, many hospital-based practitioners are not familiar with the low-profile tracheostomy tube, nor that some can be converted to a standard inner cannula with a 15-mm connector, which could result in confusion during an emergency.

Choosing a Cuffed Versus Uncuffed Tube

The earliest tracheostomy tubes were cuffless. In the 1960s, tracheostomy tubes were constructed with small-volume cuffs. These cuffs were smaller than the airway, and pressures of 160 to 300 mm Hg were required to fill the cuffs (Rumbak et al., 1997). Larger volume cuffs that required lower inflation pressure were developed in the 1970s.

The first decision when choosing the type of tracheotomy tube is whether or not the patient requires a cuffed tube. Patients who require positive-pressure ventilation almost always require a cuffed tube. If the patient is ventilator dependent, a tube with a low-pressure cuff would minimize pressure against the tracheal wall. However, the patient who is only partially dependent on positive-pressure ventilation—e.g., using nocturnal ventilation at night and a high-humidity tracheostomy collar during the day—could use a different tube. In that case, a Bivona TTS or Arcadia CTS tracheostomy tube could provide the added advantage of capping during the day. Any concerns about their high-pressure cuffs would be offset by intermittent inflation. Because the cuff lies completely against the shaft when deflated, creating no airflow obstruction, the Bivona TTS and the Arcadia CTS tubes are the only cuffed tracheostomy tubes that can be capped safely when the cuff is deflated. A properly fitted, fenestrated tube may also be capped; however, this tube has a standard high-volume, low-pressure cuff.

Positive-Pressure Ventilation and Choice of Tube. Whenever positive-pressure ventilation is required, a cuffed tracheostomy tube is necessary to ensure the set tidal volume is delivered. If a cuffless tube is used with a ventilator-dependent patient, there will be a large leak of air around the tube because of the significant difference in delivered to returned tidal volume. This difference can be problematic—not only in ventilator alarms sounding, but also in terms of respiratory distress, hypoxemia, and hemodynamic instability. Occasionally, however, some ventilator-dependent patients with cuffless tracheostomy tubes use what is called "leak speech" in order to phonate. (See chapter 6 for a detailed discussion about leak speech.) However, if these patients become unstable or critically ill, a cuffed tube is always advisable. In this circumstance, patients will need the benefit of receiving the entire tidal volume. Until a cuffed tracheostomy tube can be placed, ventilator settings should be adjusted by increasing flow and/or minute ventilation to compensate for the large deficit in returned volumes.

The success of managing a ventilator-dependent patient with a tracheostomy revolves around several factors: volume delivered versus volume returned, adequate seal of the cuff within the airway, and resistance to gas delivered. When the volume returned is much less than the tidal volume delivered, ventilator alarms will sound with an alert indicator for a system leak. This leak could be in one of three main locations: the ventilator circuit, the seal of the cuff against the airway, or within the cuff itself. See chapter 5 for a comprehensive discussion about leaks.

If it has been determined that there is sufficient air in the cuff and a leak remains, tracheomalacia is the presumed cause. Tracheomalacia is commonly caused by chronic overinflation of the cuff. This added pressure against the elastic tracheal tissue causes it to weaken and balloon out in the area of the cuff. Like overstretched elastic, the tracheal tissue appears to stretch in the area of increased pressure. This stretch is limited, however, and can result in tracheal erosion if the pressures are too great over a prolonged period of time. Tracheoscopy can be used to visualize the extent of the defect.

The method to resolve a leak due to tracheomalacia is to place the cuff in a different location within the trachea. This is usually done by placing a tracheostomy tube with a slightly longer length so as to place the cuff inferior to the area of tracheomalacia (see Figure 4.1).

4.1

Tracheomalacia and repositioning the tracheostomy tube. On the left, tracheomalacia has developed around the inflated cuff. On the right, a longer tracheostomy tube has been placed, allowing the cuff to be positioned below the level of tracheomalacia.

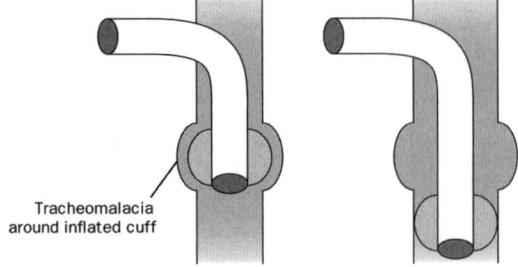

Airway Protection. Another important factor in determining the proper type of tracheostomy tube is airway protection. If the patient is able to protect his or her airway, then a cuffless tube usually offers the most benefits. However, without adequate intrinsic reflex airway protection, a cuffed tube must be chosen. Following this decision, other features can then be considered, such as phonation and single- versus dual-cannula tubes.

Airway protection is primarily influenced by intact swallow and adequate cough. The epiglottis closes over the trachea during swallowing in order prevent food and fluid from entering the trachea. A study on normal adults by Mendell and Logemann (2007) showed that the sequence of events in the pharyngeal swallow varied depending on the age of the patient and the volume and consistency of the bolus. The dominant sequence was hyoid and laryngeal elevation, followed by posterior tongue retraction and then laryngeal vestibular closure. On a larger bolus, laryngeal vestibule closure occurred before the tongue base movement—and it was thought this would add to airway protection. The sequence of events during the swallow was dependent on other factors such as age and comorbidities. Normal participants in their 60s and 70s had longer time differences between hyoid elevation and upper esophageal sphincter opening than younger subjects (Mendell & Logemann; Robbins, Hamilton, Lof, & Kempster, 1992). Neurological injury or disease may greatly influence a patient's ability to swallow, so it is advisable to obtain a swallow evaluation from a speech pathologist whenever the patient's swallow is in question. A detailed discussion on the physiology of swallow is provided in chapter 1.

Strength of Cough. Strength of cough can be subjectively observed at the bedside; however, a more objective measure is called vital capacity. Normal vital capacity is 50–70 ml/kg of body weight (Douce, 2003). However, after days or weeks of oral intubation, the ability to cough can be compromised because the glottic mechanism is bypassed. The lowest acceptable vital capacity that determines adequacy of cough is 15 ml/kg of body weight—or approximately 1 liter for most adults (Shapiro et al., 1985). Another measure of cough strength is the peak cough flow, which should be at least 360 liters per minute (Bach, 1993). Lower than this indicates poor cough strength. The primary danger of poor cough strength is the inability to clear secretions, which can result in the retention of secretions, respiratory distress, and hypoxemia.

Usually the best way to improve cough strength is vigorous exercise. In an unpublished case series by this author, a program of deep breathing and arm exercises was prescribed to tracheostomy patients who were able to independently move at least one of their upper extremities. Exercises were demonstrated to the patient, the primary nurse, and the family when available, and the patient was encouraged to do 10 (or more) repetitions per hour. All the patients who complied, even partially, demonstrated improvement in vital capacity after only 2 days—often by at least 100%, and in one case by 700%. These results are the foundation of a more robust, randomized, and controlled trial to compare this simple exercise program with standard care for tracheostomy patients and evaluate other outcomes.

Incentive spirometry is ideal for tracheostomy patients who have the manual dexterity to use it. However, it can only be used for patients who are capped and breathing through their native airway, as it requires use of a mouthpiece.

Deep breathing *and* arm exercises result in the enhanced early mobilization of secretions.

Swallowing. An intact swallow is essential for ensuring airway protection. The swallowing mechanism is disrupted by the prolonged presence of an endotracheal tube, and tracheotomy patients, particularly those with an inflated cuff, sometimes report discomfort with swallowing. Furthermore, the frequency of silent aspiration and reduced laryngeal elevation is increased with cuff inflation (Ding & Logemann, 2005).

Mental Status. Unresponsive patients usually present more of a challenge and often require a cuffed tracheostomy tube. However, unresponsive patients are sometimes able to protect their airway to a certain degree. Mental status alone is not a determining factor in fitting or downsizing a tracheostomy tube. If an unresponsive patient has an effective spontaneous cough and swallow, the patient can be considered for downsizing. The primary factors to be considered are swallow, cough, and secretions.

Choosing a Dual- Versus Single-Cannula Tracheostomy Tube

Another consideration is the choice between a dual- or single-cannula tube. The amount and thickness of secretions determines whether or not a dual-cannula tube is desirable. The primary advantage of a dual-cannula tube is that the inner cannula can be removed, inspected, and cleaned or replaced if necessary. Single-cannula tubes do not have this feature. Secretions accumulate and collect within the inner lumen of the tracheostomy tube, which results in a narrowing of the inner diameter of the tube and can contribute to increased resistance, work of breathing, or, worse, tube obstruction.

If other factors (such as the desire to speak, ventilator dependency, or altered anatomy) are considered, a single-cannula tracheostomy tube may be the better choice. Precautionary measures should be taken for patients who have large amounts of thick secretions, including offering optimal fluids to thin secretions and vigorous physical therapy to facilitate the mobility of secretions.

Secretions and Tube Obstruction. The amount and thickness of secretions are factors in the choice of tracheostomy tube. When the consistency of secretions is thin, it is easier for them to be coughed or suctioned out. Not all patients who have a large amount of secretions will require a cuffed tracheostomy tube. However, patients who cannot manage their secretions will require a cuffed tube. Thick secretions in a patient with a poor cough are the most worrisome because mucus plugs can readily develop. *Unresponsive patients who do not cough may be retaining secretions.* Patients with a poor cough reflex or who are unresponsive should be regularly stimulated. Frequent turning and increasing the patient's range of motion will help mobilize secretions. Other bronchial hygiene maneuvers—such as percussion and vibration, postural drainage, and bronchodilators—may be necessary to mobilize secretions, but they are applied on an individual basis. All efforts to mobilize secretions should be followed by tracheal suctioning to remove secretions from the airway.

Suctioning. Suctioning a patient on a regular schedule is not recommended, but it is vital to prevent mucus plugging and ensure patency of the airway (St. John & Malen, 2004). Patients with a weak or absent cough will require the most suctioning, regardless of the consistency of their secretions, as suctioning is one effective way to stimulate secretions. Passing a suction catheter will ensure patency of the tube, but there is no evidence to determine the optimal frequency of this maneuver. Patients with a strong cough will usually require less suctioning unless their secretions are very thick and they are unable to fully expectorate them.

The technique of suctioning has been described in several studies. Some authors suggest the suction catheter should not go past the tip of the tracheostomy tube to avoid causing unnecessary stimulation and possible damage to the tracheal wall. This shallow suctioning may be adequate in patients with a strong cough. However, the potential danger is to patients without a strong cough reflex. These patients are unable to effectively produce secretions and will require stimulation, often in the form of deep tracheal suctioning. The failure to provide effective stimulation and secretion mobilization in patients who are unresponsive can result in the inspissation of secretions, mucus plug formation, and obstruction of the tube—all of which have potentially serious consequences. See chapter 7 for further discussion of mobilization of secretions.

Choosing Optimal Tube Size

The choice of tracheostomy tube size goes hand in hand with determining the need for cuffed versus uncuffed and single- versus dual-cannula tubes. The appropriate size and type of tube for each patient are determined by the goal of the care plan, which takes the following factors into consideration: need for positive-pressure ventilation, phonation, amount and viscosity of secretions, hemodynamic stability, airway anatomy, and coexisting medical disorders. The initial step is to identify the inner diameter, outer diameter, and length of the current tube and compare with the available choices. Tables 4.1, 4.2, and 4.3 list the inner and outer diameters and lengths of tracheostomy tubes. This information will facilitate the optimal choice of tube for each patient.

If the patient is breathing exclusively through the tube, the largest inner diameter is recommended; however, if the patient is breathing at least partially around the tube, he or she could likely tolerate a tube with a much smaller outer diameter. The process of downsizing should enable the patient to breathe easier around the tube. Figure 4.2 shows the difference in airflow through a larger versus a smaller tube. Refer to chapter 11 for a discussion about downsizing tracheostomy tubes.

Proper sizing will also ensure a low-pressure seal to the cuff. A tube that is too small will not adequately seal the airway and, thus, will create numerous problems (Figure 4.3A), including loss of airway pressures and overinflation of the cuff. This can lead to the development of ventilator-associated pneumonia (Guyton, Banner, & Kirby, 1991; Rumbak et al., 1997). A tube that is too large can damage the tracheal mucosa, leading to granulation tissue or stenosis of the trachea (Figure 4.3B). In this case, inflating the cuff will produce high cuff pressures. Thus, the ratio of size of cuff to size of trachea is an important factor for properly fitting a tracheostomy tube (Rumbak et al.).

4.1 Tracheostomy Diameters (Adult)

Air-Lon Tracheostomy Tube

Air-Lon (also Inhalation Set)

Size	ID	OD	Length
3	4.0	7.0	70
4	5.0	8.0	76
5	7.0	9.0	83
6	8.0	10.0	89
7	9.0	11.0	95
8	10.0	12.0	102

Arcadia Tracheostomy Tubes

Arcadia Silicone Cuffless

Size	ID	OD	Length
6	6.0	9.0	51
7	7.0	10.4	67
8	8.0	11.5	78
9	9.0	12.7	91
9.5	9.5	13.9	95

Arcadia Silicone Air Cuff

Size	ID	OD	Length
6	6.0	9.0	51
7	7.0	10.4	67
8	8.0	11.5	78
9	9.0	12.7	91
9.5	9.5	13.9	95

Arcadia Silicone Foam Cuff

Size	ID	OD	Length
6	6.0	9.0	51
7	7.0	10.4	67
8	8.0	11.5	78
9	9.0	12.7	91
10	10.0	13.9	95

Arcadia Silicone Air Cuff Adjustable Neck

Size	ID	OD	Length
6	6.0	8.7	110
7	7.0	10.0	120
8	8.0	11.0	130
9	9.0	12.3	140

Arcadia Silicone Cuff (CTS)			
Size	ID	OD	Length
5	5.0	7.3	60
6	6.0	8.7	70
6.5	6.5	9.4	70
7.0	7.0	10.0	80
7.5	7.5	10.4	80
8.0	8.0	11.0	88
8.5	8.5	11.8	88
9.0	9.0	12.3	98
9.5	9.5	13.3	98

Bivona Tracheostomy Tubes

Bivona Fome-Cuff

Size	ID	OD	Length
5	5.0	7.3	60
6	6.0	8.7	70
7	7.0	10.0	80
8	8.0	11.0	88
9	9.0	12.3	98
9.5	9.5	13.3	98

Bivona Hyperflex—Adjustable Neck (Aire-Cuf, TTS Cuff)

Size	ID	OD	Length
6	6.0	8.7	110
7	7.0	10.0	120
8	8.0	11.0	130
9	9.0	12.3	140

Bivona Hyperflex—Fixed Neck (Aire-Cuf, Cuffless)

Size	ID	OD	Length
6	6.0	8.7	100
7	7.0	10.0	110
8	8.0	11.0	120
9	9.0	12.3	130

Bivona Hyperflex—Fixed Neck (TTS Cuff)

Size	ID	OD	Length
6	6.0	8.7	70
7	7.0	10.0	80
8	8.0	11.0	88
9	9.0	12.3	98

(continued)

4.1 Tracheostomy Diameters (Adult) (Continued)

Bivona Mid-Range Aire-Cuf

Size	ID	OD	Length
5	5.0	7.3	60
6	6.0	8.7	70
7	7.0	10.0	80
8	8.0	11.0	88
9	9.0	12.3	98
9.5	9.5	13.3	98

Bivona Uncuffed

Size	ID	OD	Length
5	5.0	7.3	60
6	6.0	8.7	70
7	7.0	10.0	80
8	8.0	11.0	88
9	9.0	12.3	98
9.5	9.5	13.3	98

Bivona TTS

Size	ID	OD	Length
5	5.0	7.3	60
6	6.0	8.7	70
6.5	6.5	9.4	70
7	7.0	10.0	80
7.5	7.5	10.4	80
8	8.0	11.0	88
8.5	8.5	11.8	88
9	9.0	12.3	98
9.5	9.5	13.3	98

Bivona Sleep Apnea

Size	ID	OD	Length
6	6.0	9.0	68
6.5	6.5	10.0	73
7.5	7.5	11.0	79

Moore Tracheostomy Tube

Moore

Size	ID	OD	Length
6	6.5	11	115
8	7.5	12	115

Portex Tracheostomy Tubes
Portex DIC (Cuffed and Uncuffed)

Size	Color	ID	OD	Length
6	orange	6.0	8.5	64
7	green	7.0	9.9	70
8	white	8.0	11.3	73
9	blue	9.0	12.6	79
10	yellow	10.0	14.0	79

Portex Flex DIC (Cuffed and Uncuffed)

Size	Color	ID	OD	Length
6	orange	6.0	8.2	64
7	green	7.0	9.6	70
8	white	8.0	10.9	73
9	blue	9.0	12.3	79
10	yellow	10.0	13.7	79

Portex Fenestrated DIC (Cuffed and Uncuffed)

Size	Color	ID	OD	Length
6	orange	6.0	8.5	64
7	green	7.0	9.9	70
8	white	8.0	11.3	73
9	blue	9.0	12.6	79
10	yellow	10.0	14.0	79

Portex Blue Line (Cuffed and Uncuffed)

Size	ID	OD	Length
6	6.0	8.3	55
7	7.0	9.7	65
8	8.0	11.0	76
9	9.0	12.4	87
10	10.0	13.8	98

Portex Blue Line Fenestrated (Cuffed)

Size	ID	OD	Length
7	7.0	9.7	65
8	8.0	11.0	76
9	9.0	12.4	87

(continued)

4.1 Tracheostomy Diameters (Adult) (Continued)

Portex Blue Line, Extra Horizontal Length (Cuffed and Uncuffed)

Size	ID	OD	Vertical Length	Adjustable Horizontal Length
6	6.0	8.3	23	11–31
7	7.0	9.6	26	16–36
8	8.0	11.0	35	17–37
9	9.0	12.4	38	22–42
10	10.0	13.8	41	26–46

Portex Per-Fit

Size	ID	OD	Length
7	7.0	9.6	82
8	8.0	10.9	86
9	9.0	12.3	93

Portex Blue Line, Extra Vertical Length (Double Cuff)

Size	ID	OD	Length
7	7.0	9.7	83
8	8.0	11.0	93
9	9.0	12.4	103
10	10.0	13.8	113

Portex Corrugated Inner Cannula for Standard Blue Line Trachs

ID	To Fit Size
5.0	7
6.0	8
7.0	9

Portex Blue Line Ultra (Cuffed and Uncuffed)

Size	ID	OD	Length
6	6.0	9.2	64.5
7	7.0	10.5	70.0
8	8.0	11.9	75.5
9	9.0	13.3	81.0
10	10.0	14.0	87.5

Portex Blue Line Ultra Fenestrated (Cuffed and Uncuffed)

Size	ID	OD	Length
6	6.0	9.2	64.5
7	7.0	10.5	70.0
8	8.0	11.9	75.5
9	9.0	13.3	81.0
10	10.0	14.0	87.5

Portex Blue Line Ultra Suctionaid

Size	ID	OD	Length
6	6.0	9.2	64.5
7	7.0	10.5	70.0
7.5	7.5	11.3	73.0
8	8.0	11.9	75.5
8.5	8.5	12.6	78.0
9	9.0	13.3	81.0

Portex Corrugated Inner Cannulas for Blue Line Ultra Trachs

ID	To Fit Size
5.0	6
6.0	7
7.0	8
8.0	9

Portex Lo-Profile (Cuffed and Uncuffed, Fenestrated and Nonfenestrated)

Size	ID	OD	Length
6	6.0	8.5	67
7	7.0	9.9	71
8	8.0	11.3	75
9	9.0	12.6	83
10	10.0	14.0	83

Shiley Tracheostomy Tubes

Shiley Cuffed (DCT)

Size	ID	OD	Length
4	5.0	9.4	62
6	6.4	10.8	74
8	7.6	12.2	79
10	8.9	13.8	79

(continued)

4.1 Tracheostomy Diameters (Adult) (Continued)

Shiley Cuffless (CFS)

Size	ID	OD	Length
4	5.0	9.4	65
6	6.4	10.8	76
8	7.6	12.2	81
10	8.9	13.8	81

Shiley Low-Pressure Cuffed (LPC)

Size	ID	OD	Length
4	5.0	9.4	65
6	6.4	10.8	76
8	7.6	12.2	81
10	8.9	13.8	81

Shiley Disposable Cuffless (DCFS)

Size	ID	OD	Length
4	5.0	9.4	62
6	6.4	10.8	74
8	7.6	12.2	79
10	8.9	13.8	79

Shiley Fenestrated Cuffed (FEN)

Size	ID	OD	Length
4	5.0	9.4	65
6	6.4	10.8	76
8	7.6	12.2	81
10	8.9	13.8	81

Shiley Disposable Cuffed Fenestrated (DFEN)

Size	ID	OD	Length
4	5.0	9.4	62
6	6.4	10.8	74
8	7.6	12.2	79
10	8.9	13.8	79

Shiley Cuffless Fenestrated (CFN)

Size	ID	OD	Length
4	5.0	9.4	65
6	6.4	10.8	76
8	7.6	12.2	81
10	8.9	13.8	81

Shiley Disposable Cuffless Fenestrated (DCFN)

Size	ID	OD	Length
4	5.0	9.4	62
6	6.4	10.8	74
8	7.6	12.2	79
10	8.9	13.8	79

Shiley XLT* (Extra Length, Dual-Cannula)

Size	ID	OD	Length
5	5.0	9.6	90
6	6.0	11.0	95
7	7.0	12.3	100
8	8.0	13.3	105

*Extra length can be either distal or proximal. Comes in cuffed and cuffless.

Shiley Single-Cannula (SCT)

Size	ID	OD	Length
5	5.0	7.0	58
6	6.0	8.3	67
7	7.0	9.6	80
8	8.0	10.9	89
9	9.0	12.1	99
10	10.0	13.3	105

Shiley Percutaneous (PERC)

Size	ID	OD	Length
6	6.4	10.8	74
8	7.6	12.2	79

Shiley Disposable Inner Cannulas (DIC)

Size	For Use With				
4	4 DCT	4 DFEN	4 DCFN	4 DCFS	
6	6 DCT	6 DFEN	6 DCFN	6 DCFS	6 PERC
8	8 DCT	8 DFEN	8 DCFN	8 DCFS	8 PERC
10	10 DCT	10 DFEN	10 DCFN	10 DCFS	

TRACOE Tracheostomy Tubes

TRACOE Twist (Cuffed or Cuffless)

Size	ID	OD	Length
4	4.0	7.2	56
5	5.0	8.6	66
6	6.0	9.2	72
7	7.0	10.4	74
8	8.0	11.4	76
9	9.0	12.5	78
10	10.0	13.8	80

(continued)

4.1 Tracheostomy Diameters (Adult) (Continued)

TRACOE Comfort

Size	ID	OD	Length
3	3.5	6.4	46
4	4.0	7.3	55
5	5.0	8.7	57
6	6.0	10.0	60
7	7.0	10.5	65
8	8.0	11.3	70
9	9.0	12.6	75
10	10.0	13.7	85
11	11.0	15.0	87
12	12.0	16.2	90
13	13.0	17.2	100
14	14.0	18.2	105

TRACOE Vario

Size	ID	OD	Length
6	6.0	8.2	70
7	7.0	9.7	80
8	8.0	11.2	90
9	9.0	12.3	100
10	10.0	13.7	110
11	11.0	14.8	110

TRACOE Comfort Extra Long

Size	ID	OD	Length
5	5.0	9.0	92
6	6.0	9.8	95
7	7.0	10.5	100
8	8.0	12.2	105
9	9.0	13.0	110
10	10.0	14.5	115
11	11.0	15.5	120
12	12.0	16.4	125
13	13.0	18.0	130
14	14.0	18.2	135

Metal Tracheostomy Tubes

Jackson Original (Stainless Steel or Silver, Regular or Short Length)

Size	ID	OD	Length
00	2.4	4.5	33
0	2.8	5.0	36, 38
1	3.0	5.5	44, 51
2	3.4	6.0	48, 58
3	4.3	7.0	48, 58
4	5.3	8.0	52, 62
5	6.2	9.0	56, 68
6	7.2	10.0	56, 69
7	8.3	11.0	56, 69
8	9.2	12.0	56, 69
9	9.9	13.0	56, 69
10	10.6	14.0	56, 69
11	12.3	15.3	56, 69
12	12.7	16.3	56, 69

Jackson Extra Long (Stainless Steel)

Size	ID	OD	Length
5	6.2	9.0	72
6	7.2	10.0	72
7	8.3	11.0	72
8	9.2	12.0	72
9	9.9	13.0	72

Tucker (Silver)

Size	ID	OD	Length
00	2.4	4.5	31
0	2.9	5.0	36
1	3.0	5.5	48
2	3.3	6.0	50
3	4.4	7.0	53
4	5.3	8.0	55
5	6.1	9.0	60
6	7.1	10.0	60
7	8.1	11.0	60
8	9.1	12.0	60
9	10.1	13.0	60
10	11.2	14.0	60

(continued)

4.1 Tracheostomy Diameters (Adult) (Continued)

Luer

Size	ID	OD	Length
00	2.4	4.5	33
0	2.9	5.0	34
1	3.0	5.5	35
2	3.3	6.0	36
3	4.4	7.0	37
4	5.3	8.0	39
5	6.1	9.0	42
6	7.1	10.0	42
7	8.1	11.0	42
8	9.1	12.0	42
9	10.1	13.0	42
10	11.2	14.0	42

Martin

Size	ID	OD	Length
6	7.1	10.0	69
7	8.1	11.0	69
8	9.1	12.0	69
8	9.1	12.0	56

Mayo Clinic

Size	ID	OD	Length
3	4.3	7.0	33
4	5.3	8.0	33, 40, 58
5	6.2	9.0	56, 69
6	7.2	10.0	56, 69, 85
7	8.3	11.0	56, 69, 85
8	9.2	12.0	56, 69, 85
9	9.9	13.0	56, 69
10	10.6	14.0	56, 69
12	12.7	16.4	56, 69

Holinger (Silver)

Size	ID	OD	Length
000	2.1	4.1	26, 27, 30, 33, 40, 46
00	2.4	4.5	24, 25, 26, 27, 30, 33, 40, 46
0	2.9	5.0	25, 27, 30, 33, 40, 46
1	3.0	5.5	33, 40, 46
2	3.3	6.0	33, 40, 46, 50
3	4.4	7.0	33, 40, 50, 55, 60
4	5.3	8.0	40, 50, 55, 60
5	6.4	9.0	50, 63, 68
6	7.4	10.0	63, 68, 73
7	8.3	11.0	68
8	9.2	12.0	78

Talking Tracheostomy Tubes

Portex Blue Line Trach Talk

Size	ID	OD	Length
7	7.0	9.7	75
8	8.0	11.0	82
9	9.0	12.4	87

Bivona Fome-Cuff With Talk Attachment

Size	ID	OD	Length
5	5.0	7.3	60
6	6.0	8.7	70
7	7.0	10.0	80
8	8.0	11.0	88
9	9.0	12.3	98
9.5	9.5	13.3	98

Bivona Mid-Range Aire-Cuf With Talk Attachment

Size	ID	OD	Length
5	5.0	7.3	60
6	6.0	8.7	70
7	7.0	10.0	80
8	8.0	11.0	88
9	9.0	12.3	98
9.5	9.5	13.3	98

Blom System

Size	ID	OD	Length
4	5.0	9.4	62
6	6.4	10.8	74
8	7.6	12.2	79
10	8.9	13.8	79

(continued)

4.1 Tracheostomy Diameters (Adult) (Continued)

TRACOE Twist With Air Supply Line

Size	ID	OD	Length
4	4.0	7.2	56
5	5.0	8.6	66
6	6.0	9.2	72
7	7.0	10.4	74
8	8.0	11.4	76
9	9.0	12.5	78
10	10.0	13.8	80

ID = inner diameter; OD = outer diameter. Length = neck flange to tip. All measurements expressed in millimeters.

4.2 Laryngectomy Diameters

Air-Lon Laryngectomy (also Inhalation Set)

Size	ID	OD	Length
8	10.0	12.0	63
10	12.0	14.0	63

Bivona Laryngectomy

Size	ID	OD	Length
9.5	9.5	12.0	55
9.5	9.5	12.0	85
11	11.0	14.0	55
11	11.0	14.0	105
13	13.0	16.0	55
13	13.0	16.0	85

Holinger Laryngectomy

Size	ID	OD	Length
7	9.0	12.0	50
8	10.0	13.6	50
9	10.6	14.0	50
10	11.2	14.3	50

Jackson Laryngectomy

Size	ID	OD	Length
00	2.4	4.5	33
0	2.8	5.0	38
1	3.0	5.5	44
2	3.4	6.0	51

Martin Laryngectomy (Regular or With Dressing Extension)

Size	ID	OD	Length
8	9.0	12.0	42
10	11.0	14.0	42
12	12.7	16.3	42

Portex DIC Laryngectomy

Size	Color	ID	OD	Length
8	white	8.0	11.3	50
9	blue	9.0	12.6	50
10	yellow	10.0	14.0	50

Provox LaryTube (Standard)

Size	ID	OD	Length
8 / 27	9.5	12.0	27
8 / 36	9.5	12.0	36
8 / 55	9.5	12.0	55
9 / 27	10.5	13.5	27
9 / 36	10.5	13.5	36
9 / 55	10.5	13.5	55
10 / 27	12.0	15.0	27
10 / 36	12.0	15.0	36
10 / 55	12.0	15.0	55
12 / 27	13.5	17.0	27
12 / 36	13.5	17.0	36
12 / 55	13.5	17.0	55

Provox LaryTube Fenestrated

Size	ID	OD	Length
8 / 36	9.5	12.0	36
8 / 55	9.5	12.0	55
9 / 36	10.5	13.5	36
9 / 55	10.5	13.5	55
10 / 36	12.0	15.0	36
10 / 55	12.0	15.0	55
12 / 36	13.5	17.0	36
12 / 55	13.5	17.0	55

(continued)

4.2 Laryngectomy Diameters (Continued)

Provox LaryTube With Ring

Size	ID	OD	Length
8 / 36	9.5	12.0	36
8 / 55	9.5	12.0	55
9 / 36	10.5	13.5	36
9 / 55	10.5	13.5	55
10 / 36	12.0	15.0	36
10 / 55	12.0	15.0	55
12 / 36	13.5	17.0	36
12 / 55	13.5	17.0	55

Shiley Laryngectomy (LGT)

Size	ID	OD	Length
6	6.4	11.1	50
8	7.0	12.6	50
10	8.9	13.7	50

Singer Laryngectomy (SLT)

Size	ID	OD	Length
8 x 18	9.5	12.0	18
8 x 27	9.5	12.0	27
8 x 36	9.5	12.0	36
8 x 55	9.5	12.0	55
9 x 18	10.5	13.5	18
9 x 27	10.5	13.5	27
9 x 36	10.5	13.5	36
9 x 55	10.5	13.5	55
10 x 18	12.0	15.0	18
10 x 27	12.0	15.0	27
10 x 36	12.0	15.0	36
10 x 55	12.0	15.0	55
11 x 18	13.0	16.0	18
11 x 27	13.0	16.0	27
11 x 36	13.0	16.0	36
11 x 55	13.0	16.0	55
12 x 18	13.5	17.0	18
12 x 27	13.5	17.0	27
12 x 36	13.5	17.0	36
12 x 55	13.5	17.0	55
14 x 18	16.5	20.0	18
14 x 27	16.5	20.0	27
14 x 36	16.5	20.0	36
14 x 55	16.5	20.0	55
16 x 18	20.5	24.0	18
16 x 27	20.5	24.0	27
16 x 36	20.5	24.0	36
16 x 55	20.5	24.0	55

TRACOE Twist Laryngecomy			
Size	ID	OD	Length
5	5.0	9.0	47
6	6.0	9.4	50
7	7.0	10.6	52
8	8.0	11.6	55
9	9.0	12.8	57
10	10.0	14.2	60

TRACOE Comfort Laryngectomy			
Size	ID	OD	Length
7	7.0	10.5	50
8	8.0	11.3	53
9	9.0	12.6	57
10	10.0	13.7	60
11	11.0	15.0	63
12	12.0	16.2	66

ID = inner diameter; OD = outer diameter. Length = neck flange to tip. All measurements expressed in millimeters.

4.3 Tracheostomy Diameters (Neonatal and Pediatric)

Arcadia Neonatal & Pediatric Tracheostomy Tubes

Arcadia CTS Pediatric

Size	ID	OD	Length
2.5	2.5	4.0	38
3.0	3.0	4.7	39
3.5	3.5	5.3	40
4.0	4.0	6.0	41
4.5	4.5	6.7	42
5.0	5.0	7.3	44
5.5	5.5	8.0	46

Arcadia CTS Neonatal

Size	ID	OD	Length
2.5	2.5	4.0	30
3.0	3.0	4.7	32
3.5	3.5	5.3	34
4.0	4.0	6.0	36

(continued)

4.3 Tracheostomy Diameters (Neonatal and Pediatric) (Continued)

Arcadia Cuffless Pediatric (Standard V-Neck or Perfect Fit)

Size	ID	OD	Length
2.5	2.5	4.0	38
3.0	3.0	4.7	39
3.5	3.5	5.3	40
4.0	4.0	6.0	41
4.5	4.5	6.7	42
5.0	5.0	7.3	44
5.5	5.5	8.0	46

Arcadia Cuffless Neonatal (Standard V-Neck or Perfect Fit)

Size	ID	OD	Length
2.5	2.5	4.0	30
3.0	3.0	4.7	32
3.5	3.5	5.3	34
4.0	4.0	6.0	36

Arcadia Cuffless Extended Connect Pediatric (Standard V-Neck or Perfect Fit)

Size	ID	OD	Proximal Length	Distal Length
2.5	2.5	4.0	20	38
3.0	3.0	4.7	20	39
3.5	3.5	5.3	25	40
4.0	4.0	6.0	25	41
4.5	4.5	6.7	30	42
5.0	5.0	7.3	30	44
5.5	5.5	8.0	30	46

Arcadia Extended Connect Neonatal (Standard V-Neck or Perfect Fit)

Size	ID	OD	Proximal Length	Distal Length
2.5	2.5	4.0	15	30
3.0	3.0	4.7	17	32
3.5	3.5	5.3	20	34
4.0	4.0	6.0	22	36

Bivona Neonatal & Pediatric Tracheostomy Tubes

Bivona Aire-Cuf Neonatal

Size	ID	OD	Length
2.5	2.5	4.0	30
3.0	3.0	4.7	32
3.5	3.5	5.3	34
4.0	4.0	6.0	36

Bivona Aire-Cuf Pediatric

Size	ID	OD	Length
2.5	2.5	4.0	38
3.0	3.0	4.7	39
3.5	3.5	5.3	40
4.0	4.0	6.0	41
4.5	4.5	6.7	42
5.0	5.0	7.3	44
5.5	5.5	8.0	46

Bivona Fome-Cuf Neonatal

Size	ID	OD	Length
2.5	2.5	4.0	30
3.0	3.0	4.7	32
3.5	3.5	5.3	34
4.0	4.0	6.0	36

Bivona Fome-Cuf Pediatric

Size	ID	OD	Length
2.5	2.5	4.0	38
3.0	3.0	4.7	39
3.5	3.5	5.3	40
4.0	4.0	6.0	41
4.5	4.5	6.7	42
5.0	5.0	7.3	44
5.5	5.5	8.0	46

Bivona Hyperflex, Adjustable Neck (Uncuffed)

Size	ID	OD	Length
2.5	2.5	4.0	55
3.0	3.0	4.7	60
3.5	3.5	5.3	65
4.0	4.0	6.0	70
4.5	4.5	6.7	75
5.0	5.0	7.3	80
5.5	5.5	8.0	85

(continued)

4.3 Tracheostomy Diameters (Neonatal and Pediatric) (Continued)

Bivona TTS Cuffed Neonatal

Size	ID	OD	Length
2.5	2.5	4.0	30
3.0	3.0	4.7	32
3.5	3.5	5.3	34
4.0	4.0	6.0	36

Bivona TTS Cuffed Pediatric

Size	ID	OD	Length
2.5	2.5	4.0	38
3.0	3.0	4.7	39
3.5	3.5	5.3	40
4.0	4.0	6.0	41
4.5	4.5	6.7	42
5.0	5.0	7.3	44
5.5	5.5	8.0	46

Bivona Uncuffed Neonatal

Size	ID	OD	Length
2.5	2.5	4.0	30
3.0	3.0	4.7	32
3.5	3.5	5.3	34
4.0	4.0	6.0	36

Bivona Uncuffed Pediatric

Size	ID	OD	Length
2.5	2.5	4.0	38
3.0	3.0	4.7	39
3.5	3.5	5.3	40
4.0	4.0	6.0	41
4.5	4.5	6.7	42
5.0	5.0	7.3	44
5.5	5.5	8.0	46

Bivona Uncuffed Neonatal FlexTend Plus

Size	ID	OD	Proximal Length	Distal Length
2.5	2.5	4.0	15	39
3.0	3.0	4.7	17	32
3.5	3.5	5.3	20	34
4.0	4.0	6.0	22	36

Bivona Uncuffed Pediatric FlexTend Plus Extra Length

Size	ID	OD	Proximal Length	Distal Length
3.5	3.5	5.3	38	40
4.0	4.0	6.0	40	44
4.5	4.5	6.7	43	48
5.0	5.0	7.3	45	50
5.5	5.5	8.0	48	52

Portex Neonatal & Pediatric Tracheostomy Tubes

Portex FlexTend Plus Neonatal

Size	ID	OD	Proximal Length	Distal Length
2.5	2.5	4.0	30	15
3.0	3.0	4.7	32	17
3.5	3.5	5.3	34	20
4.0	4.0	6.0	36	22

Portex FlexTend Plus Standard Pediatric

Size	ID	OD	Proximal Length	Distal Length
2.5	2.5	4.0	38	20
3.0	3.0	4.7	39	20
3.5	3.5	5.3	40	25
4.0	4.0	6.0	41	25
4.5	4.5	6.7	42	30
5.0	5.0	7.3	44	30
5.5	5.5	8.0	46	30

Portex FlexTend Plus Pediatric

Size	ID	OD	Proximal Length	Distal Length
3.5	3.5	5.3	40	38
4.0	4.0	6.0	44	40
4.5	4.5	6.7	48	43
5.0	5.0	7.3	50	45
5.5	5.5	8.0	52	48

Shiley Neonatal & Pediatric Tracheostomy Tubes

Shiley Cuffed Pediatric (PDC)

Size	ID	OD	Length
4.0	4.0	5.9	41
4.5	4.5	6.5	42
5.0	5.0	7.1	44
5.5	5.5	7.7	46

(continued)

4.3 Tracheostomy Diameters (Neonatal and Pediatric) (Continued)

Shiley Cuffed Long Pediatric (PLC)

Size	ID	OD	Length
5.0	5.0	7.1	50
5.5	5.5	7.7	52
6.0	6.0	8.3	54
6.5	6.5	9.0	56

Shiley Neonatal (NEO)

Size	ID	OD	Length
3.0	3.0	4.5	30
3.5	3.5	5.2	32
4.0	4.0	5.9	34
4.5	4.5	6.5	36

Shiley Pediatric (PED)

Size	ID	OD	Length
3.0	3.0	4.5	39
3.5	3.5	5.2	40
4.0	4.0	5.9	41
4.5	4.5	6.5	42
5.0	5.0	7.1	44
5.5	5.5	7.7	46

Shiley Long Pediatric (PDL)

Size	ID	OD	Length
5.0	5.0	7.1	50
5.5	5.5	7.7	52
6.0	6.0	8.3	54
6.5	6.5	9.0	56

TRACOE Neonatal & Pediatric Tracheostomy Tubes

TRACOE Mini (Neonatal)

Size	ID	OD	Length
2.5	2.5	3.6	30
3.0	3.0	4.3	32
3.5	3.5	5.0	34
4.0	4.0	5.6	36

TRACOE Mini (Pediatric)			
Size	ID	OD	Length
2.5	2.5	3.6	32
3.0	3.0	4.3	36
3.5	3.5	5.0	40
4.0	4.0	5.6	44
4.5	4.5	6.3	48
5.0	5.0	7.0	50
5.5	5.5	7.6	55
6.0	6.0	8.4	62

ID = inner diameter; OD = outer diameter. Length = neck flange to tip. All measurements expressed in millimeters.

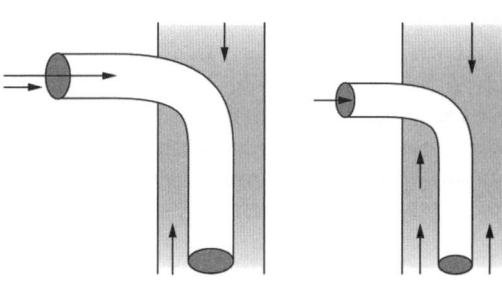

4.2 Airflow through a smaller tube compared with one that is larger. Note less resistance with breathing through a larger tube. As the tube gets smaller, resistance (hence, work of breathing) will increase.

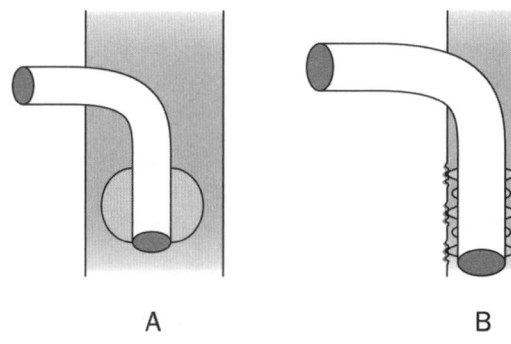

4.3 Improperly sized tubes. (A) A tracheostomy tube that is too small, despite hyperinflation of the cuff. (B) A tracheostomy tube that is too large; it leaves no room for the cuff and abuts the tracheal wall.

Choosing the Best Tube Construction

One consideration regarding the optimal tracheostomy tube is the tube's construction. For example, a patient with a tumor extrinsically compressing his or her airway might benefit from a tracheostomy tube with a more rigid shaft so the airway is not compromised. However, a patient with unusual airway anatomy might benefit from a more flexible tube. Generally speaking, tracheostomy tubes with less rigid construction tend to be more comfortable because they conform to the morphology of the airway.

Polyvinyl chloride tubes can be either rigid or flexible. Silicone is known for its flexible properties, and secretions tend to adhere less to a silicone inner lumen; however, silicone does not prevent the accumulation of secretions. Changing a tracheostomy tube that is more flexible can be a challenge because it can change shape during insertion. The obturator is necessary to maintain the position of the tube during insertion. Once the tube is in place, the obturator is removed and the tube is allowed to conform to airway anatomy.

Choosing Optimal Tube Length

When the tracheostomy tube used is too short, it can easily slip out of the airway, exert excessive pressure on the anterior tracheal wall, create backward pressure against the posterior tracheal wall, and make suctioning difficult (Mallick, Bodenham, Elliot, & Oram, 2008). In fact, one study suggested that the standard tracheostomy tube should be longer with a redesigned angle. The basis for this European study was recurrent problems with too short tubes in critically ill patients. The study was conducted both in vitro and in vivo. Measurements from a variety of standard tracheostomy tubes were compared in vivo with measurements of the depth from the skin surface to the tracheal wall as well as the angle of the tracheal stoma. Results suggested that tracheostomy tubes should be lengthened by 1 cm and the angle redesigned to 110–120 degrees in order to facilitate proper placement within the airway (Mallick et al.).

Longer tubes can be used in a variety of cases, including for patients with thick or obese necks or unusual anatomy. Ventilator-dependent patients with tracheomalacia will benefit from the placement of longer tubes where the cuff rests below the area of the tracheomalacia. By contrast, a longer tube can also act as a stent past an airway obstruction.

Matching Shape of Tube and Airway

The curvature of the tracheostomy tube will affect airway integrity and the work of breathing over time. A tube with too wide an angle can create erosion of the dorsal trachea where the shaft abrades the posterior wall. A tube with too narrow an angle can also create increased work of breathing (Pierson, 2005) and potential erosion of the anterior wall (Figure 4.4).

A patient with an irregular shape to his or her airway can develop increased airway resistance and work of breathing. For example, a neck mass can press against the airway, distorting its curvature and narrowing its diameter. In this example, it would be important to reinforce the airway to prevent narrowing and allow laminar airflow, thus optimizing the work of breathing.

Phonation and Tube Choice

There are numerous considerations involved in speech with tracheostomy patients. The details of phonation with a tracheostomy are discussed in chapter 6.

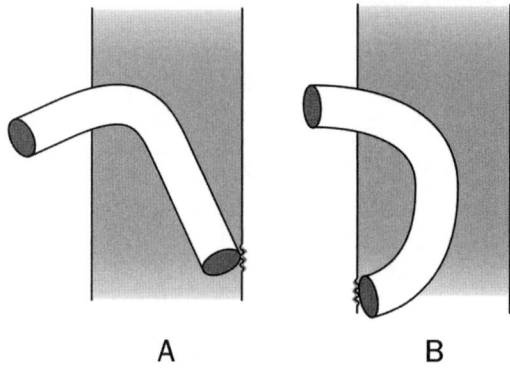

4.4

Tubes of different angles creating tracheal erosion. (A) Poorly fitting wide-angle tube shows erosion of the posterior tracheal. (B) Poorly fitting narrow-angled tube shows erosion of the anterior wall.

Tracheostomy Tube Changes

A tracheostomy tube change is not a benign procedure. The loss of the airway is a primary concern, especially in the early postoperative period. During the first postoperative week, the stomal tissue tract is not mature, and removal of the tube can result in the collapse of the tissue planes, making replacement within the airway difficult. Furthermore, attempts to replace the airway prematurely within the stoma can create a false passage if the tube is forced into the stoma and an initial caudal turn is applied. Continued efforts to insert the tube, inflate the cuff, and ventilate the patient will enlarge this false passage, compress the trachea, and potentially result in life-threatening pneumopericardium, pneumothorax, or widespread subcutaneous emphysema (Mirza & Cameron, 2001). Figure 4.5 shows the placement of a tracheostomy tube into a false passage within the pretracheal tissue.

Tabaee, Lando, Rickert, Stewart, and Kuhel (2007) conducted a survey of chief residents of accredited otolaryngology programs to determine their practice patterns related to tracheostomy tube changes. Ninety-three percent of respondents indicated they used sutures to secure the tracheostomy tube. Seventeen percent reported they changed the tube before the fifth day, 55% changed the tube on the fifth postoperative day, and 28% changed the tube after the fifth day. The mean time interval between the tracheotomy procedure and the first tube change was 5.3 days, with a range of 3–7 days. Participants were asked if they were aware of any loss of airway or death as a result of the first tube change; 42% of respondents were aware of a loss of airway, and 15% were aware of a death. A higher percentage of respondents indicated there was a significantly higher incidence of loss of airway on the wards compared to the ICU, and the investigators suggested that tube changes might be delayed for patients on the wards in order to allow for a more mature stoma, but they could not conclude that tube changes on the wards are always problematic.

Factors that complicate a tracheostomy change include obesity; a short or edematous neck; anatomical anomalies; granulation tissue; copious tracheal secretions; and lack of patient cooperation due to pain, hypoxia, or neurological

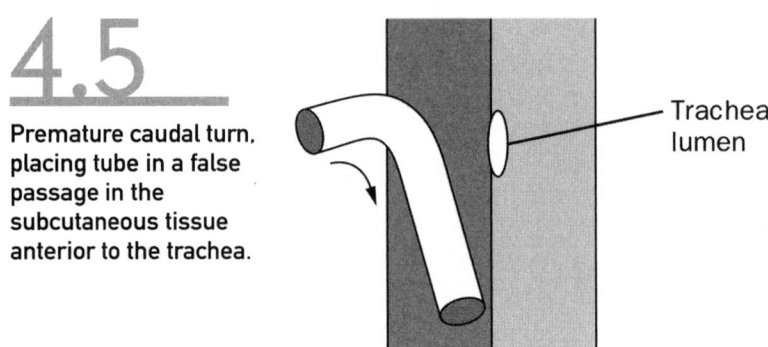

4.5 Premature caudal turn, placing tube in a false passage in the subcutaneous tissue anterior to the trachea.

issues (Mirza & Cameron, 2001). Before implementing the tracheostomy tube change procedure, it is advisable to determine what type of tube to place. This may be difficult to determine because a visual exam of the stoma and anterior airway without the tube in place plays into the decision. In any case, it is wise to have at least one type of tracheostomy tube ready, and perhaps an alternate or two nearby.

Before beginning the procedure, it is important to gain the cooperation of the patient and/or his or her family by explaining the plan and the need for the tube change. A tube change may be fraught with anxiety for the patient and family. It is important to explain that the patient will feel a pulling sensation while the tube is being removed but that this is usually momentary. Patients should also be aware that coughing is common during the procedure. If the replacement tube has a smaller outer diameter, there is usually much less discomfort—especially with a cuffless tube. However, if the new tube has a larger outer diameter, it is usually more painful and traumatic. A small amount of limited bleeding should be expected after most tube changes.

One phenomenological study conducted by Donnelly and Wiechula (2006) determined that patients were quite anxious and experienced varying degrees of discomfort with the tube change despite the fact that many clinicians consider it a routine procedure. Patients who express anxiety may be offered premedication with a low dose of intravenous opioid or benzodiazepine. One can also premedicate the stoma—with 2% Xylocaine gel several minutes prior to the procedure—to lessen sensation at the site. Patients are less anxious when they know the entire procedure usually takes less than 1 minute.

Before the procedure, it is important to gather all the necessary supplies: tracheostomy tube and alternates, lubricating gel, new tracheostomy tube holder, precut tracheostomy dressing, a dampened cloth to cleanse the stoma of dried secretions and other debris, and a suture removal tray. Sometimes skin stay sutures are present under the neck flange but not otherwise readily visible. Lighting should be adequate, and suction and oxygen should be available. A variety of tracheostomy tube sizes and types should be available. In a critically ill patient, it is also advisable to have other equipment and supplies available, including pulse oximetry, capnography, tube exchangers, and tracheal dilators (Mirza & Cameron, 2001).

If the patient is hemodynamically unstable, or if there is concern the procedure may be difficult, preoxygenation with 100% oxygen for 10 minutes prior to the procedure will provide denitrogenation and maximize the patient's oxygen reserve. In these cases, it is also advisable to have an assistant at the bedside in case a difficult situation occurs.

A bedside tracheostomy tube change is done as a clean procedure unless there are extenuating circumstances requiring sterile conditions. After thorough hand washing, the tube itself is prepped. It is usually packaged with the inner cannula in place and the cuff deflated. (One exception is the Bivona Fome-Cuf tracheostomy tube, and the procedure for that tube will be discussed separately.) The inner cannula is removed from the outer cannula. The obturator is placed within the outer cannula, and the entire distal tip of the tube is well lubricated. If the tracheostomy tube is a single-cannula tube, the obturator is placed inside it and prepped with lubricating gel. Xylocaine gel can also be used as a local anesthetic at this point. Mirza and Cameron (2001) also recommend lidocaine spray into the stoma prior to the procedure to provide added local anesthesia within the trachea.

The patient is positioned with his or her neck fully exposed and lying flat unless otherwise contraindicated. If the patient is in a cervical collar, it must be removed, and in-line stabilizjion must be maintained at all times by an assistant. There is no evidence that specifies nil per os (NPO) guidelines prior to the procedure, so prudence should be a guide. If there is any concern, patients should be asked to refrain from food and fluids for a period of time prior to the procedure. Continuous tube feedings should be turned off prior to the procedure, primarily because of the risk of aspiration while in the supine position.

Deep subglottic suctioning should always be done prior to cuff deflation. Secretions collect above the cuff and can be a source of respiratory distress and potential pneumonia if not removed prior to deflation. A soft, flexible suction catheter should be used for deep oropharyngeal suctioning, as it will create less trauma and discomfort than a rigid suction catheter. The patient should be cautioned that the procedure is likely to cause gagging but that it is vital to collect the pooled secretions prior to deflation of the cuff.

Even though most secretions are removed with this maneuver, some often remain above the cuff. The best way to prevent these remaining secretions from being aspirated is to actively engage the patient during this procedure. Ask the patient to take a deep breath and cough. The cuff can be quickly deflated following complete inhalation, when the patient begins to cough up the remaining secretions. An unresponsive or uncooperative patient should have this cuff deflation timed with exhalation, and a suction catheter should be used to remove the secretions. Another approach is to use the manual resuscitation bag to provide an "inspiratory push" during cuff deflation to clear any remaining pooled secretions above the cuff (Kazandjian & Dikeman, 2008).

Cuff deflation may be timed to occur during exhalation, or it can be extended over a longer period of time. Rapid cuff deflation can sometimes promote patient discomfort due to coughing, which may be a reaction to airflow returning through the glottis (Kazandjian & Dikeman, 2008), so it may be helpful to give the patient a few moments to adjust to the sensation of breathing through the upper airway.

There are two primary methods of changing the tracheostomy tube: the classical method and the tube exchanger method, also known as the "railroad" method (Mirza & Cameron, 2001). Both methods will be described here.

The Classic Method

The classic method involves the complete removal of the old tracheostomy tube before placing a new tube. Patient and operator positioning is important. The person changing the tube should stand on the same side of the bed as his dominant hand. In other words, if the operator is left-handed, he should stand on the patient's left when changing or manipulating the tracheostomy.

The tracheostomy tube holder should be loosened and the ties removed. After ensuring the cuff is deflated completely, the tracheostomy tube should be pulled out using a smooth, continuous motion. The cuff of the tube creates the most resistance and difficulty in replacement. Cuffless tubes offer less resistance and are easiest to remove and insert.

Examination of the Stoma. Tube replacement is an opportune time to assess the stoma and examine the free airway. The color of the stoma should be noted, along with the presence and color of any secretions. A moistened cloth can cleanse away encrusted secretions. The stoma and the definition of the edges should be noted. The stoma should be covered with a gauze pad to determine ease of ventilation, and the patient should be asked to phonate. The inability to breathe comfortably or phonate could be a sign of future difficulty with capping due to airway obstruction. The orientation of the internal tracheal lumen to the cutaneous stoma should be appraised. Horizontal, caudad, or, less commonly, cephalad orientations will determine the approach of the tube change.

The new lubricated tube is inserted by initially directing it into the stoma at a 90-degree angle and then turning caudad (Figure 4.6). An initial caudal approach or a premature caudal turn risks missing the tracheal lumen and creating a false passage within the tissues anterior to the trachea.

4.6

Illustration of proper 90-degree initial approach, followed by caudal turn.

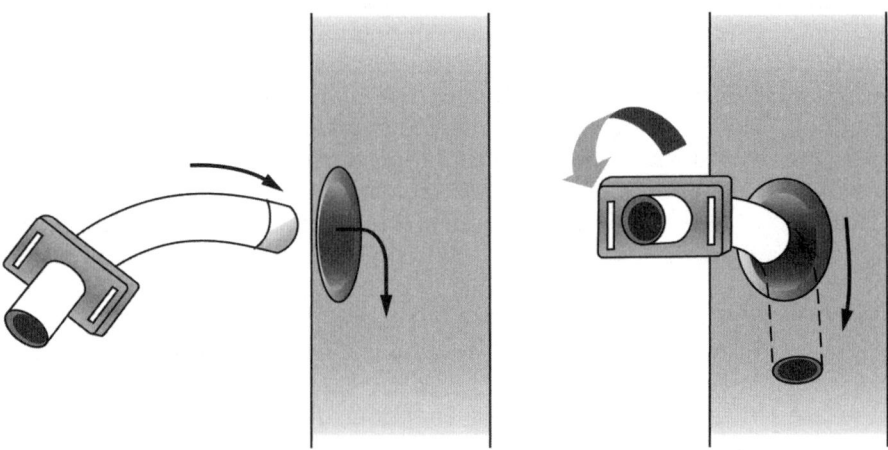

1. 90 degree approach   2. Rotate into position

4.7

Illustration of cephalad location of internal tracheal lumen when the cutaneous stoma and tracheal lumen are not aligned. The tracheal lumen can sometimes be visualized through the cutaneous stoma high in a cephalad orientation.

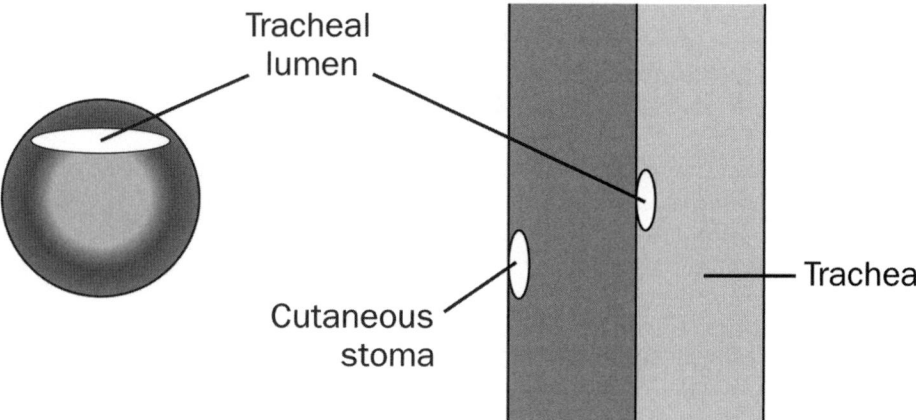

Figure 4.7 shows the misalignment of the cutaneous stoma with the tracheal lumen, which can be recognized if the tracheal lumen is high and small in the 12-o'clock position when looking into the stoma. When inserting a tube into a cephalad orientation of the internal tracheal lumen, it is often necessary to begin with the tip of the tracheostomy tube pointed upward. During insertion, it is then possible to engage the internal tracheal lumen with the tip of the tube. Once engaged, one could then make the caudal turn. However, a cephalad location of the internal tracheal lumen may not initially be evident. If the tube is not easily inserted on the first attempt, the clinician must reassess the stoma and consider if a cephalad approach is warranted. Indication for a cephalad approach can be confirmed by inserting the little finger in the stoma to palpate the location of the tracheal lumen.

After proper placement of the tube, the obturator is removed and replaced with the inner cannula. Proper placement should be confirmed by the presence of tracheal secretions, bilateral breath sounds, capnometry, and the ability to pass a suction catheter.

Patients who are hemodynamically unstable may require additional monitoring during the tube change, including electrocardiography, blood pressure, pulse oximetry, and capnography. In these patients, one must weigh the need for the tube change against the risk of hemodynamic embarrassment. Routine tracheostomy tube changes can and should be postponed until the patient is more stable.

The Tube Exchanger/Railroad Method

The tube exchanger technique is also known as the "railroad" method. If a tracheostomy tube must be changed during a period of hemodynamic instability or full mechanical ventilator support, caution is required. An additional assistant to manage the ventilator and the use of a tube exchanger can minimize the risk of loss of airway during the procedure.

Mimicking the Seldinger technique, the tube exchanger is used as a guide wire to maintain access to the airway as the old tube is removed and the new tube is inserted. Two types of tube exchangers are available: solid and hollow. An example of a solid tube exchanger is the bougie. It has the advantage of maintaining its shape when placed at a specific angle, which can be especially helpful if necessary to find the tracheal lumen for an inadvertent decannulation. However, El-Orbany and Salem (2004) suggested the bougie is not intended as an airway exchange device because it does not allow for oxygenation or ventilation.

Several hollow tube exchangers are available and have the added advantage of using 15-mm connectors to which manual resuscitation bags can be applied for ventilation and supplemental oxygen. Other reports have described using suction catheters or nasogastric tubes as tube exchangers; however, these alternate tubes require modification before use.

Prior to initiating the tube exchanger method, the patient should be preoxygenated for several minutes. The inner cannula should be removed from both tracheostomy tubes: the one to be inserted and the one in situ. The tube exchanger will then be placed through the outer cannula of the tube in situ with at least 3 cm of the exchange catheter protruding past the distal end of the tube. The tube exchanger should be held in position by an assistant while the operator removes the old tracheostomy tube. The distal end of the tube exchanger should be placed through the outer cannula of the tube to be inserted, and the new tube can be guided into position over the tube exchanger. The tube exchanger is then removed, the inner cannula replaced, and ventilation resumed. With a hollow tube exchanger, the 15-mm connector can be quickly applied for manual ventilation in case there is a delay or difficulty at any point during the procedure. The proper placement of the tube should be confirmed by any of the aforementioned measures.

Placement of Nonstandard Tracheostomy Tubes

Foam Cuff Tracheostomy Tube. A foam cuff tube is different from the other tubes because its cuff remains inflated at all times unless actively deflated. To insert a foam cuff tracheostomy tube (Bivona Fome-Cuf or Arcadia Foam Cuff), a 60-ml syringe fitted to a stockcock is used to deflate the large cuff. Complete deflation of the cuff is confirmed by observing the collapse of the pilot port. To prevent passive reinflation, the port is plugged with the attached stopper. The tip is lubricated with a water-based lubricant and inserted into place with its own obturator. The insertion of a foam cuff tracheostomy tube generally takes more pressure exertion because the cuff is larger and bulkier. Once the foam cuff tube is in place, the pilot port should be unclamped and remain open to air, allowing the cuff to self-expand to fit the trachea. No additional air should be injected into this port.

The foam cuff tracheostomy tube should be power deflated at regular intervals in order to prevent moisture accumulation within the cuff. There is no recommended frequency for this power deflation, but failure to do so often results in the ventilator alarm indicating low returned volumes. Power deflation once every 8 hours is usually enough to prevent this accumulation of moisture. Before deflating any cuff, it is important to perform deep oropharyngeal suctioning to remove all secretions above the cuff.

Fenestrated Tracheostomy Tube. A fenestration provides an added flow of air up to the vocal cords to lessen resistance to airflow, facilitating phonation. Fenestrated tracheostomy tubes are available in cuffed and cuffless versions.

An in-vitro study by Hussey and Bishop (1996) showed that fenestrated tracheostomy tubes provided significantly less resistance to airflow than non-fenestrated tubes of equal size. Their bench study on a tracheal model compared Shiley fenestrated tracheostomies in sizes 4, 6, 8, and 10 with the cuff deflated and the external opening occluded (simulating capping) while obtaining pressure measurements. They compared these airway pressure measurements to comparably sized Shiley cuffless tracheostomies in which capping was also simulated. They found that in an average-sized trachea, all tube sizes greater than 4 substantially increased work of breathing while the fenestration returned the pressure to acceptable levels. They reported that the fenestration reduced resistance by allowing airflow not only around the tube, but also through the lumen of the tube. Because of this substantial decrease in resistance, they recommended a fenestrated tracheostomy be used for all patients able to breathe through their native airway, except those with a size 4 tube. In theory, the fenestrated tracheostomy tube decreases resistance, but this depends on many factors, primarily the proper placement of the fenestration within the airway. Figure 4.8 shows the proper placement of the fenestration within the airway.

The position of the fenestration is affected by the curvature of the tube. The standard position of the fenestration on any tracheostomy tube is one-third of the way down the shaft from the neck flange, but this one-size-fits-all approach rarely produces a proper fit. The tracheas of most people are either too anterior or posterior to ensure a proper fit with a standard fenestrated tube.

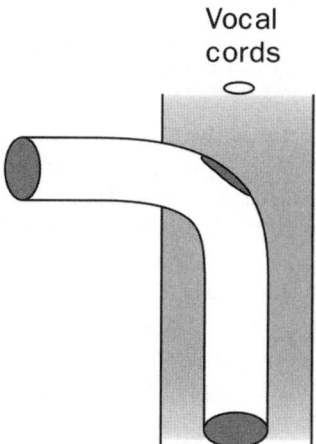

4.8

The proper placement of a fenestration centrally within the airway. Note the fenestration is placed to avoid contact with anterior or posterior tracheal walls.

One of the most troubling problems with fenestrated tubes is the growth of granulation tissue within the fenestration, which was originally reported in tubes with one large fenestration. Since that time, fenestrated tubes with different designs have been developed. For example, the Shiley FEN and CFN tubes typically have one large oval fenestration, while the Shiley DCFN and DFEN as well as the Portex tubes have several elongated channels. However, no matter what the design of the fenestration, *the risk of granulation tissue is greatest when the fenestration is not centered in the airway.* For this reason, many centers choose not to place fenestrated tracheostomy tubes. If a fenestrated tube remains the best option for phonation and ventilation, however, it is imperative to ensure a proper fit.

The procedure to fit a fenestration involves measuring the distance from the stoma to the anterior and posterior tracheal walls. One technique was originally reported by Cane, Woodward, and Shapiro (1982); however, they further described lengthening the established fenestration, which is no longer a recommended practice. To measure the tracheal depth, one can use a probe, a cotton-tipped swab, or a bent pipe cleaner to mark the distance between the anterior and posterior walls. As shown in Figure 4.9, the "handle" of a cotton-tipped swab is placed at the anterior tracheal wall and a mark is made at the stomal opening. Then the applicator is placed further within the airway until it reaches the posterior wall. A second mark is made on the applicator at the stomal skin level.

The two marks should be aligned with the intended fenestrated tube by placing the tip of the applicator on the neck flange of the tube to determine the ideal location of the fenestration. The fenestration should lie completely between the two marks to ensure proper fit. If the fenestration does not fit within these marks, a custom fenestration should be ordered, rather than cutting the shaft oneself. A cut tube may have irregular edges, which could result in inflammation or an even greater risk of granuloma. The Moore tracheostomy tube is the only one that can be modified, as small fenestration holes can be punched into the shaft with an awl that comes with the kit.

Great caution must be taken when removing a fenestrated tracheostomy tube. When granulation tissue has grown within the fenestration(s), manual removal is potentially dangerous. The mobility of a fenestrated tube should always be assessed by exerting gentle pressure to determine if it moves easily within the stoma. Shining a light within the tube itself will reveal a pinkish hue in the presence of granulation. In this case, an otolaryngologist should conduct a visual examination of the trachea. The forceful removal of a fenestrated tracheostomy tube can result in hemorrhage, leading to a surgical emergency.

Granulation tissue is not the only complication of a fenestrated tracheostomy tube. Subcutaneous emphysema has also been reported when the inner cannula is not properly aligned with the outer cannula and air escapes through the tissue planes. For this reason, a fenestrated tracheostomy tube should not be placed within an immature stoma (Orme & Welham, 2006).

Criner, Make, and Celli (1987) reported a case of a woman who experienced increased airway resistance and chronic airflow obstruction when using a fenestrated tracheostomy tube for nocturnal ventilation. The tube was confirmed to be in the correct position within the airway and the cuff was deflated, but her pressure measurements continued to be elevated. Upon decannulation and a return to mouth breathing, her minute ventilation and resultant exercise

4.9

Fitting a fenestrated tracheostomy tube. The anterior and posterior tracheal walls are measured with a probe. These measurements are then compared to the fenestration on the tube. If the markings do not line up with the fenestration, a custom tube (ideal fenestration) should be ordered.

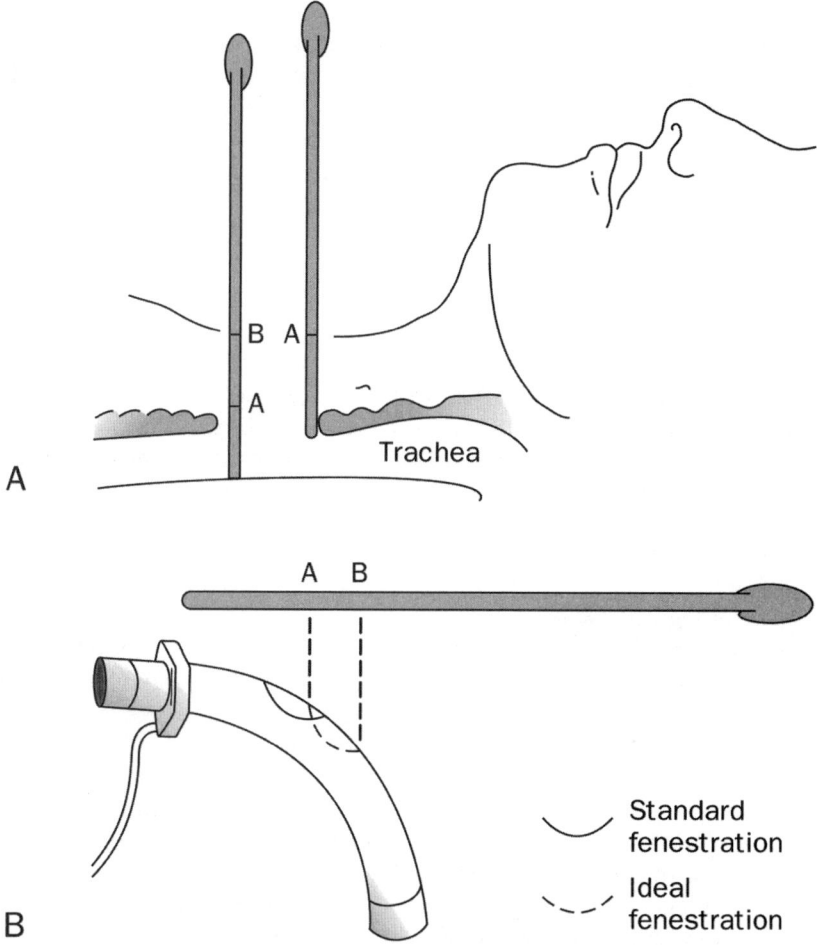

endurance dramatically increased. The investigators concluded that a deflated cut on a fenestrated tracheostomy tube significantly increases airway resistance and can further limit ventilatory muscle performance in patients with compromised ventilatory reserve.

Upsizing

Occasionally, there is a need to place a tracheostomy tube that is larger than the one in place. Typical conditions that require upsizing include a hemodynamically unstable patient who is exhibiting high airway pressures on the ventilator and a patient who has been in the process of downsizing and breathing around the tube who is currently presenting with respiratory distress. Either the tube itself or secretions within the tube can increase resistance within the respiratory system and manifest as respiratory distress. For example, it is unreasonable to expect an average-sized adult to breathe through a size 4 cuffed tube; it is simply too small. If positive-pressure ventilation is applied to a small tube, the problem will become immediately apparent.

When possible, it is advisable to provide some analgesic premedication and/or benzodiazepine prior to upsizing a tracheostomy tube. Placing a larger tube often involves some degree of resistance and discomfort. In addition, lidocaine gel can serve a dual purpose as a local anesthetic and lubricant. Occasionally, it may be necessary to dilate the stoma in order to allow the placement of a larger tube. The cuff of the tracheostomy tube in situ can be used to dilate the opening of the stoma by maneuvering the tube in several positions and hyperinflating the cuff.

Fitting a Tracheostomy Button

A tracheostomy button is used as a stent to maintain patency of the stoma. It is intended for temporary use and is indicated in patients who may require repeated tracheostomies such as those who have myasthenia gravis, spinal cord injuries, or sleep apnea. It can also be used with patients who are undergoing rehabilitation while working toward decannulation or in patients for whom a future surgery is planned. Olympic Medical recommends that their tracheostomy buttons are not intended for permanent use, as the Teflon material will fatigue and deteriorate over time.

When properly placed, the tracheostomy button fits solely within the stoma, eliminates resistance within the airway, and allows the patient to breathe entirely through his or her upper airway. The tracheostomy button consists of three primary parts: the cannula, the closure plug, and a range of spacers that can be used to ensure a snug fit against the anterior tracheal wall. Spacers included are one each of the following: 1 mm, 2 mm, 4 mm, 7 mm, and 10 mm.

The length of the stoma is determined by measuring the distance from the cutaneous stoma to the anterior tracheal wall. The Olympic tracheostomy button comes in two standard lengths: 27 mm and 40 mm. If the distance between the cutaneous stoma and the anterior tracheal wall is less than 27 mm, the 27-mm length should be used. If this distance is between 28–40 mm, the 40-mm length should be used. Combinations of spacers are then used to ensure the exact stomal length is achieved. For example, if the measured stomal length is 20 mm, the 27-mm cannula should be used with the 7-mm spacer. If the stomal length is 32 mm, the 1-mm and 7-mm spacers should be used on the 40-mm cannula. Prior to insertion, the spacers should be placed on the distal end of the cannula and the tip lubricated.

The cannula should be inserted into the stoma until a give is felt when the distal tip clears the anterior tracheal wall. The closure plug is then inserted into the cannula, which splays the petals on the tip of the cannula, locking it into place against the anterior tracheal wall. When positioned properly (Figure 4.10), the

4.10

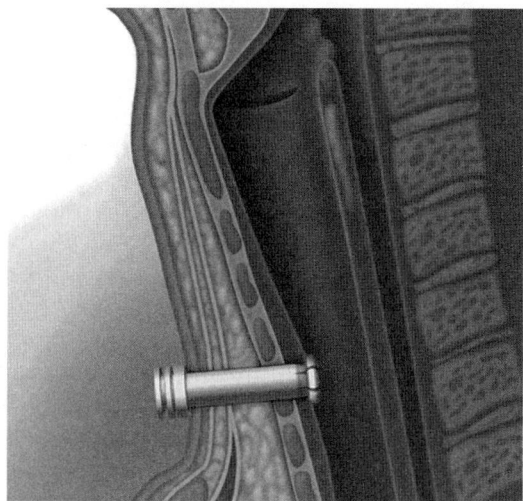

Tracheostomy button in place. Note that a properly fit tracheostomy button creates no obstruction within the airway. Image courtesy of Natus Medical Incorporated.

4.11

Fitting a tracheostomy button. (A) A tracheostomy button with proper fit. (B) A button fitted too short, allowing closure of the tracheal lumen. (C) A button fitted too long, creating an obstruction within the airway.

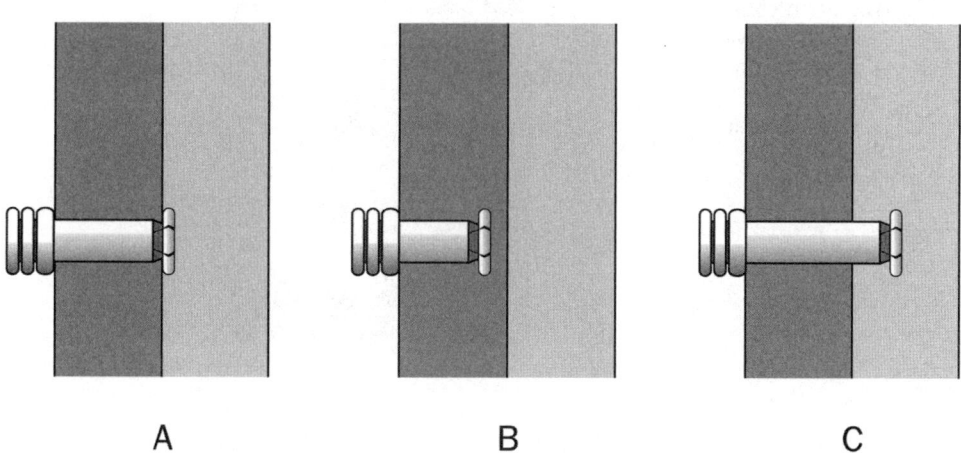

button should resist gentle pulling against the cannula. The closure plug should always remain in place in order to ensure the security of the button. If immediate access to the airway is required, the closure plug can be replaced with a separate ventilator adapter that provides a standard 15-mm connector. However, if long-term access to the airway is required such as for frequent suctioning, replacement of the button with a standard tracheostomy tube is recommended.

When a tracheostomy button is properly placed, there is no obstruction within the airway. Figure 4.11 illustrates a tracheostomy button that is properly placed (A); one that is too short (B), allowing the tracheal lumen to close; and one that is too long (C), creating an obstruction within the airway. There are two conditions that prevent proper fit of the tracheostomy button: irregular shape of the stoma and posterior angling of the trachea. When the stoma is irregular, a separate flange can be used to prevent irritation of the cannula against the stoma. The flange is placed next to the skin of the neck between the cannula and the spacers, where it stabilizes the cannula and prevents its movement within the stoma.

Another condition that prevents proper fit of the tracheostomy button is a posterior angle to the trachea (see Figure 4.12). In this case, the length of the stoma varies between its superior and inferior aspects. Because of this difference, the tracheostomy button will not fit properly because the shaft of the cannula has uniform length. The best solution for this condition is a tracheal stent with an angle to the internal flange that abuts the anterior tracheal wall. The Montgomery cannula and the Hood stoma stent have special internal angles designed for the posteriorly angled trachea (Figure 4.13).

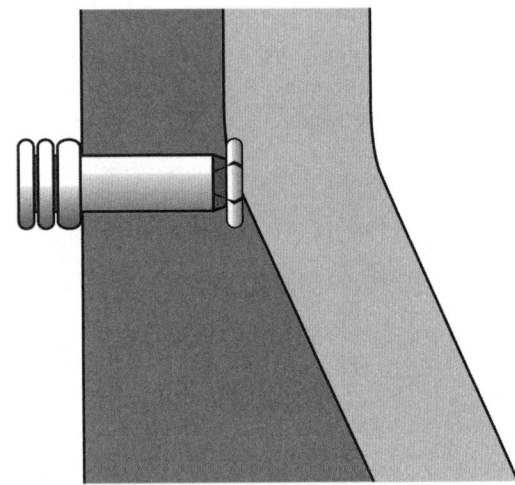

4.12 Posterior angulation of the trachea, showing a difference in superior and inferior stomal length and an improperly fitting a tracheostomy button.

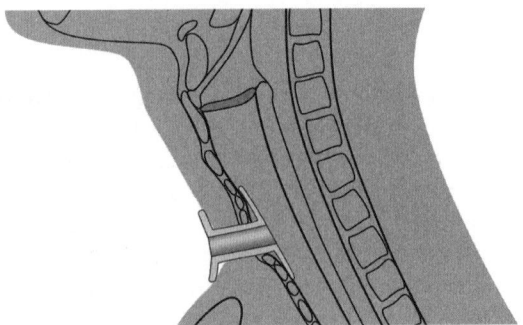

4.13 Hood stoma stent in place. Note that the stent is angled at the posterior flange to fit properly against a posteriorly angled trachea. Hood Labs (Pembroke, MA).

Summary

The process of sizing and fitting a tracheostomy tube requires planning and consideration of goals. The tube should be long enough for the patient's anatomy and large enough to provide adequate ventilation. There are several factors that must be considered when fitting and changing a tracheostomy tube. These include determining whether a cuff is necessary in addition to assessment of airway protection and secretions. Identifying goals is the first step toward a determination of the proper tube.

Key Points

- The first decision when fitting a tracheostomy tube is if the patient requires a cuffed tube.
- A dual-cannula tube should be chosen for a patient who has a large amount of thick secretions.
- A larger tube size is optimal for a patient who is breathing through the tube; whereas, a smaller tube size is more appropriate for a patient who is breathing around the tube.
- The tracheostomy tube can be changed by using either the classic method or the tube exchanger method; the latter is used when the patient is hemodynamically unstable or there is concern about loss of the airway.
- Fenestrated tracheostomy tubes must be fitted carefully to prevent granulation growth in the aperture.

References

Bach, J. R. (1993). Mechanical insufflation-exsufflation comparison of peak expiratory flows with manually assisted and unassisted coughing. *Chest, 14,* 1553–1562.

Beachey, W. (2007). *Respiratory care anatomy and physiology.* St. Louis, MO: Mosby.

Cane, R. D., Woodward, C., & Shapiro, B. A. (1982). Customizing fenestrated tracheostomy tubes: A bedside technique. *Critical Care Medicine, 10*(12), 880–881.

Criner, G., Make, B., & Celli, B. (1987). Respiratory muscle dysfunction secondary to chronic tracheostomy. *Chest, 91*(1), 139–141.

Ding, R., & Logemann, J. A. (2005). Swallow physiology in patients with trach cuff inflated or deflated: A retrospective study. *Head and Neck, 27*(9), 809–813.

Donnelly, F., & Wiechula, R. (2006). The lived experience of a tracheostomy tube change: A phenomenological study. *Journal of Clinical Nursing, 15,* 1115–1122.

Douce, F. H. (2003). Pulmonary function testing. In R. L. Wilkins, J. K. Stoller, & C. L. Scanlan (Eds.), *Egan's fundamentals of respiratory care* (8th ed., pp. 391–425). St. Louis, MO: Mosby.

El-Orbany, M., & Salem, M. R. (2004). The Eschmann tracheal tube is not an airway exchange device. *Anesthesia and Analgesia, 99*(4), 1269–1270.

Epstein, S. K. (2005). Anatomy and physiology of tracheostomy. *Respiratory Care, 50*(3), 476–482.

Guyton, D., Banner, M. J., & Kirby, R. R. (1991). High-volume, low-pressure cuffs: Are they always low? *Chest, 100,* 1076–1081.

Hussey, J. D., & Bishop, M. J. (1996). Pressures required to move gas through the native airway in the presence of a fenestrated vs. a nonfenestrated tracheostomy tube. *Chest, 110*(2), 494–497.

Kazandjian, M. S., & Dikeman, K. J. (2008). Communication options for tracheostomy and ventilator-dependent patients. In E. N. Myers & J. T. Johnson (Eds.), *Tracheostomy: Airway management, communication, and swallowing.* San Diego, CA: Plural Publishing.

Mallick, A., Bodenham, A., Elliot, S., & Oram, J. (2008). An investigation into the length of standard tracheostomy tubes in critical care patients. *Anaesthesia, 63,* 302–306.

Mendell, D. A., & Logemann, J. A. (2007). Temporal sequence of swallow events during the oropharyngeal swallow. *Journal of Speech, Language, and Hearing Research, 50,* 1256–1271.

Mirza, S., & Cameron, D. S. (2001). The tracheostomy tube change: A review of techniques. *Hospital Medicine, 62*(3), 158–163.

Orme, R. M., & Welham, K. L. (2006). Subcutaneous emphysema after percutaneous tracheostomy—time to dispense with fenestrated tubes? *Anaesthesia, 61,* 911–912.

Pierson, D. J. (2005). Tracheostomy and weaning. *Respiratory Care, 50*(4), 526–533.

Robbins, J., Hamilton, J. W., Lof, G. L., & Kempster, G. B. (1992). Oropharyngeal swallowing in normal adults of different ages. *Gastroenterology, 103,* 823–829.

Rumbak, M. J., Graves, A. E., Scott, M. P., Sporn, G. K., Walsh, F. W., Anderson, W. M., et al. (1997). Tracheostomy occlusion protocol predicts significant obstruction to air flow in patients requiring prolonged mechanical ventilation. *Critical Care Medicine, 25*(3), 413–417.

Shapiro, B. A., Harrison, R. A., Kacmarek, R. M., & Cane, R. D. (1985). *Clinical application of respiratory care* (3rd ed.). Chicago: Yearbook Medical Publishers.

St. John, R. E., & Malen, J. F. (2004). Contemporary issues in adult tracheostomy management. *Critical Care Nursing Clinics of North America, 16*(3), 413–430.

Tabaee, A., Lando, T., Rickert, S., Stewart, M. G., & Kuhel, W. I. (2007). Practice patterns, safety, and rationale for tracheostomy tube changes: A survey of otolaryngology training programs. *Otolaryngology, 117,* 573–576.

Special Considerations for the Tracheostomy Patient

Linda L. Morris

Each patient with a tracheostomy is unique, and individual circumstances must be taken into account during assessment, planning, and management. Some of these special circumstances deserve discussion. When a critically ill patient on mechanical ventilation develops high airway pressures, one must assess whether there is increased resistance within the tracheostomy tube or whether lung compliance is decreasing. The cough is the primary defense mechanism against retained secretions, and efforts to mobilize secretions are vital in tracheostomy patients. Leaks may develop within the cuff, around the cuff, or within the tube itself, and a plan for the management of cuff leaks is presented. A discussion is also included of pistoning and the management of cuff changes that occur at altitude and with anesthesia. Complex tracheostomy wounds can also be a challenging management issue. The chapter concludes with a discussion of tracheostomy as a lived experience and dealing with tubes with defects or missing parts.

The Critically Ill Patient on Mechanical Ventilation

Critically ill patients on mechanical ventilation present a challenge. There are numerous conditions that require intubation and maintenance when on mechanical ventilation. These include acute respiratory failure; airway obstruction; and neurological conditions rendering the patient without sufficient respiratory drive, adequate spontaneous endurance, or the ability to protect his or her airway. All these factors must be evaluated when planning for a long-term artificial airway. The majority of patients in ICUs receive tracheostomies because of prolonged mechanical ventilation and failure with the weaning process. The reasons for this difficulty in weaning vary according to the patient's underlying conditions. Like endotracheal intubation, the conditions that require a tracheostomy fall into four broad categories: difficulties with ventilation, obstruction, airway protection, and secretions (Shapiro, Harrison, Kacmarek, & Cane, 1985)—remember VOPS for a mnemonic. Current practice in critical care reports a varied lifespan for the placement of an endotracheal tube in an adult that ranges from a few short days up to 2 weeks. A tracheotomy should be considered when the expected need for an artificial airway outlasts that time frame.

Time to Tracheotomy

When patients cannot be weaned soon after intubation, the practitioner must determine whether to place a tracheostomy or whether efforts to wean should continue. Tracheotomy is performed more frequently than in years past due to several factors, including increased use of percutaneous techniques. Numerous studies have attempted to identify the optimal time to place a tracheostomy; however, no definitive recommendations have been developed. The difficulty lies in the interpretation of results because different studies use different time frames as well as different outcome measures. Several authors have shown no mortality rate benefit with early tracheotomy (Arabi et al., 2009; Marsh, Gillespie, & Baumgartner, 1989), while other studies have shown a decreased mortality rate (Rumbak et al., 2004; Scales & Kahn, 2008). The definitions of early tracheotomy in these studies have included those done within 48 hours to 1 week of intubation and mechanical ventilation.

Kluge and colleagues (2008) used a questionnaire to survey physician directors of ICUs in Germany. They found that 67.2% of tracheostomies were performed during the second week of mechanical ventilation, while only 21.7% were performed within 7 days of initiation of mechanical ventilation.

Blot and others (2008) recruited patients from 25 ICUs in France to show the benefit of early tracheostomy compared to prolonged intubation. They recruited patients on mechanical ventilation and randomized them into two groups: early tracheostomy within 4 days of intubation versus patients with prolonged intubation. The sample size of the early tracheotomy group was calculated to be 470 patients; however, the study was stopped early because there was no difference in the study's primary endpoint of mortality. They concluded that the sole benefit of the tracheostomy was greater comfort as self-reported by patients.

Other studies have examined the benefit of tracheostomy on weaning from mechanical ventilation. However, this is also difficult to study because of the numerous factors that affect the weaning process, including work of breathing, dead space, secretions, sedation, and an aggressive weaning protocol. Pierson (2005) and Scales and Kahn (2008) suggest that perhaps the benefit of tracheostomy on weaning can be appreciated in less dramatic ways, such as by decreasing complications from overexposure to mechanical ventilation, facilitating improved removal of secretions, and improved comfort leading to reduced sedation requirements.

Project IMPACT, a multi-institutional database adopted by the Society of Critical Care Medicine (SCCM), attempted to identify not only optimal time to tracheotomy but also to evaluate clinical and nonclinical factors on tracheostomy practice. With a database of nearly 44,000 patients, they found the median time to tracheotomy was 9 days and that prolonged intubation led to increased duration of mechanical ventilation, increased ICU length of stay, and increased hospital length of stay (Freeman, Borecki, Coopersmith, & Buchman, 2005). Currently, the recommended critical care practice is withholding sedation and initiating a weaning trial with spontaneous breathing on a daily basis. When the patient is unable to be weaned after 7–10 days, a tracheotomy is usually considered. See chapter 2 for further discussion on time to tracheostomy.

Airway Pressures and Work of Breathing

The tracheostomy patient on a ventilator presents a special challenge. It is important to minimize airway pressure and resistance and maximize the mobilization of secretions. A mechanical ventilator provides the power to insufflate the lungs, aerate the alveoli, and remove carbon dioxide. Numerous modes are used to adjust a graded work of breathing. Whenever a patient is mechanically ventilated, the clinician monitors the trend in compliance of the respiratory system (the balance between pressure and volume). Often the progression of mechanical ventilation and the mode, whether on volume-limited ventilation (e.g., synchronized intermittent mandatory ventilation, SIMV) or pressure-limited ventilation (e.g., pressure support ventilation, PSV), are driven by changes in lung compliance. Empirically, in a volume-limited ventilation mode, a preset tidal volume is delivered to the patient, and lung pressure is dependent on compliance. With a pressure-limited ventilation mode, the ventilator delivers a flow of gas to the patient until a preset pressure is achieved, and the generated tidal volumes are dependent on compliance. Of particular concern to the tracheostomy patient is the development of high airway pressures, and this concern is magnified as the tube caliber gets smaller or airway secretions accumulate.

Peak and Plateau Pressures. The peak pressure, or peak inspiratory pressure (P_{peak}), is the highest pressure in the system during inspiration. It is a dynamic pressure reflecting changes in compliance due to changes within the lung itself, secretions, obstruction, and other factors that affect driving pressure. When tidal volume is constant, an increased peak pressure can reflect reduced lung compliance or increased airway resistance (Pilbeam, 1998). Because peak pressure is measured during airflow, it consists of both lung and chest wall recoil plus the resistance created by the tracheostomy tube and the airway itself. Lung compliance is the change in volume (V) as a function of a change in pressure (P). The formula is as follows (Gomella & Haist, 2006):

$$\text{Compliance} = \Delta V \div \Delta P$$

Dynamic compliance varies per breath and is a function of the tidal volume (V_t), peak inspiratory pressure (P_{peak}), and PEEP. The formula for dynamic compliance is as follows:

$$\text{Dynamic compliance} = V_t \div (P_{peak} - \text{PEEP})$$

The plateau pressure (P_{plat}) is measured in the absence of airflow and reflects static compliance. The absence of airflow is created by adding an inspiratory pause at the end of inspiration. The formula for static compliance is as follows:

$$\text{Static compliance} = V_t \div (P_{plat} - \text{PEEP})$$

Factors that change compliance include level of PEEP, the compliance of ventilator tubing, and all of the conditions that cause changes in the density and distensibility of lung tissue. Compliance can also be affected by tracheostomy tubes that are constructed of more distensible materials, such as silicone. Static compliance reflects the elastic recoil of the alveolar walls and thoracic cage against the volume of air in the lungs. It also reflects the recoil of the ventilator tubing on the volume of air in the circuit. It is difficult to measure accurately in spontaneously breathing patients because it cannot be measured when a patient is making active respiratory efforts. Decreased static compliance implies ventilation is less effective and can be caused by air trapping, pulmonary edema, pneumothorax, atelectasis, and other conditions that limit the compliance of the chest wall and abdominal wall such as pneumomediastinum and abdominal compartment syndrome (Pilbeam, 1998).

Because dynamic compliance consists of both compliance and resistance, it is actually a measure of elastance (Bone, 1983). Lung problems can be differentiated from airway problems by monitoring changes between the peak and plateau pressure. If P_{peak} and P_{plat} are both increasing while volume stays constant, then lung compliance is decreasing (Pilbeam, 1998).

Assessing peak and plateau pressures is especially important in the mechanically ventilated patient with a tracheostomy. When peak or plateau pressures are high, the clinician must first ensure the patency and proper positioning of the tube. High peak pressure in the presence of normal plateau pressure indicates an airway problem such as an obstruction due to secretions or a tracheostomy tube that is too small.

Work of Breathing. Work is required to overcome the forces in opposition to lung inflation. High airway resistance contributes to work of breathing. The formula for work of breathing is calculated as follows:

$$\text{Work of breathing (in joules)} = (P \times V) \div 10$$

The product of P and V is expressed as cm H_2O; however, mechanical work is usually not expressed in cm H_2O, but rather kg/m, or joules. To convert cm H_2O into joules, divide the product by 10 (Beachey, 2007).

There are significant changes in aerodynamics associated with both tracheostomy and return to breathing through the native airway. Factors involved in the decision to place a tracheostomy tube are often complex, especially when attempting liberation from mechanical ventilation. It is often difficult to discern the causes for a failure to wean from mechanical ventilation, and it is even more of a mystery why many patients are able to wean shortly after the placement of a tracheostomy. Davis, Campbell, Johannigman, Valente, and Branson (1999) explored this phenomenon by studying the effects of tracheostomy and work of breathing in a group of surgical patients who had failed two attempts at weaning from mechanical ventilation. Patients had an esophageal balloon inserted transnasally to monitor esophageal pressure 6 to 10 hours before tracheotomy. Balloon placement was confirmed, and patients were disconnected from the ventilator and allowed to breathe with a continuous flow of gas at an oxygen concentration equal to that of the ventilator. After 10 minutes of stabilization, measurements were made of tidal volume, respiratory rate, airway pressure, flow, and esophageal pressure, and work of breathing was calculated. Allowing for elimination of anesthetic gases, the same measurements were repeated 10 hours after tracheotomy. They found that all patients were successfully weaned to a high-humidity tracheostomy collar within 24 hours of tracheostomy placement. There was a statistically significant decrease in work of breathing and PEEP after tracheotomy, but the authors suggest these changes do not fully explain the facilitated weaning. The investigators proposed that facilitated weaning is promoted by the decreased length, rigid structure, and curvature of the tracheostomy tube, as well as its less tortuous path compared to an endotracheal tube.

Retained Secretions

Effective bronchial hygiene is of paramount importance to a patient with a tracheostomy. Normally, there is a continuous blanket of mucus covering the epithelial lining of the large airways. The forward motion of cilia propels this mucus lining toward the hilus of the lung, moving toward the larynx and the pharynx, where it is eventually swallowed. This mucus blanket moves at a rate of 1 to 2 cm per minute and can completely cleanse the entire lung in 20 minutes in a normal, healthy adult. Ciliary activity is diminished in conditions such as smoking, positive-pressure ventilation, high levels of inspired oxygen, dehydration, general anesthesia, and tracheal foreign bodies such as tracheostomy tubes (Shapiro et al., 1985).

The cough is the primary defense mechanism against retained secretions. The purpose of the cough is to provide high-velocity airflow on expiration. The cough mechanism consists of five components: deep breath, inspiratory pause, glottic closure, increased thoracic pressure, and glottic opening. Without adequate inspiration, a cough is ineffective. Vital capacity must be at least 15 ml/kg of ideal body weight to produce an adequate cough. Following deep inspiration, the breath-holding maneuver provides time for maximal distribution of air, followed by glottic closure. With the glottis closed, the primary mechanism for increasing intrathoracic pressure is to increase intra-abdominal pressure. This pushes the diaphragm upward and decreases the volume of the thoracic cavity. The primary muscles involved in increasing intra-abdominal pressure are the anterior abdominal wall muscles, which force the diaphragm up against the closed glottis. Suddenly, the glottis opens and allows high-velocity airflow from the lungs—as high as 300 liters per minute (Shapiro et al., 1985).

Retained secretions can be caused by dehydration, pulmonary disease, artificial airways, generalized muscular weakness, central nervous system disorders causing bulbar malfunction, and limitation of the abdominal musculature as in spinal cord injury or abdominal surgery. Efforts to mobilize retained secretions should be directed to the cause(s), but the importance of the mobilization of secretions cannot be overstated. Specific measures to mobilize secretions are discussed further in chapter 7.

Cuff Leaks

One of the most common occurrences with a tracheostomy is a cuff leak. In order to provide proper management, the clinician must first determine whether the leak is coming from within the cuff, around the cuff, or within the tube itself.

Leak Within the Cuff

The tight quality-control process of companies that produce airway appliances makes a defect within a tube cuff a rare occurrence. Nonetheless, cuff integrity should always be checked prior to the insertion of any tracheostomy tube. The simplest maneuver is to ensure the cuff sustains inflation against digital pressure. A second maneuver is to place an air-inflated cuff into a small basin of sterile water, where bubbling will indicate a leak within the cuff.

It is possible for a leak within a cuff to develop over time. Leaks in endotracheal tube cuffs are more common due to damage from the teeth and other airway appliances as tubes are introduced through the oropharynx. When the tracheostomy tube is in place, the easiest way to check for a leak within the cuff is to attach a syringe and deflate the cuff. If air can be continuously withdrawn, there is a leak in the cuff. Another easy way to check for a leak is to inflate the cuff with air and check for an adequate seal by ensuring delivered tidal volume on the ventilator and the integrity of measured cuff pressure. If the cuff does not seem to hold air, damage to the pilot balloon valve, inflation line, or cuff should be suspected. The definitive treatment for any of these concerns is to change the tracheostomy tube.

Cuff leaks have also been reported following the percutaneous approach to tracheotomy, which presents a unique dilemma. With percutaneous placement, the tracheostomy tube is snug within the stoma. In fact, less bleeding has been reported with the percutaneous approach than with the surgical approach due to its tamponade effect within the stoma. Cuff leaks occurring after a percutaneous approach could be due to pressure applied during insertion. For this reason, some practitioners prefer to delay the first tube change with a percutaneous tracheotomy until a more mature stoma has developed. Although the definitive treatment for a cuff leak is to change the tube, if a cuff leak is detected soon after the placement of a percutaneous tracheostomy, the advisable approach is to maintain constant close monitoring of the patient's gas exchange and hemodynamic status and later replace the tube in the presence of a specialized airway team, possibly in a controlled environment such as the operating room.

Leak Around the Cuff

Leaks around the cuff are much more common than leaks within the cuff and result from a less than adequate seal within the airway. Unless there is a risk for aspiration, a leak around the cuff is not usually a concern, nor is it even noticeable, in a patient free from mechanical ventilation. In fact, an imperceptible leak around the cuff might be an incidental advantage in minimizing pressure against the trachea. Patients with a cuff leak can often talk, indicating they are able to comfortably pass air not only through the tube but also to reach the vocal cords.

When the patient is ventilator dependent, however, a cuff leak can be quite exasperating for the nurse or respiratory care practitioner due to frequent ventilator alarms indicating low pressure. Naturally, a cuff leak in a mechanically ventilated patient who is hemodynamically unstable would require immediate exploration of the cause of the leak. There are numerous causes for a leak around the cuff, including the following:

- Cuff is not fully inflated to seal the airway.
- Cuff is inflated, but the tube is too small for the airway.
- Cuff is inflated, but air and secretions are leaking past the cuff.
- Leak is associated with changes in patient position.
- Patient is on high levels of PEEP.
- An area of tracheomalacia has developed.

Cuff Is Not Fully Inflated. In some cases, there is a very simple solution to a leak around the cuff. Sometimes all that is required is to put more air in the cuff. This can be assessed by palpating deeply on the pilot balloon. This maneuver is equivalent to adding air to the cuff because it pushes air from the pilot balloon into the cuff itself. The pilot balloon provides an indicator of cuff inflation but has no bearing on cuff pressure. It has been demonstrated that an estimation of cuff pressure with balloon palpation is often inaccurate (Fernandez, Blanch, Mancebo, Bonsoms, & Artigas, 1990; Hoffman, Parwani, & Hahn, 2006). However, palpation of the cuff can provide information about the presence of air in the cuff. A flat pilot balloon indicates there is no air in the cuff, whereas a tense pilot balloon indicates there is a large volume of air in the cuff relative to the diameter of the trachea. If the leak disappears with deep palpation of the pilot balloon, then more air should be added to the cuff. However, cuff inflation should not always be an automatic response to a leak. For a cuff that repeatedly loses air, the clinician should explore further to determine the cause of the leak.

Cuff Is Inflated, but the Tube Is Too Small for the Airway. The pilot balloon should first be palpated for the presence of air when investigating a cuff leak in an inflated cuff. If the pilot balloon is tense, the cuff is probably overinflated. Frequently, the cuff may be overinflated in an attempt to create an adequate seal. However, an overinflated balloon with a continued leak is indicative of a tracheostomy tube that is too small to create an adequate seal within the airway (see Figure 5.1). Besides palpation, the manufacturer's recommendations regarding inflation volumes should be reviewed. For example, Shiley provides leak test inflation volumes for its cuffed tracheostomy tubes that list the maximum volume that should be added to the cuff to seal the airway. For the Shiley LPC and FEN tracheostomy tubes, the leak test inflation volumes are 11, 14, 17, and 20 ml for the size 4, 6, 8, and 10 tubes, respectively. When these volumes are exceeded, the cuff can be considered overinflated. An optimal treatment in this case is to place a larger tracheostomy tube. (See discussion on upsizing in chapter 4.)

Cuff Is Inflated, but Air and Secretions Are Leaking Past the Cuff. Up to 150 ml of secretions can be aspirated per day from ICU patients. From patients in the prone position, over 50 ml of secretions per hour have been reported (Young, Rollinson, Downward, & Henderson, 1997).

Longitudinal channels can occur in high-volume, low-pressure cuffs, and these folds appear upon inflation of the cuff because the diameter must be greater than that of the trachea for intracuff pressure to equal tracheal wall pressure. Winklmaier, Wüst, Schiller, and Wallner (2006) studied leakage around the cuffs of three different tracheostomy tubes: Rüsch Ultra-Tracheoflex, TRACOE

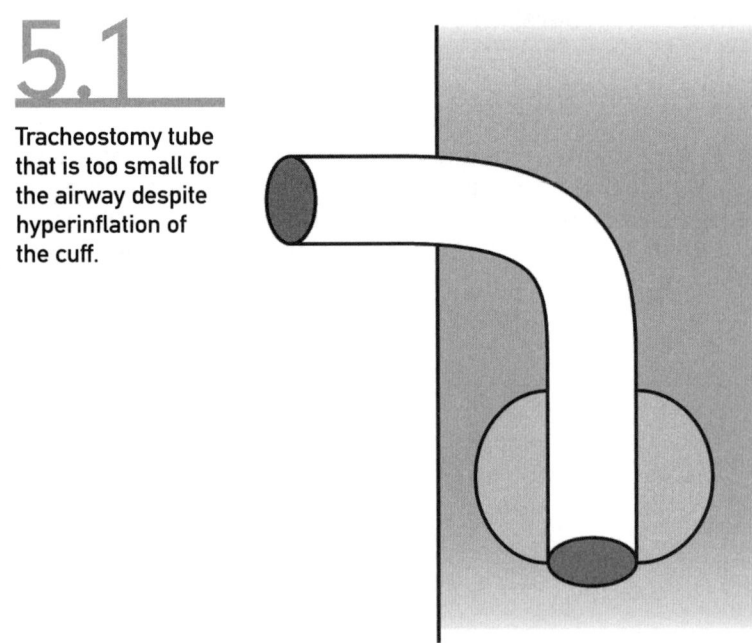

5.1

Tracheostomy tube that is too small for the airway despite hyperinflation of the cuff.

Vario, and Portex Blue Line Ultra. They injected 6 ml of water or artificial saliva into a pig model and measured the volumes that leaked past the cuff after 5, 10, and 15 minutes. They studied these conditions with and without artificial ventilation. They found that when water runs into the subglottic space, it disappears almost completely down the longitudinal channels. The increased viscosity of saliva reduced this leakage significantly compared to water.

The investigators found that the Portex Blue Line Ultra was the most effective of the tubes studied in preventing leakage of fluid and that leakage was higher without artificial ventilation. An interesting observation was that cuff pressure in all three tubes dropped significantly after 15 minutes. All tubes were initially measured at 25 cm H_2O; after 15 minutes, the pressure dropped to an average of 18.76 cm H_2O in the TRACOE tube, 19.54 in the Rüsch tube, and 19.07 in the Portex tube. The researchers concluded that leakage of fluid was associated with the thickness of the cuff membrane, and they projected that ultrathin polyurethane might be the cuff material of the future. Interestingly, both Covidien and Kimberly-Clark have recently launched new ultrathin polyurethane cuffs on endotracheal tubes, and preliminary testing is promising. Future studies will determine the potential clinical benefit of polyurethane cuffs with tracheostomy tubes.

Young and colleagues (1997) performed similar testing in a model lung and trachea and found that leakage occurred down the longitudinal folds in all cuffs tested. They found that the application of lubricant around the cuff helped protect it from leakage, and the use of PEEP and CPAP also protected against leakage.

The leakage of secretions around the cuff may not be clinically evident. The normal response to the leakage of secretions around the cuff is continued coughing, but sedation blunts this response. Normal glottic function is impaired with prolonged intubation. Silent aspiration is common in certain patients who have been orotracheally intubated for mechanical ventilation and in those with neurologic deficits.

Leak Is Associated With Changes in Patient Position. In some cases, the leak is present when the patient is in a certain position but disappears when the patient's position is changed. Tracheostomy and endotracheal tubes can move within the airway when the patient's head is moved in different positions, which can then move the position of the cuff within the airway. Sometimes simple repositioning will solve the problem. Frequently, leaks result not only from head movement and repositioning of the cuff within the airway but also from external forces on the tube. The presence of added weight on the tracheostomy tube from filters, in-line suctioning systems, or unsupported circuit tubing will cause traction or torque on the tracheostomy tube. If this is the case, the added weight should be removed, and the ventilator tubing should be adequately supported. If the leak remains after these maneuvers, the tracheostomy tube should be changed to a longer tube for improved placement in the airway.

Patient Is on High Levels of PEEP. When the level of PEEP is high, it is sometimes difficult to maintain an adequate seal because air that is pushed through the tube can also push against the cuff. With higher levels of PEEP (usually greater than 10 cm H_2O), the tracheostomy tube can be nearly displaced outward. The movement of the tube in the airway with the respiratory cycle is called pistoning, which will be discussed further later in this chapter. A patient on high levels of PEEP should be closely monitored not only for hemodynamic stability and evidence of barotrauma but also for proper tube placement.

An Area of Tracheomalacia Has Developed. If the tube is of adequate size for the patient's airway and the leak remains following full inflation of the cuff, one can assume tracheomalacia has developed. Tracheomalacia can be definitively diagnosed by endoscopy. Chronic overinflation of the tracheostomy tube cuff can create an area of tracheal ischemia, which later becomes a localized softening of the tracheal tissue known as tracheomalacia (see Figure 5.2). Upon direct visualization, a floppy area moves freely with breathing; depending on the location of the defect, it can result in a severe narrowing of the trachea. Extrathoracic tracheomalacia can cause collapse during spontaneous inspiration, while intrathoracic tracheomalacia can collapse the airway on exhalation (Zur & Schilero, 2006). While on mechanical ventilation, the short-term correction of the leak associated with tracheomalacia is to place a longer tracheostomy tube to position the cuff in a lower area within the trachea. However, surgical resection of the trachea is the long-term solution to this problem. See chapter 10 for more discussion about tracheomalacia.

Though it is not clinically feasibly to continually place progressively longer tracheostomy tubes, one can alternate placing a longer, then a shorter, tube. Another alternative is to use an adjustable-neck flange tracheostomy tube, though it is not recommended for long-term use. A third option is to use a

5.2

Tracheomalacia and repositioning the tracheostomy tube. On the left is an area of tracheomalacia around an inflated cuff. On the right, a longer tracheostomy tube has been inserted, allowing the cuff to be positioned below the level of tracheomalacia.

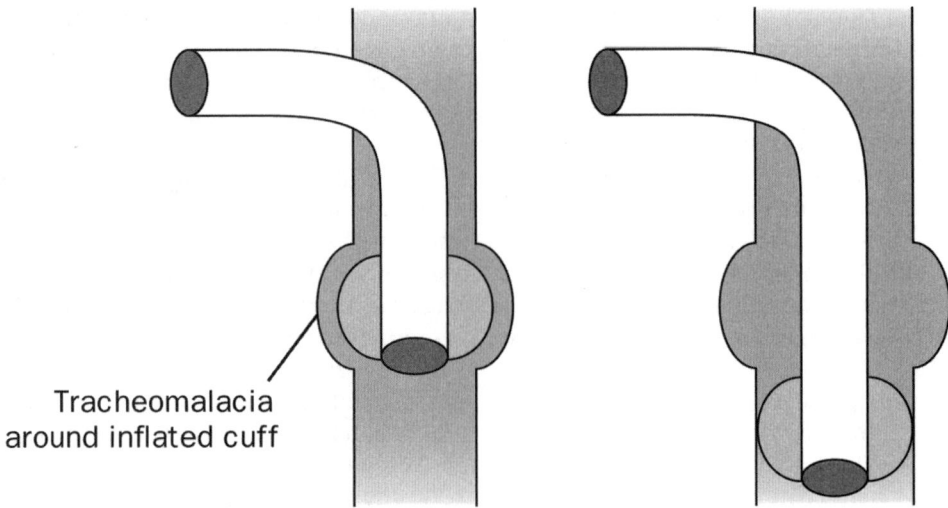

Tracheomalacia around inflated cuff

double-cuffed tube and alternate inflation of the cuffs. Portex currently manufactures a double-cuffed tube; however, it is scheduled to be discontinued.

Leak Within the Tube

Rarely, a leak can occur within the tracheostomy tube itself and can result from several factors: a poor fit of the inner cannula into the outer cannula, imperfect connections, or damage during placement. A leak caused by poor fit occurs when there is a size difference between the inner cannula and the outer cannula. When a smaller inner cannula is placed into a larger outer cannula, air will leak between them. Similarly, a leak can be caused when a properly sized inner cannula is not locked into place and air escapes around it. Rarely, a leak can be caused as a result of a manufacturing defect, such as a nonfitting connection between the inner cannula and the outer cannula. More often, a leak within a tube occurs as a result of damage to the tube during insertion, such as during percutaneous insertion, where a higher degree of force is necessary to insert the tube. Any suspected defects in a tube must be reported promptly to the manufacturer and, in some cases, to the Food and Drug Administration (FDA).

Managing cuff leaks can be challenging; therefore, it is important to evaluate them following a systematic method. Figure 5.3 shows an algorithm for detecting the cause of a cuff leak.

Pistoning

During positive-pressure ventilation, a tube with an inflated cuff tends to move up and down within the airway as the ventilator cycles while the cuff remains fixed in place. Pistoning describes the movement of the tracheostomy tube inside the trachea with the fully inflated cuff fixed in place (see Figure 5.4). Pistoning is more apparent with the larger cuff of the endotracheal tube, but it frequently occurs with the tracheostomy tube as well. Over time, this action creates weakness within the integrity of the cuff and adds pressure against the tracheal mucosa as it drags along the walls of the trachea. Though it is suggested that teardrop-shaped cuffs may prevent this pistoning action, there are no studies to support this claim.

Cuff Changes at Altitude

The patient with a tracheostomy presents significant complications when traveling by air. During ascent to altitude, ambient pressure decreases. As altitude increases, pressure within the cuff also increases. Boyle's law states that a fixed volume of gas will expand as pressure decreases (Henning, Sharley, & Young, 2004), so as barometric pressure decreases with altitude, tracheal tube cuffs will expand.

Air-filled cuffs expand with increasing altitude at a rate of 30 mbar/1,000 feet. The critical perfusion pressure of the tracheal mucosa is exceeded at 1,820 feet, so it is important to control for cuff volume expansion in aeromedical transport (Mann, Parkinson, & Bleetman, 2007). Commercial airlines tend to

5.3

Algorithm for cuff leak.

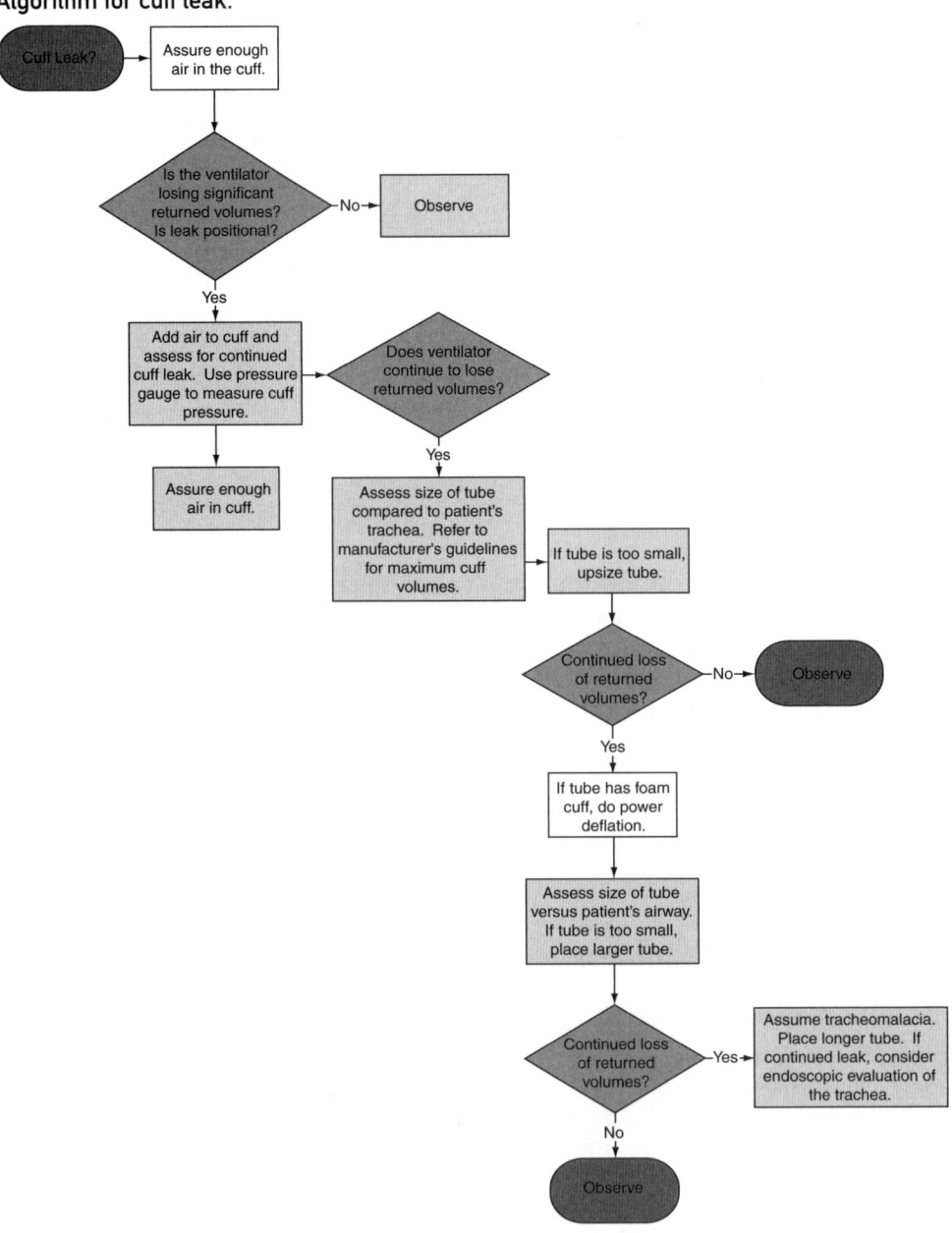

5.4

Pistoning of tracheostomy tube against the tracheal wall. Note the cuff stays fixed in place.
(A) Tube at rest. (B) Downward movement of tube with positive-pressure ventilation.
(C) Upward movement of tube with positive-pressure ventilation.

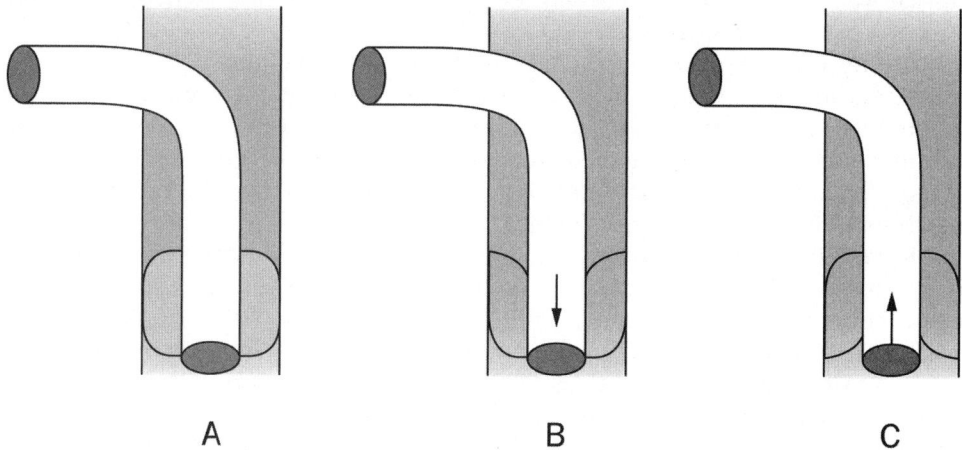

pressurize cabins to 6,000 to 8,000 feet. Helicopters are unpressurized and fly at approximately 5,000 feet (Henning et al., 2004).

Several studies have been done to demonstrate the deleterious effect of pressure on tracheal tube cuffs. Stoner and Cooke (1974) conducted an early study of endotracheal tube cuffs in anesthetized dogs. At ground level, the cuff pressure was 45 torr in a Portex tube and 78 torr in a Rüsch tube. However, at 8,000 feet, the pressures measured 64 torr in the Portex tube and 130 torr in the Rüsch tube. Upon decompression to 35,000 feet, pressures in the cuffs exceeded 135 and 230 torr, respectively. Interestingly, at compression back to ground level, both cuffs were 60% and 45% of their original pressures, respectively.

Henning and colleagues (2004) measured cuff pressures of 10 patients during aeromedical flights in helicopters and fixed-wing aircraft. All patients began the flight with a cuff pressure of 22 cm H_2O at ground level, and pressure was measured again at 3,000 feet. The investigators found that all pressures had significantly increased, ranging from 40 to 51 cm H_2O.

Normally, it is possible to determine adequate cuff inflation by using either the minimal occlusive volume or the minimal leak technique. (See chapter 7 for a description of methods to minimize pressure in the cuff.) In air transport, however, the noise level is too high to use these methods effectively. Current evidence in the aeromedical transport literature supports the use of cuff inflation with saline, an alternate balloon to vent air from the cuff, or deflation of the cuff at altitude (Mann et al., 2007).

Yoneda, Watanabe, Hayashida, Kanno, and Sato (1999) described a method to vent air from the cuff by using a separate balloon attached directly to the cuff of an endotracheal tube. They chose balloons of different sizes and connected them to the endotracheal tube with a roller clamp and a three-way stopcock. With no pressure-controlling device, they found the tracheal pressure rose 20.8 cm H_2O per 1,000 feet and reached 228.7 cm H_2O at 10,000 feet. Following decompression, tracheal pressure rose from 21.2 cm H_2O at 8,000 feet to 259.0 cm H_2O at 22,000 feet. With the pressure-control device, however, they found no significant increases in pressure. Upon ascent, the pressure with the controlling device was 20.9 cm H_2O at ground level and 20.3 cm H_2O at 10,000 feet. Upon descent, pressure was 19.8 cm H_2O and 20.7 cm H_2O at ground level.

Rather than using a venting device, Mann and colleagues (2007) described a formula for the removal of air from the cuff at altitude. They recommended an air-filled cuff should have 0.3 ml of air removed per 1,000 feet during ascent to control for rising pressure. During descent, the cuff should be inflated at the same rate. Smith and McArdle (2002) recommended that air be removed after reaching altitudes as low at 2,000 feet.

Kaye (2007) suggested that the use of saline in the cuffs of tracheal tubes is an easier and more effective method for controlling for gas expansion and contraction during air transport. Smith and McArdle (2002) found that replacing air with saline resulted in much smaller increases in cuff pressure. The study by Henning and colleagues (2007) reported that even with saline in the cuff, there still may be a rise in pressure with altitude, and the pressures even at ground level may be variable. While there are no products currently approved by the FDA, the use of an automatic device to continuously monitor and adjust cuff pressure might be an ideal solution to air transport with cuffed tracheostomy tubes.

Cuff Changes With Anesthesia

It is common knowledge among anesthesiologists that nitrous oxide increases cuff pressure because of easy diffusion into the cuff. This increased cuff pressure manifests as postoperative complaints of sore throat, with severity dependent on the length of the operative procedure. Numerous methods have been employed during nitrous oxide administration to prevent these high cuff pressures. These include high-volume, low-pressure endotracheal tube cuffs; balloon-limiting pressure; inflation of the cuff with a mixture of nitrous oxide and oxygen or saline; a gas barrier cuff; an ultrathin endotracheal tube; and continuous monitoring of cuff pressure (Tu et al., 1999).

Karasawa, Hamachi, Takamatsu, and Oshima (2003) tested the time required to achieve a stable cuff pressure during 67% nitrous oxide anesthesia. Air-filled cuffs of a standard endotracheal tube were aspirated every 30 minutes for the first 3 or 4 hours, and cuff pressures were monitored for an additional 3 hours. Intracuff concentrations of nitrous oxide increased during the repeated cuff deflation, and continued to increase during the additional 3-hour monitoring period, from 39.8 cm H_2O to 44.3 cm H_2O. When the cuff was deflated periodically over a 4-hour period, it was possible to maintain a stable cuff pressure, implying that cuff pressures continue to increase even after the completion of nitrous oxide anesthesia.

Dullenkopf, Gerber, and Weiss (2004) tested cuff compliance and pressure during nitrous oxide exposure with a new polyurethane material compared with standard polyvinyl chloride cuffs. They found that the ultrathin polyurethane cuff demonstrated a higher permeability for nitrous oxide and led to a rapid increase in cuff pressure when exposed to nitrous oxide.

Postaci and colleagues (2008) compared intracuff pressures during high-flow and low-flow nitrous oxide anesthesia. Cuff pressures were measured continuously with a pressure manometer, and inspired oxygen and nitrous oxide levels were noted every 10 minutes. The time required to reach maximum cuff pressure was significantly shorter in the low-flow anesthesia group.

Navarro and others (2007) studied endotracheal cuffs filled with air versus alkalinized lidocaine. In their sample of 50 patients, endotracheal cuff pressures were recorded at 30, 60, 90, and 120 minutes after starting and after ending nitrous oxide anesthesia. Patients were randomly assigned to one of two groups: one group was given a cuff inflated with air to attain a pressure of 20 cm H_2O, while the other used a cuff filled with 2% lidocaine plus 8.4% sodium bicarbonate to attain the same pressure. Pressures in the lidocaine cuffs were significantly lower than those filled with air, and postoperative complaints of sore throat also decreased.

Sato, Tanaka, and Nishikawa (2004) measured changes in intracuff pressure using a new endotracheal tube cuff, the Portex Soft-Seal Cuff. Patients were randomly selected to use a standard endotracheal tube or the Soft-Seal tube. Cuffs were inflated with air and intracuff pressure was measured during 67% nitrous oxide anesthesia. The investigators noted that cuff pressure gradually increased in both groups, but the mean pressure of the Soft-Seal cuffs was significantly lower than the standard tube. The incidence of postoperative sore throat was not significantly different between the two groups.

Combes and others (2001) randomly assigned patients to two groups—those with cuffs filled with air and those with cuffs filled with saline during nitrous oxide anesthesia—at 20–30 cm H_2O pressure. In their study of 50 patients, they found that cuff pressure gradually increased during anesthesia in cuffs filled with air but remained stable in those filled with saline. In addition, the incidence of sore throat was greater in patients whose cuffs were filled with air. At the time of extubation, tracheal lesions were seen in all patients with air-filled cuffs, compared to 32% of patients with saline-filled cuffs.

The Complex Tracheostomy Wound

Patients with complex stomal wounds require extra attention. Occasionally, traction against the stoma will create a widened area of erosion or maceration of tissue. These wounds can become inflamed or infected and turn into cellulitis. Some of the more common problems involved with these lesions and their prevention is described in this section.

Stomal Erosion

Erosion of the stoma is caused by either outward or inward traction. Outward traction is excessive outward pressure on the tracheostomy tube resulting from poorly supported ventilator tubing with devices added to the circuit (such as HMEs, in-line closed suction systems, or filters). This added traction introduces the risk of inadvertent tube dislodgement, which often results from internal erosion of the stoma. The erosion can be so severe that it widens the stoma enough for the entire shaft and cuff to be visible. The only way to prevent this type of erosion is to eliminate excess weight and traction forces. Methods to prevent this internal erosion include the following practices:

- Support the ventilator tubing with support arms, or strategically cushion it with a well-placed towel roll.
- Survey the security of the tracheostomy ties/holder frequently.
- Minimize traction/torque whenever the patient is moved. Whenever turning a patient, always turn him or her first toward the ventilator, then away from the ventilator, and avoid traction throughout the turn.
- Remove the in-line suction system when feasible.
- Replace the HME with a heated humidity unit when feasible.

Inward traction can cause stomal erosion by forcing the neck flange into the tissues of the neck. The effect can be magnified when a twisting force is applied at the pivot points of a rigid neck flange. The only way to prevent this type of stomal erosion is to remove these traction forces by eliminating all mechanisms that cause it and by ensuring proper patient positioning. Other preventive steps include supporting the ventilator tubing, generously using drain sponges to cushion the neck flange against the skin, preventing neck flexion when possible, removing excess weight from the circuit, and, if necessary, changing the tracheostomy tube to one with a soft and flexible neck flange.

Inflammation/Cellulitis

Most inflammation of the stoma is caused by moisture. The prolonged contact of secretions with the skin creates irritation and inflammation of the skin—not unlike diaper rash—and can lead to the maceration of tissue and the development of cellulitis. These complications can be prevented by keeping the stoma dry, particularly in patients who produce copious amounts of secretions. If frequent changes of the gauze dressing are not enough to keep the stoma dry, then absorbent dressings may be required. One example of an absorbent dressing is Lyofoam, which comes in a precut form for use as a drain sponge.

Infected, erosive wounds present a greater challenge. Systemic antibiotics may be indicated if the patient exhibits signs of systemic infection, including fever, elevated white blood cell count, tachycardia, and so forth. In most cases, adequate local treatment is effective in preventing systemic infection. Hotter and Warfield (1997) described an approach to care for deep, erosive, infected wounds. They used a product called Mesalt, a thin cloth ribbon impregnated with 15% sodium chloride. The wound was gently packed with the ribbon to absorb excess secretions and bacteria and was changed every 2 to 3 hours. The researchers hypothesized that the hypertonicity of the product provided an osmotic effect within the wound bed to increase oxygen delivery and decrease edema. For deeply erosive wounds, they also used DuoDERM as a platform to support the neck flange from digging into the skin. DuoDERM is a hydrocolloid wafer that forms a gel when it comes in contact with moisture or exudate. The authors suggested that DuoDERM can be left in place for up to 10 days; however, the manufacturer recommends only up to 7 days. Figure 5.5 shows a complex tracheostomy wound using DuoDERM as a platform for stomal erosion.

Silver-impregnated pads have been shown to be effective on infected wounds. Direct contact with silver disrupts the bacterial cell membrane and results in a significant bactericidal effect. Aquacel Ag is one such silver-infused product, and it can be used for infected and draining wounds. It turns to a hydrocolloid gel that absorbs secretions and can be left in place for up to 7 days.

Tracheostomy as a Lived Experience

There is very little research on the patient's experience of living with a tracheostomy. Recently, however, Sherlock, Wilson, and Exley (2009) reported the results of their semistructured interviews with eight patients still in the hospital. Though their sample size was admittedly small, their results give quite a powerful message to caregivers. The study intended to shed light on the amount and

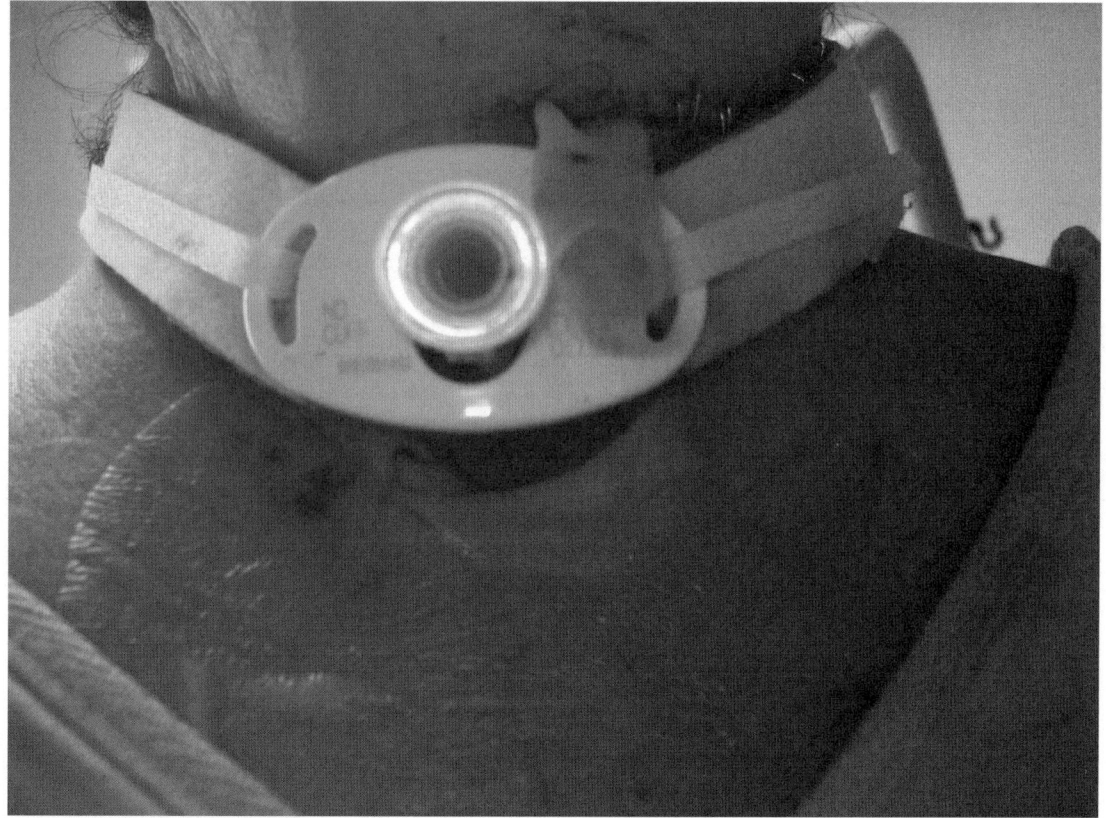

5.5

A complex tracheostomy wound. Note hydrocolloid dressing used as a platform.

quality of information provided to patients while in the hospital. The researchers found that patients are provided little information about the tracheostomy procedure and their condition in general, but they also found that patients' responses fell into several categories: physical sensations and feelings related to the tube, eating and drinking, suctioning, communication, understanding, and information provided. All the patients described the bulkiness of the tube as restricting their freedom of movement. They also reported their fears associated with the tube. One patient reported, "For a couple of days, I was really scared of moving my head, 'cos [sic] there was something new stuck in my neck." All patients who had commenced oral intake commented on the difficulty they experienced with swallowing. One patient commented, "I was uncomfortable with it because every time you tried to swallow you could feel this lump there."

All the patients understood the necessity of suctioning for removal of secretions, but they also described their fear of and discomfort with the procedure. One patient described his experience: "The worst part was when it needed to be cleaned with suction....I would panic because I couldn't breathe. I had no control over what was happening." Another patient reported, "Every time they put it (the suction catheter) down, you coughed violently. You felt as if you were going to explode and then sort of relief because they'd taken all the mucus away....It's a most uncomfortable process."

Every patient expressed frustration at his or her inability to communicate effectively. One patient expressed his frustration in this way: "That's terrible. The fact that you can't communicate. You can open, close your mouth and know what you're saying, knowing that nobody else can hear what it is that you are trying to say, so we got a board in the end and I used to have to write messages."

Patients reported they received little, if any, information about the tracheostomy and its implications. One patient reported, "They come and have a few words with you and then go on their way and not have time to sit and explain....It would have been nice to have had more (information)." Three patients reported being given information but still awoke feeling shocked that the tracheostomy tube was in place. "They tell you what's going to happen. They're going to put this tube in your throat to help you breathe; but with me it wasn't until I actually realized I'd got it there that I thought, 'What's this thing?'" (Sherlock et al., 2009).

Segaran (2006) studied the experience of eating with a tracheostomy during critical illness. The responses of the subjects fell into several categories, including regaining control, self-determination, sensory impact, and apprehensions. Patients were interviewed either while still in the ICU or within 7 days of leaving the ICU. Unstructured interviews were used, and the patients' responses were analyzed using a phenomenological approach. Patients started to develop goals in an effort to regain control over their situation. One subject reported the need to start "shedding attachments" and that his "number one goal was to get the tracheostomy out." Eating and drinking were key priorities, but many became frustrated at their inability to meet those goals. Subjects reported the difficulty they had with eating with a tracheostomy: "Eating with a tracheostomy was very cumbersome. That was frustrating, as I couldn't eat properly really, well not what I really wanted, like coke or fish and chips." Subjects also described eating as a difficult procedure that added to their frustration. When finally allowed to eat or drink, patients reported their fears about eating and drinking for the first time with a tracheostomy, especially after having been cautioned about the risks of aspiration. They also identified a restriction in their throat that they could always feel. Patients who had been decannulated reported the impact it had on their sense of taste and smell. One patient reported: "When I had the trache [sic] in, nothing tasted or smelt [sic] as it should. But I think it's getting better now the trache is out, I'm definitely starting to smell things again now" (Segaran).

Defective Tracheostomy Tubes

Manufacturing defects are relatively rare in airway devices, but they do occur. Parts that are fused may become disconnected or detached; pieces may be missing or not fit properly. It is better to discover a problem before the device is placed into a patient, but often defects are not discovered until the tube has been in place for some time. In any case, it is wise to always save the packaging for a device. The package identifies the batch number (and sometimes the serial number) so the problem can be more easily traced. Ideally, this identifying information should be recorded in the medical record when the device is placed in the patient. One company (TRACOE) provides a wallet-sized identification card for their tracheostomy tubes that includes serial number, model number, size, and length along with the company's contact information.

When a defect is identified, the manufacturer must be contacted immediately and notified of the problem. Manufacturers usually have a system in place for the return shipping of equipment for a safety inspection. Ideally, all parts of the tracheostomy tube should be returned with the package it came in. In many cases, these defects must also be reported promptly to the FDA. This is even more important if an adverse event occurred because of the defective device.

Tracheostomy tubes can also become damaged during the tracheotomy procedure itself, especially during percutaneous insertion. A tracheostomy tube inserted percutaneously creates a much tighter fit than one inserted with a standard surgical approach. Because of this tight fit, excessive pressure must sometimes be used to insert the tube. The neck flange may be weakened during insertion and may not become noticeable until hours or days later. This situation presents a unique dilemma. Ordinarily, a damaged tube must be replaced immediately. However, the replacement of any tracheostomy tube in the early postoperative period is fraught with the risk of loss of airway access. It is preferable that measures be taken to stabilize the tube until a more mature stoma can develop; however, if this is not possible, the tube should be replaced in a controlled environment using a well-developed plan.

Missing Parts

Tracheostomy tubes are packaged as a set, with all the pieces fitting together. All the parts within a set are designed to be used together. With few exceptions, these parts are not interchangeable with other tubes. For example, a missing inner cannula should not be replaced with an inner cannula from a different set; the entire tube should be changed. Frequently, lengths will be different between two identical tubes of the same size. The inner cannula may be longer than the outer cannula and may create erosion of the tracheal wall as it protrudes from the end of the outer cannula. In addition, disposable inner cannulas may not be used with nondisposable outer cannulas because of the different locking mechanisms.

Summary

There are many special considerations for the patient with a tracheostomy. Airway pressures must be closely monitored for patients who are ventilator dependent. The retention of secretions is a particular concern with a tracheostomy, and increased airway pressures are an early sign of secretion accumulation within the tracheostomy tube. Cuff leaks are a particular concern in the mechanically ventilated patient and can be managed with a methodical approach. Care should be taken to minimize pressure against the stoma, as both inward and outward traction forces can cause erosion of the stoma. This erosive action can be prevented by eliminating excessive weight from the ventilator tubing and by strategically placing a towel roll to support it. Altitude and nitrous oxide anesthesia cause large increases in cuff pressure, so paying careful attention to optimal cuff pressure and volume will prevent complications. Though rare, manufacturing defects do occur in tracheostomy tubes, and damage may be caused to the tube during the insertion procedure. With careful assessment and a methodical approach, the experienced practitioner can expertly manage all of these challenges.

Key Points

- For the patient on mechanical ventilation, high peak pressure in the presence of normal plateau pressure indicates an airway problem, including an obstruction due to secretions or a tracheostomy tube that is too small.
- Cuff leaks can occur within the cuff, around the cuff, or within the tube itself. A systematic approach should be used to determine the cause of a cuff leak.
- Stomal erosion commonly occurs from traction caused by the ventilator circuit against the tracheostomy tube.
- Cuff pressures dramatically increase at altitude and with administration of nitrous oxide anesthesia. Close attention to cuff pressure is warranted in these situations.
- To minimize apprehension and fear, patients need continued guidance and information about how to manage specific functions such as tube care, feeding, and phonation.

References

Arabi, Y. M., Alhashemi, J. A., Tamim, H. M., Esteban, A., Haddad, S. H., Dawood, A., et al. (2009). The impact of time to tracheostomy on mechanical ventilation duration, length of stay, and mortality in intensive care unit patients. *Journal of Critical Care, 24*(3), 435–440.

Beachey, W. (2007). Mechanics of ventilation. In W. Beachey, *Respiratory care anatomy and physiology* (2nd ed.). St. Louis, MO: Mosby.

Blot, F., Similowski, T., Trouillet, J. L., Chardon, P., Korach, J. M., Costa, M. A., et al. (2008). Early tracheotomy versus prolonged endotracheal intubation in unselected severely ill ICU patients. *Intensive Care Medicine, 34,* 1779–1787.

Bone, R. C. (1983). Monitoring ventilatory mechanics during respiratory failure. *Respiratory Care, 28*(5), 1287.

Combes, X., Schauvliege, F., Peyrouset, O., Motamed, C., Kirov, K., Dhonneur, G., et al. (2001). Intracuff pressure and tracheal morbidity. *Anesthesiology, 95*(5), 1120–1124.

Davis, K., Campbell, R. S., Johannigman, J. A., Valente, J. F., & Branson, R. D. (1999). Changes in respiratory mechanics after tracheostomy. *Archives of Surgery, 134,* 59–62.

Dullenkopf, A., Gerber, A. C., & Weiss, M. (2004). Nitrous oxide diffusion into tracheal tube cuffs: Comparison of five different tracheal tube cuffs. *Acta Anaesthesiologica Scandinavica, 48*(9), 1180–1184.

Fernandez, R., Blanch, L., Mancebo, J., Bonsoms, N., & Artigas, A. (1990). Endotracheal tube cuff pressure assessment: Pitfalls of finger estimation and need for objective measurement. *Critical Care Medicine, 18*(12), 1423–1426.

Freeman, B. D., Borecki, I. B., Coopersmith, C. M., & Buchman, T. G. (2005). Relationship between tracheostomy timing and duration of mechanical ventilation in critically ill patients. *Critical Care Medicine, 33*(11), 2513–2520.

Gomella, L. G., & Haist, S. A. (2006). Critical care. In L. G. Gomella & S. A. Haist, *Clinician's pocket reference: The scut monkey* (11th ed.). Columbus, OH: McGraw-Hill.

Henning, J., Sharley, P., & Young, R. (2004). Pressures within air-filled tracheal cuffs at altitude—An in vivo study. *Anaesthesia, 59*(3), 252–254.

Hoffman, R. J., Parwani, V., & Hahn, I. (2006). Experienced emergency medicine physicians cannot safely inflate or estimate endotracheal tube cuff pressure using standard techniques. *American Journal of Emergency Medicine, 24,* 139–143.

Hotter, A. N., & Warfield, K. (1997). Technique for promoting healing of complex tracheostomy wounds. *Otolaryngology—Head and Neck Surgery, 11*(6), 693–695.

Karasawa, F., Hamachi, T., Takamatsu, I., & Oshima, T. (2003). Time required to achieve a stable cuff pressure by repeated aspiration of the cuff during anesthesia with nitrous oxide. *European Journal of Anaesthesiology, 20*(6), 470–474.

Kaye, P. (2007). Effects of altitude on endotracheal tube cuff pressure. *Emergency Medicine Journal, 24,* 605–607.

Kluge, S., Baumann, H. J., Maier, C., Klose, H., Meyer, A., Nierhaus, A., et al. (2008). Tracheostomy in the intensive care unit: A nationwide survey. *Anesthesia and Analgesia, 107*(5), 1639–1643.

Mann, C., Parkinson, N., & Bleetman, A. (2007). Endotracheal tube and laryngeal mask airway cuff volume changes with altitude: A rule of thumb for aeromedical transport. *Emergency Medicine Journal, 24,* 165–167.

Marsh, H. M., Gillespie, D. J., & Baumgartner, A. E. (1989). Timing of tracheostomy in the critically ill patient. *Chest, 96*(1), 190–193.

Navarro, L. H., Braz, J. R., Nakamura, G., Llima, R. M., Silva, F.deP., & Modolo, N. S. (2007). Effectiveness and safety of endotracheal tube cuffs filled with air versus filled with alkalinized lidocaine: A randomized clinical trial. *Sao Paolo Medical Journal, 125*(6), 322–328.

Pierson, D. J. (2005). Tracheostomy and weaning. *Respiratory Care, 50*(4), 526–533.

Pilbeam, S. P. (1998). Basic patient assessment and methods to improve ventilation. In S. P. Pilbeam (Ed.), *Mechanical ventilation: Physiological and clinical applications* (pp. 244–261). St. Louis, MO: Mosby.

Postaci, A., Karabeyoglu, I., Erk, G., Ayerden, T., Sastim, H., Barcin, S., et al. (2008). A comparison of intra cuff pressures in high-flow and low-flow nitrous oxide anesthesia. *Saudi Medical Journal, 29*(12), 1719–1722.

Rumbak, M. J., Newton, M., Truncale, T., Schwartz, S. W., Adams, J. W., Hazard, P. B. (2004). A prospective, randomized study comparing early percutaneous dilational tracheotomy to prolonged translaryngeal intubation (delayed tracheotomy) in critically ill medical patients. *Critical Care Medicine, 32*(8), 1689–1694.

Sato, K., Tanaka, M., & Nishikawa, T. (2004). Changes in intracuff pressure of endotracheal tubes permeable or resistant to nitrous oxide and incidence of postoperative sore throat. *Masui, 53*(7), 767–771.

Scales, D. C., & Kahn, J. M. (2008). Tracheostomy timing, enrollment and power in ICU clinical trials. *Intensive Care Medicine, 34*(10), 1743–1745.

Segaran, E. (2006). Returning to normal: The role of eating in recovery from a critical illness. *British Journal of Neuroscience Nursing, 2*(3), 141–148.

Shapiro, B. A., Harrison, R. A., Kacmarek, R. M., & Cane, R. D. (1985). *Clinical application of respiratory care* (3rd ed.). Chicago: Yearbook Medical Publishers.

Sherlock, Z. V., Wilson, J. A., & Exley, C. (2009). Tracheostomy in the acute setting: Patient experience and information needs. *Journal of Critical Care.* (e-pub ahead of print: doi:10.1016/j.jcrc.2008.10.007).

Smith, R. P., & McArdle, B. H. (2002). Pressure in the cuffs of tracheal tubes at altitude. *Anaesthesia, 57*(4), 374–378.

Stoner, D. L., & Cooke, J. P. (1974). Intratracheal cuffs and aeromedical evacuation. *Anesthesiology, 41*(3), 302–306.

Tu, H. N., Saidi, N., Lieutaud, T., Bensaid, S., Venival., V., & Duvaldestin, P. (1999). Nitrous oxide increases endotracheal cuff pressure and the incidence of tracheal lesions in anesthetized patients. *Anesthesia and Analgesia, 89,* 187–190.

Winklmaier, U., Wüst, K., Schiller, S., & Wallner, F. (2006). Leakage of fluid in different types of tracheal tubes. *Dysphagia, 21*(4), 237–242.

Yoneda, I., Watanabe, K., Hayashida, S., Kanno, M., & Sato, T. (1999). A simple method to control tracheal cuff pressure in anaesthesia and in air evacuation. *Anaesthesia, 54,* 975–980.

Young, P. J., Rollinson, M., Downward, G., & Henderson, S. (1997). Leakage of fluid past the tracheal tube cuff in a benchtop model. *British Journal of Anaesthesia, 78,* 557–562.

Zur, K. B., & Schilero, G. J. (2006). Pulmonary physiology and mechanical ventilation. In T. R. Van de Water & H. Staecker (Eds.), *Otolaryngology: Basic science and clinical review.* New York: Thieme.

Phonation With a Tracheostomy

Linda L. Morris

Phonation is the creation of sound, and articulation is the creation of words. Sound is created as air passes through the vocal cords. Speech is the effective blending of both phonation and articulation. The ability to communicate is vital for effective overall medical care, psychological function, and social interaction. Speech allows patients to express needs, communicate with caregivers, use the telephone, and maintain personal relationships (Hoit, Banzett, Lohmeier, Hixon, & Brown, 2003). The inability to speak greatly restricts patients' abilities to participate meaningfully in their health care plan (Leder, 1990). The inability to speak is often fraught with frustration for patients and caregivers alike. Patients who cannot speak may feel an additional loss of control and powerlessness, which can often lead to depression and other behavioral concerns.

General Principles of Voice Restoration

The tracheostomy tube redirects air, and normal speech is interrupted as air bypasses the vocal cords. A tracheostomy results in a loss of subglottic air pressure, which creates many other sequelae in addition to the loss of speech. An unoccluded tracheostomy tube interferes with effective swallowing, coughing, and defecation (Kazandjian & Dikeman, 2008).

The restoration of patients' voices is often a surprising and an emotional moment for them and their loves ones. Many times, patients haven't heard their own voices for weeks or months, and the opportunity to vocalize again is a surprise. They frequently don't remember that they can use their voice and will often begin with a whisper. Hearing their own voices speak even a few words can provide great comfort and restore a sense of well-being.

There are several mechanisms to restore speech. All of them require some manipulation of the tracheostomy tube or ventilator circuit and almost all require cuff deflation.

There also are several factors that must be considered when planning for phonation with a tracheostomy. The first consideration is whether or not the patient requires cuff inflation. Most often, patients require cuff inflation because of the need for positive-pressure ventilation, airway protection, or both. Not all patients who require positive-pressure ventilation also require cuff inflation. The most challenging patient is the one who requires cuff inflation for both airway protection and continuous positive-pressure mechanical ventilation. For these reasons, it is necessary to have a clear understanding of the patient's medical status and treatment plan before attempting to restore speech.

Risk of Aspiration

There are several possible explanations for the risk of aspiration with a tracheostomy tube. The first is decreased elevation and anterior rotation of the larynx because the trachea is anchored to the strap muscles with the inflated cuff. It is also thought that esophageal compression causes the cuff to impinge against the esophageal wall. There is also an attenuation of the reflex of the vocal cords because airflow is redirected away from the upper airway. In addition, there is a reduction in subglottal air pressure (Suiter, McCullough, & Powell, 2003).

Leder and Ross (2000) examined 20 consecutive patients using a swallow study before and after tracheotomy. They found no causal relationship between tracheostomy and aspiration. All these patients had the same aspiration status before and after the test. The authors concluded that certain of these patients had multiple risk factors other than the presence of the tracheostomy tube that would predispose them to aspirate.

Requirements for Successful Phonation

Patients must be cognitively intact and attempting to communicate before phonation is initiated. Patients who are able to respond to questions appropriately may be ready to be evaluated for phonation. If a patient is not making some attempt to speak, he or she is probably not ready to do so. In order to achieve adequate voice quality, a patient must be able to generate a tracheal pressure of at least 2 cm H_2O. In normal people, tracheal pressure is 5–10 cm H_2O during speech, and airflow through the upper airway during speech is 3–18 liters per minute (Bard, Slavit, McCaffrey, & Lipton, 1992; Hess, 2005; Holmberg, Hillman, & Perkell, 1988).

6.1 Methods of Phonation for Patients Who Do Not Require Cuff Inflation

Method of Phonation	Special Considerations
Digital occlusion	Requires cuffless or cuffed tube with cuff down only.
Capping	Requires cuffless tube or TTS or CTS cuff only.
Cuffless fenestrated tube	Requires capping either by removal of the standard inner cannula or with fenestrated inner cannula.
Speaking valve	Patient must be able to tolerate cuff deflation, preferably cuffless tube. Requires sufficient air to pass around outside of tube.

Current methods to restore speech can be divided into three major groups: methods for patients who do not require mechanical ventilation, methods for those who require continuous mechanical ventilation, and methods for those who require intermittent positive-pressure ventilation. These methods are summarized in Tables 6.1 and 6.2.

It is usually relatively easy to restore speech for patients who do not require positive-pressure ventilation. Most often, all that is required is cuff deflation or a cuffless tube and capping or finger occlusion. Let us first discuss the more straightforward approaches to phonation, followed by the more complicated approaches. It may also be helpful to refer to Figure 6.1 on page 185.

Patients Who Do Not Require Mechanical Ventilation

First, phonation should not be attempted in a patient who is not cognitively aware and making an effort to speak. There are several methods that will allow speech for patients who do not require mechanical ventilation.

Digital Occlusion (Cuffless Tube or Deflated Cuff)

Digital occlusion is performed with a cuffless tracheostomy tube or with the cuff fully deflated. Prior to cuff deflation, deep oropharyngeal suctioning should always be performed to remove secretions accumulated above the cuff. In addition, cuff deflation can be timed to coincide with exhalation to further prevent secretions from being aspirated.

Digital occlusion should never be attempted with the cuff inflated and ideally should be done with a cuffless tube. After cuff deflation, a gloved finger of a caregiver or patient is placed over the opening of the tube. This redirects air to the upper airway and allows it to pass through the vocal cords, thus producing sound. If the tracheostomy tube is too large, resistance to airflow around the tube will prevent comfortable breathing as well as phonation. If the tracheostomy tube is too small, the patient's voice will be breathy as most of the air will escape through the stoma rather than through the vocal cords.

6.2 Methods of Phonation for Patients Who Require Intermittent Mechanical Ventilation

Method of Phonation	Special Considerations
Digital occlusion	■ Can be done on cuffed tube with cuff down only.
Capping trials when not on ventilator	■ TTS or CTS cuff is the ideal choice for a patient who requires intermittent cuff inflation.
Leak speech	■ Requires cuff deflation. ■ Procedure involves increasing tidal volume and adjusting to comfortable ventilation and optimal voice quality. ■ Procedure increases inspiratory time. ■ The addition of PEEP may improve voice quality and increase duration of speech time. ■ Ventilator alarms must be adjusted because exhaled volume is lost through the ventilator circuit.
Leak speech with speaking valve	■ Requires cuff deflation. ■ Procedure involves increasing tidal volume and adjusting to comfortable ventilation and optimal voice quality. ■ Procedure increases inspiratory time. ■ The addition of PEEP may improve voice quality and increase duration of speech time. ■ Ventilator alarms must be adjusted because exhaled volume is lost through the upper airway. ■ The addition of speaking valve may improve swallowing and decrease secretions. ■ HME is ineffective with the valve.
Fenestrated tracheostomy tube	■ Cuff can remain inflated. ■ Requires proper fit of fenestration. ■ Requires adjustment of ventilator settings and alarms because exhaled volume is lost through the upper airway. ■ Subcutaneous emphysema can occur if using a fenestrated tube through an immature stoma.
Speaking tracheostomy tube	■ Cuff can remain inflated. ■ Involves adjusting gas flow of 2–15 liters per minute for optimal voice quality. ■ Requires patient or caregiver to occlude port for phonation. ■ Subcutaneous emphysema can occur if using a speaking tracheostomy tube through an immature stoma.
Blom tracheostomy tube	■ Cuff can remain inflated. ■ On inhalation, air is delivered to the lungs through the flap valve. Upon exhalation, air passes through the bubble valve and the fenestration. ■ The exhaled volume reservoir helps prevent ventilator alarms from sounding due to lost returned volume through the upper airway.
Nomori ventilator talking tracheostomy	■ Cuff inflates during inhalation and deflates during exhalation. ■ Currently not available for clinical use.

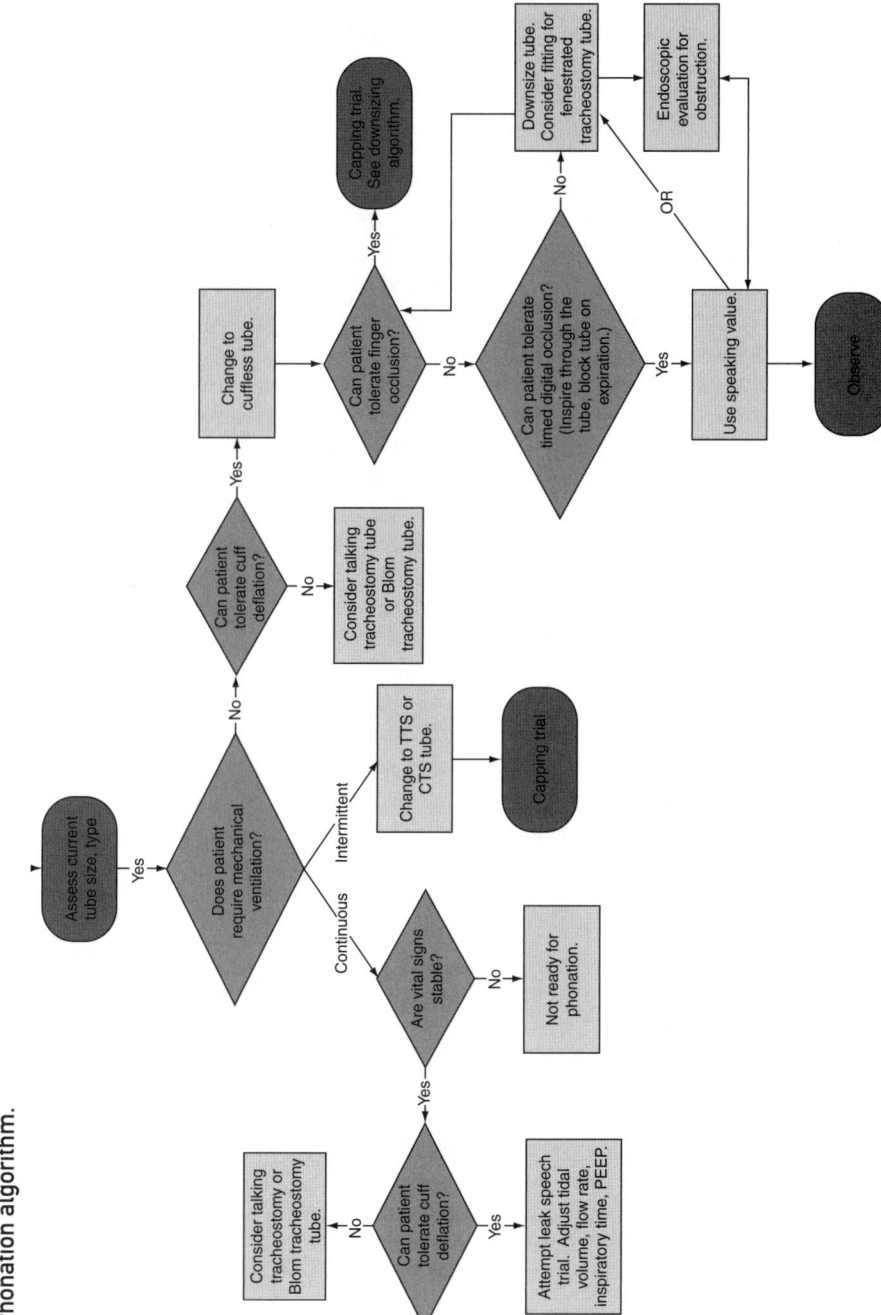

6.1 Phonation algorithm.

The biggest safety advantage of digital occlusion is that the patient must be alert and coordinated enough to perform it. Patients who are not alert can quickly develop respiratory distress and be unable to summon help. This problem is magnified when the tracheostomy tube is capped. In order for these patients to speak, an assistant must be present in the patient's room. Patients who are cognitively alert but unable to use their upper extremities may experience frustration with the digital occlusion method if they have a lot to say.

Capping, Corking, and Plugging (Cuffless Tube)

Capping is used when the opening of the tracheostomy tube is plugged with a cap, a cork, or a plug. The nuances of these devices are reviewed in chapter 3, but they are all designed to prevent air from entering and exiting through the tracheostomy itself. As a result, some or all of the airflow is redirected around the tube and up to the vocal cords.

Not all patients should be capped. Capping should not be attempted in those who cannot tolerate cuff deflation and who are at risk for aspiration. With the exception of properly fit fenestrated tubes, *capping should never be applied on a standard cuffed (low-pressure, high-volume) tracheostomy tube, even if the cuff is deflated*. If the cuff is deflated and the tube is capped, the patient is forced to breathe around the tracheostomy tube *and* the deflated cuff. The bulk of the deflated cuff adds a great deal of resistance, and it may be difficult or impossible for the patient to ventilate adequately. Additionally, the patient may be unable to effectively clear secretions around the tube and cuff. The patient may complain that when coughing, the secretions seem to "get stuck" in his or her neck. A classic example is a patient with a cuffed tracheostomy tube who had been capped at an outside hospital. She complained that, as much as she tried, she was never able to cough out her secretions. Once her tube was changed to a cuffless version, she immediately coughed out several large mucus plugs and expressed immediate relief from her symptoms. Figure 6.2 shows the airflow around a capped tracheostomy tube. Note that both inspiration and expiration are around the tube and that the outer diameter of the tube must be small enough to allow the easy passage of air around it.

The Bivona TTS and the Arcadia CTS tracheostomy tubes are the only exceptions to the general clinical rule of not capping a cuffed tube. In this case, these cuffs function exactly like cuffless tracheostomy tubes with fully deflated cuffs. The deflated cuff on both of these tubes assumes the shape of the tube around the shaft, creating no additional resistance when moving air outside of the tube. (Refer to Figure 12.4 for an illustration of the inflation and deflation characteristics of high-volume, low-pressure versus low-volume, high-pressure cuffs.)

When capping a tracheostomy tube, it is important to monitor the patient's ability to breathe comfortably around the tube. Often simply changing the tube to a cuffless version of the same size provides sufficient space to move air. However, if the patient is unable to breathe comfortably, either there is still not enough room to move air around the tube, or there is an obstruction within the airway. In this case, the tube should be downsized. If efforts to phonate are still unsuccessful, use of a speaking valve can be attempted (discussed later in this chapter); however, the patient's airway should be examined for the cause of the

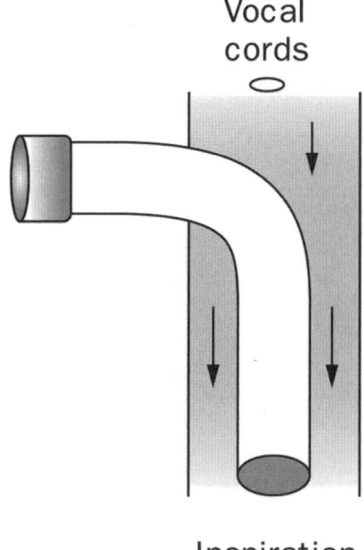
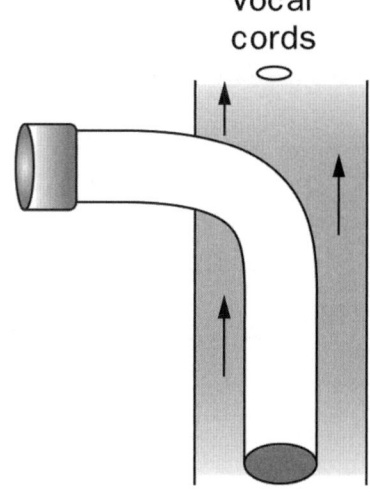

6.2

Airflow with cuffless tracheostomy tube, capped. Note both inspiration and expiration are around the outside of the tube.

obstruction. Chapters 11 and 12 provide a broader discussion of the issues associated with downsizing tracheostomy tubes.

The act of capping a tracheostomy tube not only restores phonation, but it also restores subglottal pressure and improves taste, swallow, cough, and the Valsalva maneuver. Additionally, the quantity of tracheal secretions tends to diminish after the tracheostomy tube has been capped.

Cuffless Fenestrated Tracheostomy Tube

Another option for phonation is the use of a fenestrated tracheostomy tube. The fenestrated tube provides an opening on the dorsal aspect of the shaft that should align centrally within the airway. When properly placed, it provides an additional boost of air up to the vocal cords. (See chapter 4 for a discussion of how to properly fit a fenestrated tracheostomy tube.)

Great care must be taken when using a fenestrated tracheostomy tube. These tubes can have single or dual cannulas. The dual-cannula fenestrated tube usually has both a fenestrated and nonfenestrated inner cannula; however, the outer cannula is always fenestrated. The fenestrated inner cannula is used when phonation is desired. In this case, air passes around and through the tracheostomy tube. Figure 6.3 shows airflow through a cuffless fenestrated tracheostomy tube. Note that the resistance of the tube is decreased because air also moves through the fenestration upon inspiration and expiration.

When a fenestrated tracheostomy tube is capped, quality of voice improves because all the exhaled air passes through the upper airway as shown in Figure 6.4.

When the nonfenestrated inner cannula is used, the fenestration mechanism is lost, and air cannot reach the vocal cords. However, the nonfenestrated

6.3

Airflow with cuffless fenestrated tracheostomy tube, uncapped. Note airflow around and through fenestrated tube.

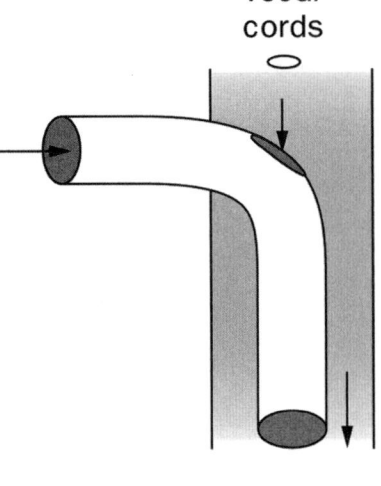

Inspiration

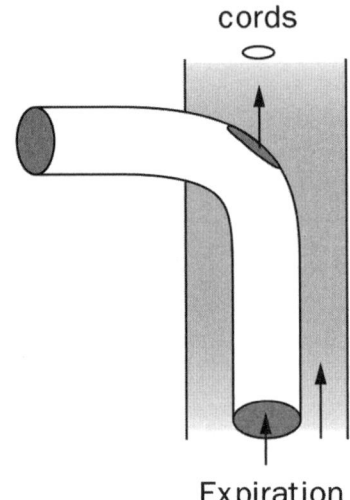

Expiration

6.4

Airflow with cuffless fenestrated tracheostomy tube, capped. Note inspiration and expiration around and through tube.

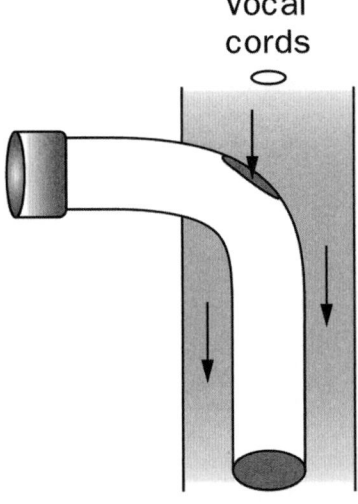

Inspiration

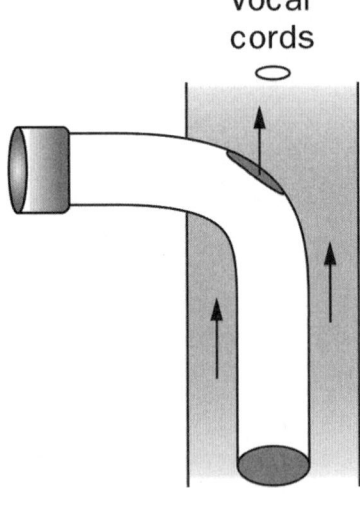

Expiration

inner cannula should be used when the patient requires suctioning so that the suction catheter does not get lodged within the fenestration.

To use the fenestrated tracheostomy tube for phonation, one can either keep the fenestrated inner cannula in place or remove it so only the fenestrated outer cannula remains. One of two occlusion methods can be used: digital occlusion or capping. When the fenestrated inner cannula is in place, digital occlusion should initially be used to ensure the patient is able to breathe comfortably. Capping can take place with a regular cap (inner cannula in place) or decannulation plug (inner cannula removed). When the cuffless fenestrated tracheostomy tube is occluded, the patient breathes around *and through* the tracheostomy tube. This action minimizes the obstruction of the tube itself within the airway. The decision about whether or not to cap the fenestrated tracheostomy tube depends on the patient's mental status. Digital occlusion should be reserved for initial and limited vocalization trials in the patient with slightly less than optimal cognitive and respiratory reserve.

When phonation is achieved without the fenestrated inner cannula in place, the inner diameter of the tube is larger, imposing less resistance to airflow and providing easier breathing. Often, 1 or 2 mm enhance the patient's ease of breathing. The inner cannula should only be removed in patients with minimal secretions.

With the fenestrated inner cannula removed, some tracheostomy models cannot be capped in the standard way. For example, the inner cannulas of the Shiley, TRACOE Twist, and Blom tracheostomy tubes provide a 15-mm connector, so a standard cap cannot be applied when it is removed. A decannulation plug is made for this purpose. After the removal of the inner cannula, the decannulation plug is attached directly to the hub of the outer cannula to allow continuous occlusion of the opening so that airflow is directed through the fenestration and to the upper and lower airway.

Speaking Valves (Cuffless Tube or Cuff Deflated)

Speaking valves are one-way valves that allow air into the tracheostomy tube but prevent it from being exhaled through the valve. Instead, exhaled air is redirected around the tracheostomy tube and through the upper airway. Ideally, a cuffless tube is used with a speaking valve; however, if using a cuffed tube, it is essential that the cuff be completely deflated and that air can move easily. The deflated cuff itself creates an obstruction, so the ability of air to move around it should be tested before a speaking valve is applied. This can be done by digitally occluding the tube and asking the patient to take a few breaths (simulating capping). If the patient is unable to breathe comfortably with this maneuver, the clinician can simulate a speaking valve by allowing the patient to inspire through the tube and occluding it during exhalation. If it is still uncomfortable for the patient to breathe with this maneuver, the clinician should consider downsizing the tracheostomy tube or evaluating the patient for upper airway obstruction.

In order to safely use a speaking valve, the patient should be awake, alert, attempting to communicate, able to tolerate cuff deflation, and medically stable. If the patient is at risk for aspiration, a speaking valve should not be used (Hess, 2005). Figure 6.5 shows airflow with a speaking valve and a cuffless tracheostomy

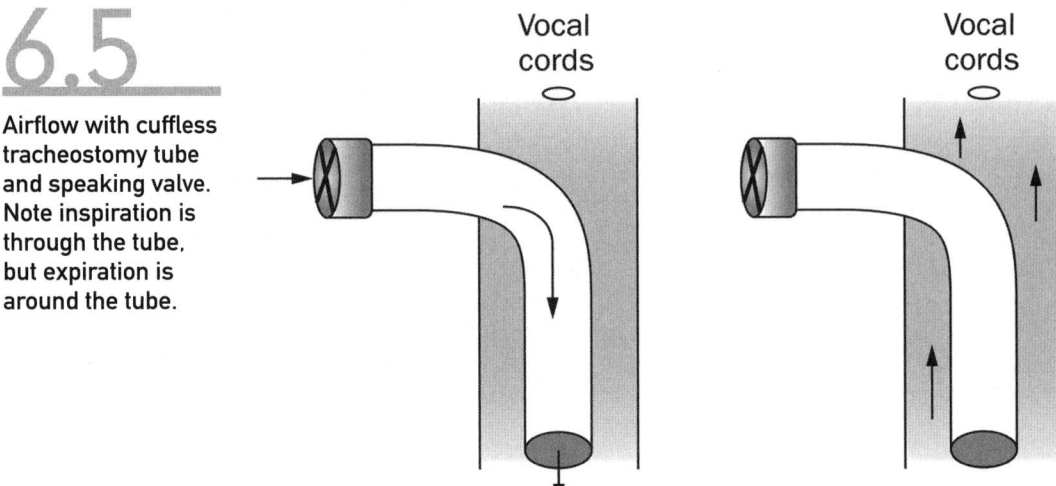

6.5 Airflow with cuffless tracheostomy tube and speaking valve. Note inspiration is through the tube, but expiration is around the tube.

tube. Air is inspired through the tube, and the valve closes upon expiration, forcing air through the upper airway. There are several different types of valves available, and they all have slightly different characteristics (see Table 6.3).

Early piston-type valves included the Toremalm valve, a flap valve by Emery, an adaptation of a Jackson tube by Cowan, and a two-way valve that could be rotated to allow inspiration only or both inspiration and expiration. When this two-way valve was used for inspiration only, it could also be used as a speaking valve (Saul & Bergstrom, 1979; Tippet & Vogelman, 2000; Toremalm, 1968). It is unclear whether any of these older valves are still in clinical use.

In 1993, Fornataro-Clerici and Zajac completed a study on the commercially available valves at that time, including those made by Kisner, Montgomery, Olympic, and Passy-Muir. They evaluated each valve's individual aerodynamic characteristics. The internal diaphragm of one-way valves is either in the open (bias open) or closed position at rest (bias closed). This position may have implications for work of breathing. The Kisner valve, which is no longer manufactured, was bias closed and attached to a metal tracheostomy tube. The Montgomery valve is bias open and has a unique "cough release" feature. This eliminates the possibility of the valve being blown off the tube. When the patient coughs, the diaphragm partially dislodges from the housing and must be pushed back into place. The Olympic valve is also bias open. It is T-shaped and can be used for oxygen delivery. It also has a removable cover that permits suctioning without removal of the valve. The Passy-Muir valve is bias closed in design, which means that the valve stays closed except when inspiratory effort is used to open the valve. None of these early valves were designed for use with a patient on a mechanical ventilator.

These valves were tested in a laboratory for their aerodynamic properties at four different flow rates. Resistance was calculated with each valve alone or with the valve attached to a tracheostomy tube. The results showed that the Kisner valve created significantly more resistance at all flow levels than the other valves

6.3 Types of One-Way Speaking Valves

Valve	Design	Unique Features
Montgomery Ventrach	Bias-open flap valve	■ For ventilator-dependent patients
Passy-Muir	Bias-closed flap valve	■ Several models are available ■ PMV 005 (white), 007 (aqua), 2000 (clear), and 2001 (purple) can be used with ventilator-dependent patients.
Olympic Trach Talk	Bias-open flap valve	■ Noticeable click with closure of valve
Shiley Phonate	Bias-closed flap valve	■ Silicone diaphragm with hinged cap; one model has oxygen port
Montgomery speaking valve	Bias-closed flap valve	■ Cough-release feature ■ Removable cover for suctioning
Eliachar speaking valve	Flap valve	■ For use with Hood stoma stent
TRACOE Phon Assist	Flap valve	■ Oxygen supply port ■ Adjustable airflow mechanism ■ With twist of housing, patients can "dial up" desired level of airflow
Shikani-French	Ball valve	■ For use with either plastic or metal tubes ■ Less inspiratory effort than others tested
Tucker	Flap valve	■ Fenestrated flap on inner cannula that opens on inhalation and closes on exhalation

available at that time. Since then, several new valves have been developed, and others have been redesigned. Zajac, Fornataro-Clerici, and Roop (1999) updated their previous study with six valves on the market in 1999—the Montgomery speaking valve, the Olympic Trach Talk, the Shiley Phonate Speaking valve, the Montgomery Ventrach (Figure 6.6), and the Passy-Muir PMV™ 007 (aqua) and PMV™ 2001 (purple; Figure 6.7).

The new Montgomery speaking valve has a bias-closed diaphragm—a change in design from its previous configuration. It was designed for use with the Montgomery cannula and comes in compatible sizes. The Olympic Trach Talk is a bias-open valve with a spring-loaded mechanism. Exhaled air forces

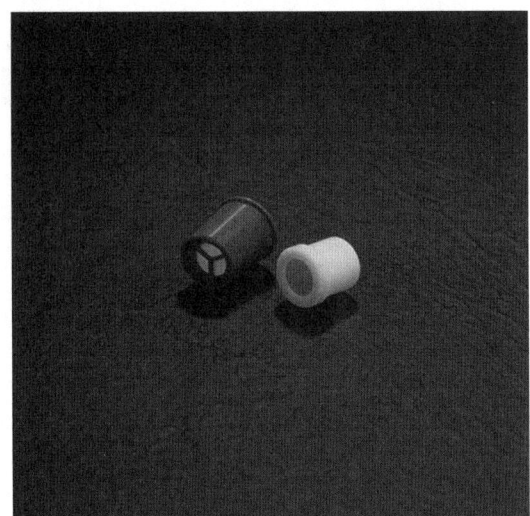

6.6 Montgomery Ventrach (left) and Montgomery valve (right). Photo courtesy of Boston Medical Products. All rights reserved.

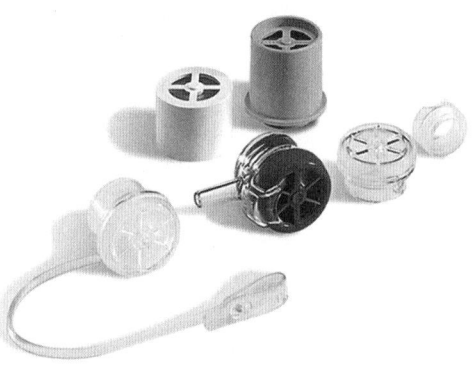

6.7 Passy-Muir valves. Clockwise from far left: PMV™ 2000, PMV™ 005, PMV™ 007, PMV™ 2020-S, PMV™ 2020, and PMA™ 2000. Photo courtesy of Passy-Muir.

closure of the valve, which is accompanied by a noticeable click. This valve was discontinued in 2000 (based on personal communication, Rachel Proctor, Olympic Medical, May 21, 2009). The Shiley Phonate speaking valve (Figure 6.8) is bias-closed with a silicone diaphragm. It has a hinged cap that makes the diaphragm available for cleaning. One model has a port to attach to an oxygen source; however, this model was not included in the study. The Montgomery Ventrach has a bias-open silicone diaphragm and can be used with ventilator-dependent patients. The Passy-Muir PMV™ 005 (white), PMV™ 007 (aqua), PMV™ 2000 (clear), and PMV™ 2001 (purple) can also be used for ventilator-dependent patients. The PMV™ 007 can be used with disposable ventilator tubing, and the others are used with rubber nondisposable tubing. All the Passy-Muir valves are bias closed (Zajac et al., 1999). The PMV™ 2020, a modified version of the PMV™ 2000, was designed for use with metal tracheostomy tubes without 15-mm adapters (Fitsimones, 2003).

Each of these valves was tested using different flow rates. The flow rates in the 1999 study were higher than in the earlier work because they were associated with patients on mechanical ventilation. Except for minor differences, all the valves exhibited similar low resistance—even those with a bias-closed design. There were some differences in manufacturing specifications between the

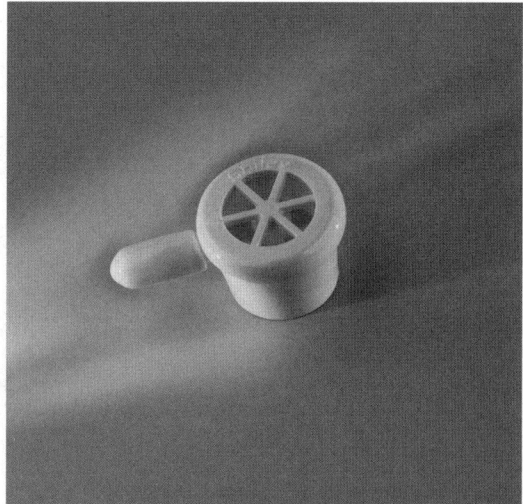

6.8

Shiley Phonate with oxygen port (SSVO). Covidien.

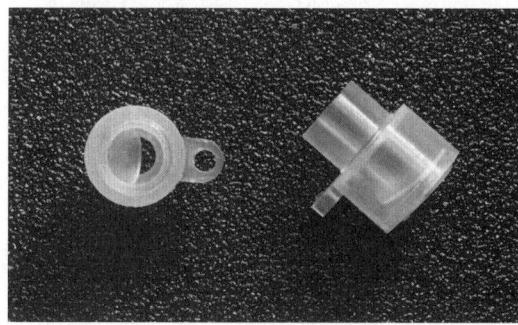

6.9

Eliachar speaking valve. Hood Labs (Pembroke, MA).

1993 and 1999 studies. The researchers measured the thickness of the PMV™ 007 and found a thinner diaphragm than in the earlier study. This could explain the finding of reduced resistance; however, they were unable to confirm a design change with the company (Zajac et al., 1999).

These six valves were also tested in vivo with the use of a mouthpiece; patients repeated the sound /pa/, and the researchers tested for leakage of air through the valve. They found that both the Olympic Trach Talk and the Montgomery Ventrach showed significant air loss during expiration when the valves should have been closed (Zajac et al., 1999).

The Eliachar speaking valve (Figure 6.9) is made of silicone and is designed for use with the Hood stoma stent. It has a low-profile appearance and flap design that provide low resistance. The Hood speaking valve (Figure 6.10) and the TRACOE Phon Assist are both flap valves. The Phon Assist has an oxygen supply port, but its most unique feature is an adjustable airflow mechanism that patients can use to dial up their desired level of airflow.

The Shikani-French valve uses a different mechanism than the other diaphragm valves—a unidirectional flow ball valve. It has lower resistance, a lower profile, and is more easily hidden under clothing than the other valves (Shikani, French, & Sievens, 2000). Originally called the Hopkins valve, the Shikani-French valve has been adapted for use with plastic as well as metal tracheostomy tubes. Figure 6.11 shows the mechanism of the Shikani-French ball valve. In the

6.10

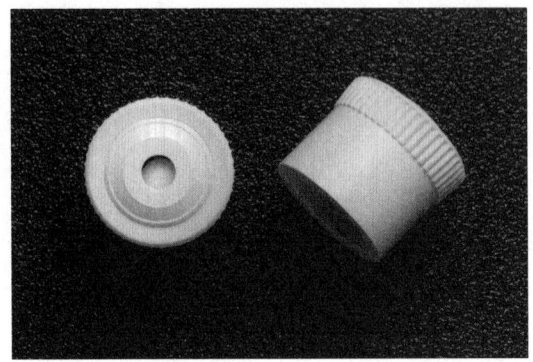

Hood speaking valve. Hood Labs (Pembroke, MA).

6.11

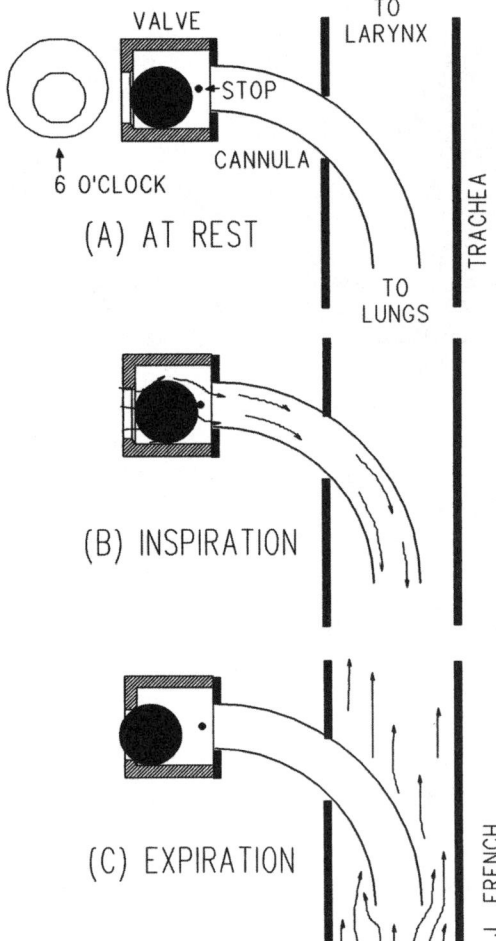

Mechanism of Shikani-French valve. Reprinted with permission from "Preserving Oral Communication in Individuals With Tracheostomy and Ventilator Dependency," by D. C. Tippett and A. A. Siebens, 1995. *American Journal of Speech Language Pathology, 4*(2), 55–61. Copyright 1995 by the American Speech-Language-Hearing Association. All rights reserved.

resting state, the ball lies on the wall of the air chamber (A). On inspiration, the ball moves toward the opening of the cannula, allowing air to enter the cannula (B). Airflow pushes the ball back, but it is prevented from entering the cannula by a wire stop. On expiration (C), the ball seals the port, forcing air into the upper airway. Because of this design, less pressure is required for valve closure, which is almost instantaneous. This is especially important in patients with very low tidal volumes and vital capacities. The valve is more compact than the other valves and can be used in the standard versions of all commercially available tracheostomy tubes. The valve can also replace the inner cannulas of these tubes and provide lower resistance (Shikani et al.).

One study compared the Shikani-French ball valve (named Hopkins at the time of the study) with the Passy-Muir valve and found less inspiratory resistance and easier cleaning with the ball valve (Tippett & Vogelman, 2000).

The Tucker valve uses a different mechanism. The Tucker tracheostomy tube is composed of metal with a fenestrated flap on the inner cannula that opens on inhalation and closes on exhalation. This action forces air up through the upper airway (Tippett & Vogelman, 2000). Airflow during inspiration rotates the flap to an open position and then to a closed position during expiration (Tippett & Siebens, 1995).

The Clinical Use of Speaking Valves. With the exception of the Tucker valve, speaking valves are externally placed on the 15-mm or low-profile connector of a cuffless or deflated-cuff tracheostomy tube. Patients and their caregivers require education to effectively use the valve and to alleviate any anxiety about shortness of breath. They also need to know how to remove the valve in the event of acute dyspnea. Patients should not be left unsupervised with the valve in place until their ability to tolerate it has been established (Tippett & Vogelman, 2000).

Initially, a schedule for using the speaking valve should be structured to target continuous wearing during daytime hours. The manufacturer recommends that the Passy-Muir valve not be used while sleeping; however, one study established its potential usefulness for one night in seriously ill tracheostomy patients without any untoward effects such as apnea, desaturation, respiratory distress, or cardiac arrhythmias. Accordingly, recommendations for testing these valves for longer night duration were concluded (Gross, Atwood, Grayhack, & Shaiman, 2003).

Studies have shown that speaking valves provide more benefits than merely verbal communication. Lichtman and colleagues (1995) studied the potential secondary benefits of speaking valves. They found that patients accumulated significantly fewer secretions with speaking valves than without. Other reported benefits include more effective swallowing, more effective coughing, a restoration of intrinsic PEEP, an enhanced Valsalva maneuver, and the prevention of aspiration.

Several studies have examined the effect of speaking valves on aspiration. Dettelbach, Gross, Mahlmann, and Eibling (1995) studied 11 patients with tracheostomies and clinical evidence of aspiration. They found that aspiration was reduced or eliminated in all patients when a speaking valve was in place. Suiter and others (2003) studied swallow physiology as well as the incidence of aspiration with tracheostomized nonventilator-dependent patients under three different conditions: cuff inflated, cuff deflated/cuffless tube, and with a Passy-Muir speaking valve. They found that cuff deflation significantly improved swallowing ability by increasing both pharyngeal transit duration as well as duration of hyoid excursion. In addition, they found that cuff status had no effect on aspiration. However, there was significantly less incidence of aspiration with the speaking valve when compared to the cuff-inflation and cuff-deflation conditions. Eight out of 10 patients who aspirated thin liquids with cuff inflation or deflation were able to safely take liquids with the valve in place. The authors concluded that the speaking valve might restore subglottal air pressure lost with use of a tracheostomy tube and that patients who are unable to tolerate thin liquids may be able to ingest them safely with the valve in place.

Elpern, Okonek, Bacon, Gerstung, and Skrzynski (2000) also studied the effect of the Passy-Muir valve on aspiration and obtained different results. In their study of 15 patients with tracheostomies and evidence of aspiration, 7 patients aspirated thin liquids, 5 patients aspirated only when the valve was off, and 2 patients aspirated with and without the valve. They found that aspiration was less frequent with the valve in place and concluded that a speaking valve can reduce, but not eliminate, aspiration in patients with a tracheostomy.

Manzano and colleagues (1993) found that the use of a speaking valve decreased the amount of secretions, improved the ability to cough, reduced the need for tracheal suctioning, and improved the sense of smell in patients. Although they did not specifically study patient mood, they also found that patients appeared to be happier and interacted better with their families and nursing staff.

Contraindications for Speaking Valves. While speaking valves provide many benefits in addition to speech, not all patients can tolerate them. Patients with poor pulmonary reserves can develop hypercarbia. Because some degree of air trapping can occur with speaking valves, patients with severe lung disease may not be able to fully exhale (Kazandjian & Dikeman, 2008). The contraindications for the use of a speaking valve are listed as follows:

- Inability to tolerate cuff deflation (risk of aspiration)
- Hemodynamic instability
- Severe pulmonary disease
- Total laryngectomy
- Vocal cord paralysis

Patients Who Require Intermittent Positive-Pressure Ventilation

It is clear that patients who require continuous positive-pressure ventilation need a cuffed tube; however, patients who use intermittent ventilation require cuff inflation only during that time. Intermittent positive-pressure ventilation is applied to patients during weaning from mechanical ventilation, for nocturnal ventilation, and for bronchial hygiene. As patients are weaned from continuous mechanical ventilation, they spend increasing amounts of time free from the ventilator at which time the cuff can be deflated. During the weaning process, altering the tracheostomy tube can accommodate the patient's changing goals.

When patients do not require continuous cuff inflation, it is usually relatively easy to restore phonation when they are without the ventilator. This can be done by simply deflating the cuff and occluding the tube to allow air up to the vocal cords, while assessing for the adequate movement of air around the deflated cuff. However, cuffed tubes should never be capped. Thus, these patients will require a different type of tracheostomy tube.

The Bivona TTS and the Arcadia CTS are ideal choices to accommodate a patient who requires intermittent cuff inflation. In contrast to standard low-pressure, high-volume cuffs, these tubes have low-volume, high-pressure cuffs. When inflated, they can exert high pressures against the tracheal wall, so careful attention to minimizing cuff pressure should guide practice. The significant advantage of this type of tube is its deflation characteristics, which allow it to lie flush against the shaft of the tube when deflated, creating no obstruction to airflow outside the tube. When deflated, the TTS and CTS tubes function as cuffless tubes, and they are the only cuffed tubes currently on the market that can be capped safely.

A TTS or CTS tube can be capped while the patient is free from the ventilator, and the cuff can be inflated when returning to the ventilator. This technique often speeds up the weaning process and frequently marks the beginning of freedom from the ventilator.

When inflating the cuff of the TTS or CTS tubes, the clinician must take care to ensure minimal pressure in the cuff. Because of the inflation characteristics of the high-pressure cuff, direct cuff pressure measurement will result in a high reading; thus, the minimal leak technique is recommended. In order to distribute pressure evenly and prevent a loss of cuff volume from the diffusion of gas, the cuff should be inflated with sterile water (not saline).

A CTS or TTS tube is also ideal for patients who require intermittent cuff inflation because of bronchial hygiene or administration of inhaled medications. The cuff can be inflated during these maneuvers and deflated after completion.

In addition to concerns with the high-pressure cuff, the primary disadvantage of the TTS and CTS tubes is that they are single-cannula tubes. Patients who have large volumes of thick secretions may be at particular risk for tube obstruction because these tubes lack an inner cannula. In this case, measures should be taken to ensure optimal mobilization of secretions, or it may be necessary to change to a tube with an inner cannula.

Patients Who Require Continuous Mechanical Ventilation

Unless there are extenuating circumstances, phonation should not be attempted in patients who are hemodynamically unstable and on mechanical ventilation. In most cases, it is best to wait until patients are more stable and can tolerate cuff deflation because most options for phonation require cuff deflation or tube change.

There is competition between airflow requirements for speech and gas exchange in the ventilator-dependent tracheostomy patient (Shea, Hoit, & Banzett,

1998). Normally, patients speak during expiration using air that has already been used for gas exchange. Competition occurs when patients "steal" air from alveolar ventilation during the inhalation phase, producing sound by diverting air around the tracheostomy tube and up to the larynx. Speech during inhalation produces relative hypoventilation.

Shea and others (1998) asked five patients with long-term tracheostomies to perform two speaking tasks. The patients read a standard text and spoke extemporaneously while the investigators measured speech ventilation volumes. All the subjects had either a fenestrated tracheostomy tube or a deflated cuff. They performed both tasks under normal conditions with 100% oxygen and under experimentally induced hypercapnic conditions using a mixture of carbon dioxide and oxygen. Normal individuals at rest will hyperventilate during speaking. The investigators noted an average loss of 14% of alveolar ventilation when speaking. During induced hypercapnia, which caused shortness of breath, all the subjects could still speak adequately. Two patients adapted to hypercapnia by reducing the amount of air used for speaking. One patient increased the airflow used per syllable during hypocapnic speech, which is a maladaptive strategy. The investigators concluded that there is complete antagonism between the airflow requirements for speaking and gas exchange during the ventilator's inspiratory phase. In their experiment, the behavioral drive to speak was modified but never fully suppressed by increasing respiratory drive.

Leak Speech (Cuff Deflated)

Leak speech involves creating a leak in the seal between the cuff and the trachea so that some air can be diverted up to the vocal cords. The ventilator provides the power behind the voice, and ventilator settings are adjusted to accommodate the leak. Leak speech is possible only when the patient uses a deflated cuff, a cuffless tube, or a fenestrated tracheostomy (MacBean et al., 2008). In addition, leak speech is possible only when airflow is sufficient to generate adequate subglottal pressure. This pressure is usually limited to the inspiratory cycle and the beginning of the expiratory cycle. For this reason, leak speech is characterized by bursts of short phrases and long pauses (Hoit et al., 2003; MacBean et al.).

Leak speech is beneficial because it improves patient quality of life by restoring communication, and the required cuff deflation reduces pressure against the trachea. However, it also involves trial and error until the optimal settings are achieved. Optimal leak speech requires ventilator adjustments to produce the best voice quality without discomfort or shortness of breath.

Inspiratory speech is something of a paradox because normal speech commences during expiration. Competition of tidal volume use between speech and ventilation varies with glottic resistance, which can be consciously controlled by the patient. When the glottis is narrowed, more tidal volume is delivered to the lungs; when there is little laryngeal resistance, less tidal volume is delivered to the lungs (Tippet & Vogelman, 2000).

Typically, the first step toward leak speech is to assess the size of the tracheostomy tube with the cuff deflated. One must ensure the patient can move enough air comfortably around the deflated cuff. If the patient is unable to move enough air, it may be necessary to downsize the tracheostomy tube. Following cuff deflation, the tidal volume should be increased up to 50% more than for resting ventilation, and the inspiratory time can also be increased to permit comfortable and longer speech. During initial trials, the patient will require some coaching to speak on inspiration when the ventilator breath is delivered. Inspiratory speech often requires some practice because it is the opposite of normal.

Some patients report anxiety or discomfort with leak speech because of the flow of air through the upper airway; this is especially common in those who have not experienced this sensation for a long time. This is often resolved by coaching the patient to time their voicing with inspiration. It may also help to instruct patients to push down, hold their breath, or tighten their throat. Patients can be taught to widen or narrow their glottic aperture in order to increase or decrease the volume delivered to the lungs (Tippet & Vogelman, 2000).

If patients become breathless during a leak speech trial, tidal volume or flow rate can be increased. Another strategy is to add PEEP. The addition of PEEP has several advantages, including lengthening the duration of tracheal pressure for voicing into the exhalation phase. Adding PEEP can allow patients to speak through 80% of the respiratory cycle (Hess, 2005; Hoit et al., 2003; Hoit & Banzett, 1997; Hoit, Shea, & Banzett, 1994; MacBean et al., 2008; Shea et al., 1998). The addition of 4–15 cm H_2O of PEEP can extend speech duration, produce higher quality speech, and allow more syllables per ventilator cycle. Patients using leak speech with PEEP have been observed to speak through the entire ventilator cycle without any pauses for breathing (Hess).

Leak Speech With a Speaking Valve. Leak speech can also be used with a speaking valve rather than PEEP. Only three speaking valves are approved by the FDA for use with ventilator-dependent patients—the Montgomery Ventrach and Passy-Muir models PMV™ 005 and PMV™ 007 (MacBean et al., 2008).

Speaking valves allow the ventilator to deliver a breath through the tracheostomy tube while the exhaled air is redirected around the tube—and so, it is essential that the cuff be completely deflated. Manzano and others (1993) used the Passy-Muir valve in their series of ventilator-dependent patients to determine its usefulness, advantages, and disadvantages during mechanical ventilation. Because cuff deflation is vital to the use of the speaking valve, they recommended that a cuffless tracheostomy tube be used while the valve is in place. The presence of a deflated cuff makes aspiration possible, and because of this, it is necessary to closely monitor tidal volume peak inspiratory pressure, thoracic movements, the elimination of secretions, and continuous airflow through the mouth and nose.

Figure 6.12 shows the placement of the valve within the ventilator circuit.

The speaking valve can be applied one of two ways. For patients with a closed suction system, the valve should be applied to the side port to allow the suction catheter to pass easily into the tracheostomy tube (Hess, 2005). For patients who are not using a closed suction system, the valve can be applied directly between the ventilator tubing and the 15-mm connector. An HME is not functional with a speaking valve because no exhaled gas will pass through when it is in place. Some patients report discomfort when initially using a speaking valve due to drying of the pharyngeal membranes or decreased tone

6.12

Proper placement of speaking valve within ventilator circuit. Valve is positioned between the tracheostomy tube and ventilator circuit to allow intake of air into the tube.

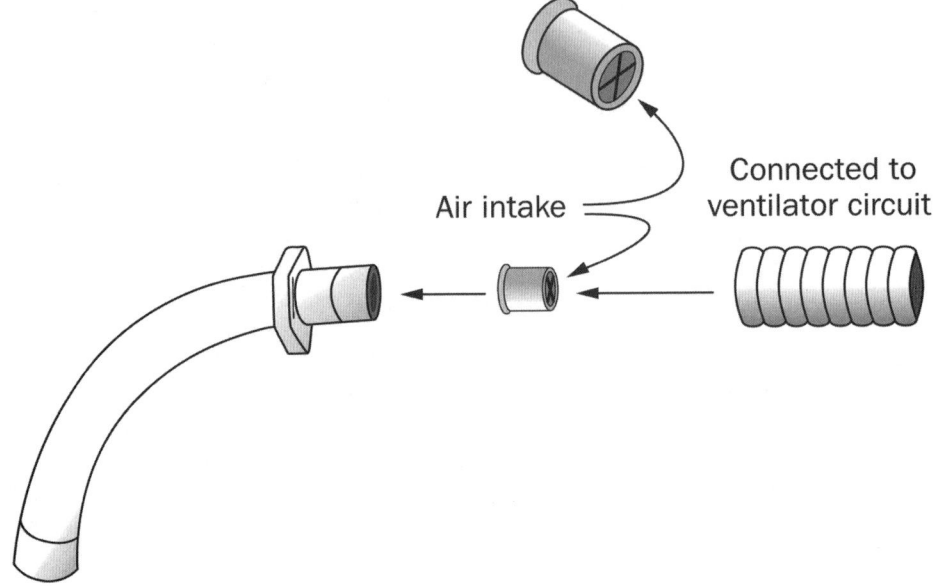

from weakness and lack of airflow through the upper airway. This effect can be mitigated by slow cuff deflation over several minutes (Hess).

In a study of 15 ventilator-dependent patients, Passy, Baydur, Prentice, and Darnell-Neal (1993) found that all the subjects using the Passy-Muir valve showed marked improvement in speech intelligibility, speech flow, elimination of speech hesitancy, and speech time. MacBean and colleagues (2008) studied the use of leak speech in two patients with cervical spinal cord injuries. They found that the use of PEEP in addition to a speaking valve provided the best quality speech.

Figure 6.13 shows airflow when a speaking valve is used with a ventilator. With a speaking valve, air will be redirected through the upper airway upon exhalation and not returned to the ventilator. Therefore, the exhaled tidal volume alarm must be adjusted accordingly. In addition, the tidal volume and high-pressure alarms must be carefully monitored to avoid excessive air trapping (Kazandjian & Dikeman, 2008).

Most critical care ventilators will not easily tolerate a speaking valve; however, the Puritan Bennett 760 has a speaking valve mode (Hess, 2005). The Respironics Esprit and the new Respironics V200 ventilator also have speaking modes in which the exhalation valve is closed, allowing gas flow past the vocal cords. In speaking modes, exhaled gas pressure is measured to evaluate whether the tube has become disconnected or obstructed.

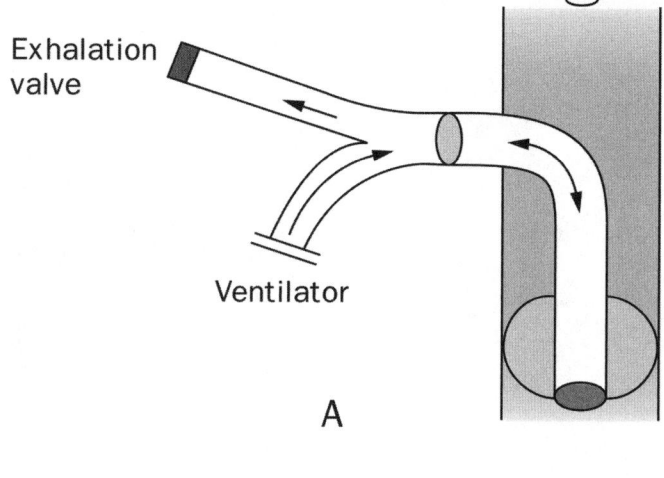
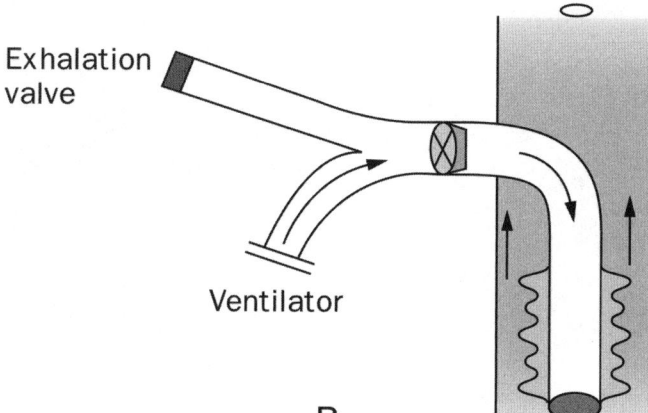

6.13

Airflow with valve and ventilator circuit. (A) Normal ventilator circuit. Note inflation of the cuff with inflow of air from the ventilator and exhaled air through exhalation valve. (B) Ventilator circuit with speaking valve. Note deflation of the cuff, with all exhaled air passing through the upper airway and bypassing the ventilator.

Cuffed Fenestrated Tracheostomy Tube (Cuff Inflated)

Patients who are ventilator dependent will usually require a cuffed tracheostomy tube. In order for these patients to phonate, one option is a cuffed fenestrated tracheostomy tube. The proper fit of the fenestration within the airway is vital for the proper functioning of the tube as well as preventing complications such as granulation tissue. See chapter 4 for a discussion of the proper fitting of a fenestrated tracheostomy tube.

Figure 6.14 shows airflow through fenestrated tracheostomy tubes. View A shows inspiration and expiration through a cuffless fenestrated tracheostomy tube. Air moves through the upper airway and through the tube. In View B, when the cuff is inflated on a cuffed fenestrated tube, inspiration and expiration occur primarily through the tube; however, a small amount of air moves through the upper airway. In View C, the cuff is deflated on a cuffed fenestrated tube. Inspiration is primarily through the tube; however, a small amount of air is inspired though the upper airway. On exhalation, air must pass around the deflated cuff and though the fenestration to reach the upper airway.

6.14

Airflow of fenestrated tracheostomy tubes on inspiration and expiration. (A) Cuffless fenestrated tracheostomy tube. Note inspiration around and through tube and expiration around and through tube, with boost of air up to vocal cords. (B) Cuffed fenestrated tracheostomy tube with cuff inflated. Note inspiration and expiration through (but not around) the tube. A small amount of air is directed to the vocal cords on expiration. (C) Cuffed fenestrated tracheostomy tube with cuff deflated. Note inspiration is through the tube and around the deflated cuff. A small amount of air is directed to the vocal cords on expiration.

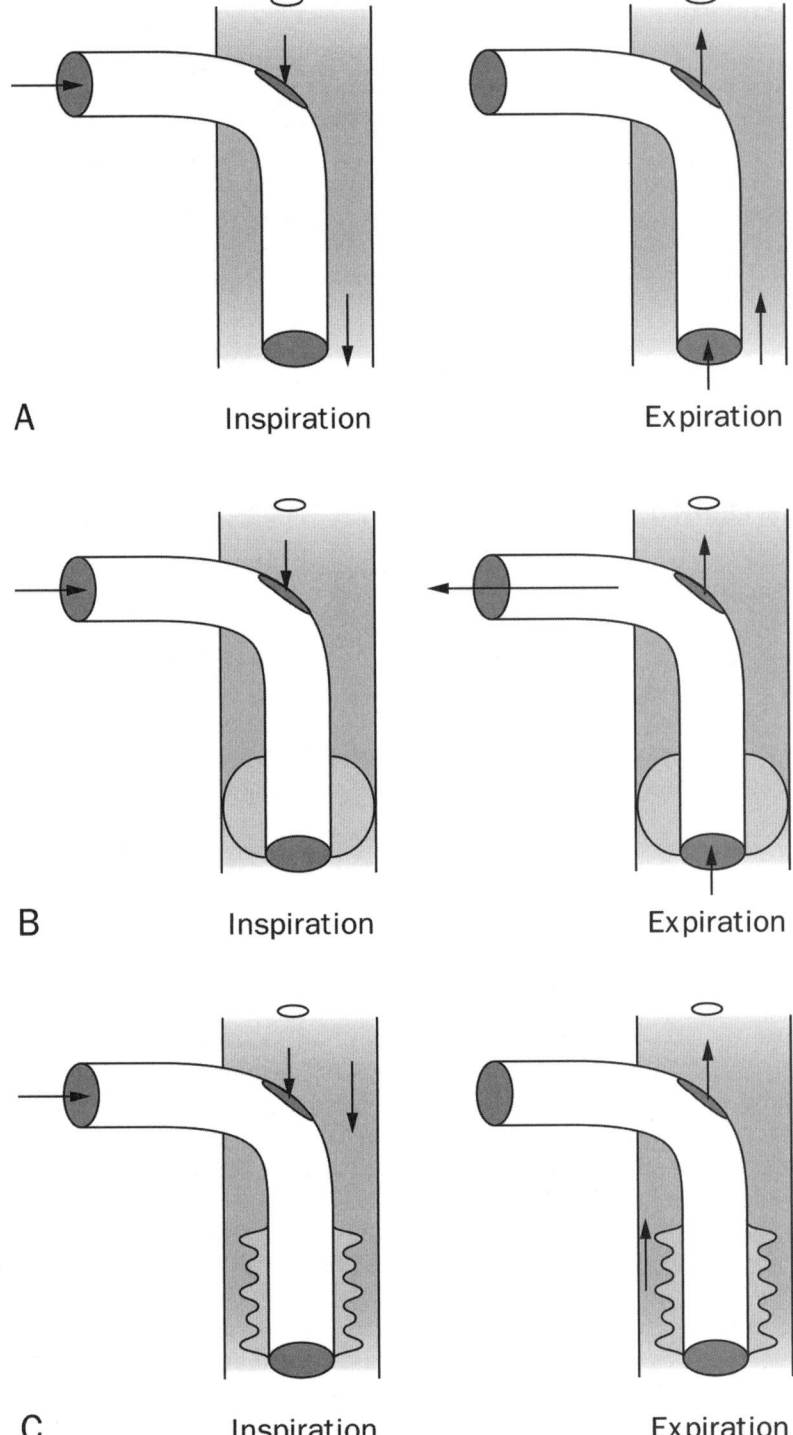

Several authors have reported cases of subcutaneous emphysema with the use of fenestrated tracheostomy tubes (Mozart & Stuart, 2001; Orme & Welham, 2006). Orme and Welham reported a case of massive subcutaneous emphysema shortly after the percutaneous placement of a fenestrated tracheostomy tube. Later these clinicians were directed to the manufacturer's instructions, which directed that a fenestrated tube should not be used in the early postoperative period and that the position of the fenestration should be checked once placed. Prior to the maturation of the stoma, air can become displaced into the pretracheal tissues with the use of a fenestrated tube.

Talking Tracheostomy Tube (Cuff Inflated)

A talking tracheostomy is a tube that allows a ventilator-dependent patient to speak; unlike other methods, it does not require cuff deflation. This tube was designed for the ventilator-dependent patient who is at high risk for aspiration or cannot otherwise tolerate cuff deflation. An additional air supply line provides an extra source of air independent of ventilation. This supply line carries air from a regulated compressed source and terminates with an opening just above the cuff. When connected to a source of compressed air or oxygen, occlusion of the air control port allows gas flow to be directed to the vocal cords. Figure 6.15 shows airflow with a talking tracheostomy tube.

For optimal use of the talking tracheostomy, airflow must be adjusted. Starting at 4 liters per minute, the flow can be increased up to 12–15 liters per minute until optimum voice quality is reached. However, one author (Hess, 2005) cautioned that high flow rates could be associated with a greater risk of airway injury. At these high flow rates, humidification is important to prevent drying of laryngeal tissues (Kazandjian & Dikeman, 2008). Because of the continuous independent flow of air, talking tracheostomy tubes allow speech throughout the entire respiratory cycle (Tippet & Siebens, 1995).

Tippet and Vogelman (2000) suggested that the adjustment of airflow is a delicate balance between patient comfort and clarity of speech. A flow rate between 2–15 liters per minute is compatible with speech. A rate of 5 liters per minute is necessary to produce a whisper, and 8–10 liters per minute is necessary for speech with normal volume. Flow rates above 10 liters per minute have been reported to be uncomfortable and may necessitate warming and humidifying the airflow to make it more comfortable and reduce the drying effect.

Talking tracheostomy tubes have some disadvantages. Speaking is dependent on a caregiver and a source of compressed gas. The air supply line frequently becomes clogged with secretions and prevents airflow above the cuff. In this case, it is acceptable to flush the air supply line with 5 ml of sterile water (Shahvari, Kigin, & Zimmerman, 1977). A source of suction should be provided to remove the secretions from above the cuff. The accumulation of secretions is a persistent complication of speaking tracheostomy tubes, and deep subglottic suctioning above the cuff may be necessary before beginning speaking trials (Tippet & Vogelman, 2000).

The production of speech with talking tracheostomy tubes requires some trial and error in order to produce optimal voice quality. Patients need time to adjust to the new sensation of airflow and practice occlusion of the airflow port. Theoretically, patients can speak throughout the entire respiratory cycle

6.15

Illustration of airflow with talking tracheostomy tube. Reprinted with permission from "Preserving Oral Communication in Individuals With Tracheostomy and Ventilator Dependency," by D. C. Tippet and A. A. Siebens, 1995. *American Journal of Speech Language Pathology,* 4(2), 55–61. Copyright 1995 by the American Speech-Language-Hearing Association. All rights reserved.

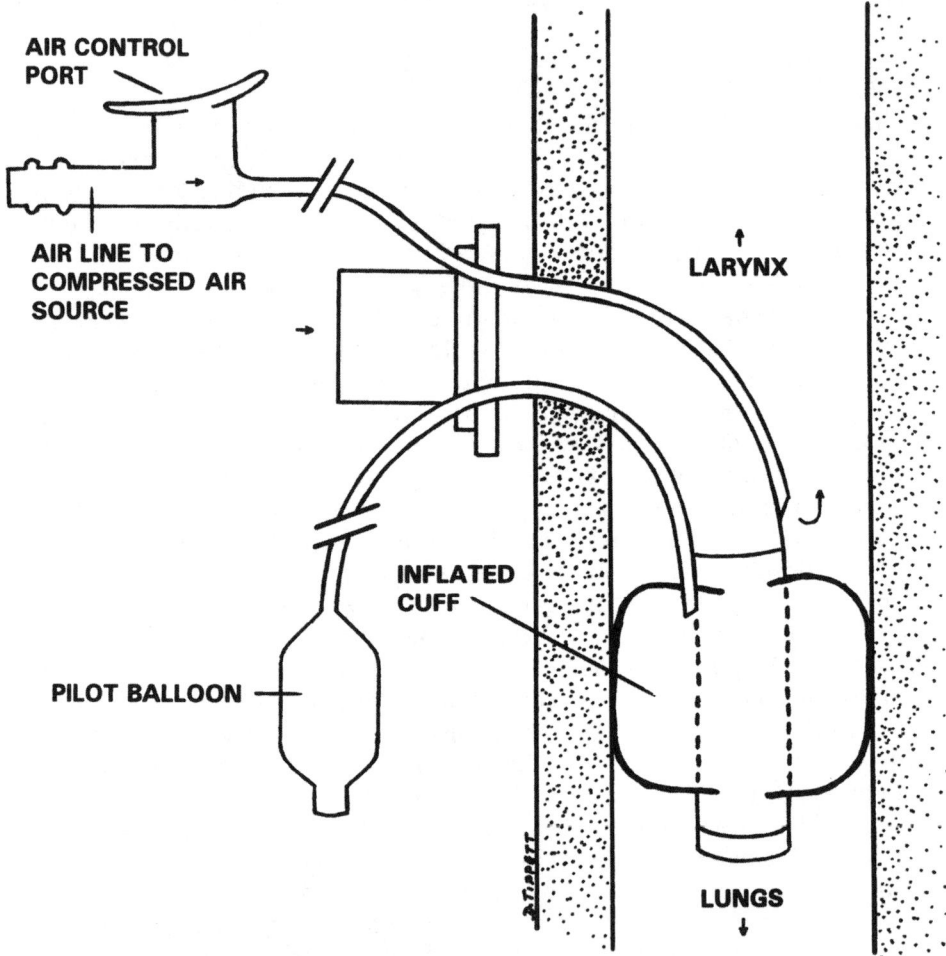

with this tube; however, Leder and Traquina (1989) reported that some patients have difficulty speaking through inspiration because it feels unnatural. They recommended that tube occlusion be timed for the expiratory phase of the ventilator.

Some difficulty has been reported with positioning the tube so its openings are unobstructed. Positioning is also an issue because of the weight of the ventilator circuit, which can pull the tube down and away from the stoma, resulting in an air leak. The weight of the ventilator tubing can also cause the rotation of the tube and the blockage of air vents coming in contact with the tracheal wall (Tippet & Vogelman, 2000). A malpositioned tube leaks air around the stoma and makes loud gurgling sounds. In addition, voice quality with this type of tracheostomy tube may not reach more than a whisper (Hess, 2005; Shahvari et al., 1977). For these reasons, the use of talking tracheostomy tubes with rehabilitation patients may be limited (Tippett & Siebens, 1995).

The speaking tracheostomy tube has also been used to provide continuous suction above the cuff in patients at risk for aspiration from a large amount of oropharyngeal secretions. When connected to suction, the removal of up to 600 ml of secretions per day has been reported (Shahvari et al., 1977).

A waiting period of 3–5 days is recommended after the initial tracheotomy procedure before using a talking tracheostomy tube. The waiting period allows the tract to heal and prevents air leaks through the fresh tissue planes, which could lead to subcutaneous or mediastinal emphysema (Tippett & Vogelman, 2000).

Nomori Ventilator Talking Tracheostomy Tube. A Japanese physician developed a new talking tracheostomy tube specifically for patients on mechanical ventilation. The tube has slits along the sides of the shaft and an elastic cuff that inflates and deflates in synchrony with respirations. The cuff expands on inspiration with positive pressure from the ventilator and deflates on expiration.

Sixteen patients with a variety of underlying conditions used the prototype tube with excellent results. All patients except one were able to speak with strong voice quality. The one patient who was not able to vocalize had a conspicuously bent trachea from long-standing tuberculosis. Two patients with particularly weak voice quality due to COPD and spinal cord injury used the Passy-Muir valve, which improved the loudness of their voices.

One of the most notable factors from this initial clinical trial is that there were no complications from this tracheostomy tube. It never became occluded with secretions, and no cuff problems developed (Nomori, 2004). Many of us eagerly anticipate its production for clinical use, hopefully in the near future. However, Hiroaki Nomori recently reported that the new tube has not yet been approved by the Japanese Ministry of Health and Welfare (based on personal communication, December 30, 2008).

Blom Tracheostomy Tube System. Eric Blom, a speech and language pathologist, developed the Blom tracheostomy tube system; it has recently been introduced to the market and clinical trials are in progress. Its unique design is intriguing, and initial clinical trials will determine its clinical usefulness. The tube comes in four sizes: 4, 6, 8, and 10. The fenestrated aperture on the outer cannula is located only 1 mm above the cuff. This unique placement is intended to prevent contact with the tracheal mucosa when the cuff is inflated. In addition, it has a subglottic suctioning port to reduce the incidence of ventilator-associated pneumonia when connected to continuous suction.

In addition to a standard inner cannula and a subglottic suctioning cannula, the Blom tracheostomy tube system (Figure 6.16) also has two additional cannulas that can provide speech. The speech cannula is designed to allow speech to those patients who require a fully inflated cuff, while the low-profile cannula is designed for use with patients who can tolerate cuff deflation. The

6.16

Blom tracheostomy tube system. Note fenestration of outer cannula just above the cuff, speech cannula, and inner cannula with subglottic suctioning port. Reprinted with permission of Pulmodyne (Indianapolis, IN).

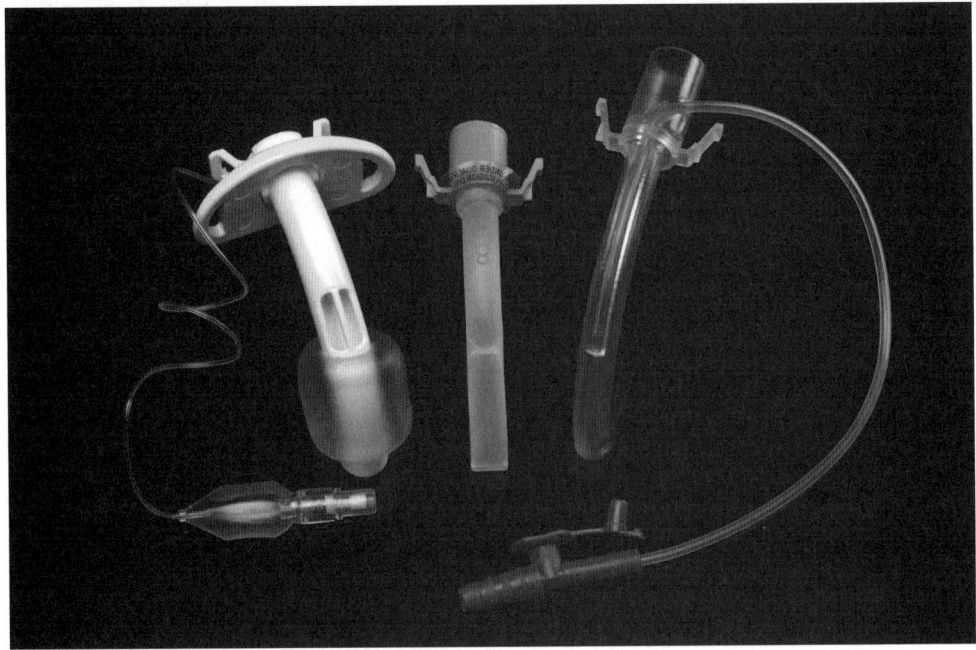

speech cannula is very soft and floppy, fits within the outer cannula, and has two unique valves—a flap valve and a bubble valve—that function at different parts of the respiratory cycle.

Figure 6.17 shows the airflow with the Blom tracheostomy tube system. The flap valve, located at the tip of the speech cannula, opens during inhalation, allowing air to flow through the tube and into the trachea. At the same time, the bubble valve, located along the dorsal aspect of the speech cannula, expands into the fenestration and seals it, preventing air from escaping into the upper airway. On exhalation, the flap valve closes and the bubble valve collapses, exposing the fenestration and directing the airflow through it and up to the vocal cords. Another unique feature of this tracheostomy tube is the exhaled volume reservoir, which prevents the ventilator from recognizing false low-volume readings as air is redirected through the upper airway rather than through the ventilator. This feature is likely to be appealing to practitioners who manage ventilators, because, to date, there are no described methods to prevent low-volume alarms as exhaled air is diverted from the expiratory limb of the ventilator. The manufacturer recommends that use of laser or electrosurgery electrodes should be avoided with this tube to prevent the release of toxic gases and fire in an oxygen-rich environment.

6.17

Airflow with Blom tracheostomy tube on inspiration and expiration. As air is inspired through the tube, the flap valve (located at the distal tip of the tube) opens. The flexible bubble valve (located on the dorsal shaft of the tube) also expands, covering the fenestration in the outer cannula. On exhalation, the flap valve closes, allowing airflow around it and collapsing the bubble valve to allow air through the fenestration and to the vocal cords. Reprinted with permission of Pulmodyne (Indianapolis, IN).

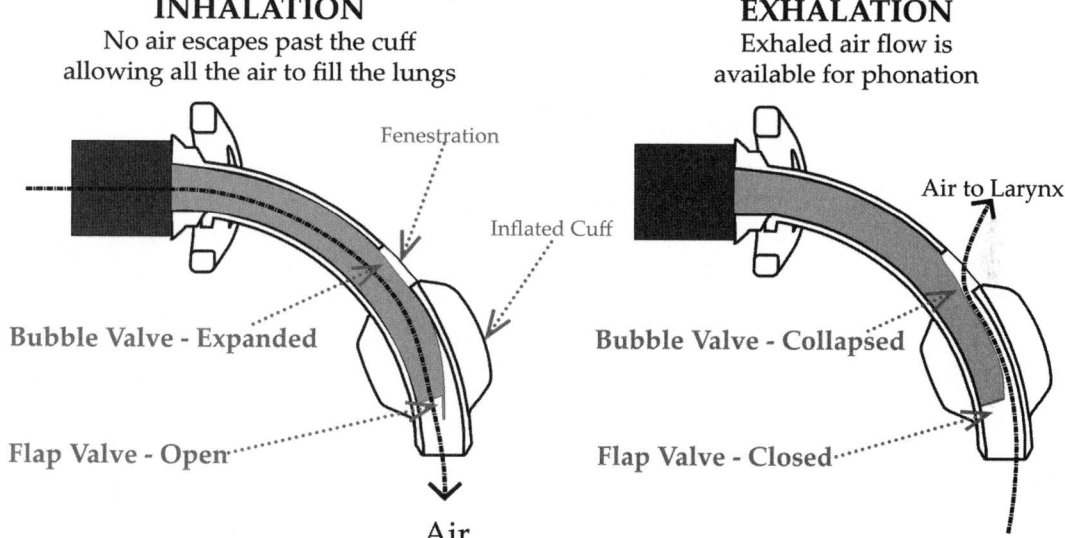

Summary

The many options available to restore phonation make it difficult at times to determine the best method for a particular patient. The best method is often the simplest, but numerous factors must be considered. The first factor in determining the optimal choice for phonation is if the patient requires mechanical ventilation. The second factor is whether the patient can tolerate cuff deflation. When continuous mechanical ventilation is not required, a cuffless tube with capping trials works well for the majority of patients. For patients who require intermittent mechanical ventilation, a TTS or CTS tube with capping trials allows the flexibility of a cuff and provides minimal resistance to airflow. Patients on continuous mechanical ventilation who can tolerate cuff deflation can be managed with leak speech. Those patients who are on continuous mechanical ventilation and require cuff inflation usually provide the greatest challenge. Available options are talking tracheostomy tubes and the Blom tracheostomy tube system. Fenestrated tracheostomy tubes are rarely used and must be fit individually to ensure the central placement of the fenestration within the airway.

Health professionals must recognize the importance of a patient's voice to his or her well-being and for effective communication with the health care team. The restoration of a patient's voice is often an emotional moment and can represent the beginning of a return to normal for the patient. It requires patience and an individual, methodical approach to determine the best strategy for each individual patient.

Key Points

- Speaking valves are ideally used with a cuffless tracheostomy tube but may be used with a completely deflated cuff as long as the patient's ability to breathe comfortably has been thoroughly assessed.
- For patients who do not require continuous mechanical ventilation, a cuffless tube with capping trials allows phonation for the majority of patients.
- For patients who require intermittent mechanical ventilation, a TTS or CTS tube with capping trials allows the flexibility of a cuff and offers minimal resistance to airflow when deflated.
- Ventilator-dependent patients who can tolerate cuff deflation can be managed with leak speech, but those who are on continuous mechanical ventilation and who require cuff inflation usually provide the greatest challenge.

References

Bard, M. C., Slavit, D. H., McCaffrey, T. V., & Lipton, R. J. (1992). Noninvasive technique for estimating subglottic pressure and laryngeal efficiency. *Annals of Otology, Rhinology, and Laryngology, 101*(7), 578–582.

Dettelbach, M. A., Gross, R. D., Mahlmann, J., & Eibling, D. E. (1995). Effect of the Passy-Muir valve on aspiration in patients with tracheostomy. *Head & Neck, 17*(4), 297–302.

Elpern, E. H., Okonek, M. B., Bacon, M., Gerstung, C., & Skrzynski, M. (2000). Effect of the Passy-Muir tracheostomy speaking valve on pulmonary aspiration in adults. *Heart and Lung, 29*(4), 287–293.

Fitsimones, L. (2003). Tracheostomy and ventilator speaking valves: Benefits beyond speech. *Vital Signs*. Retrieved October 27, 2009, from http://www.passy-muir.com/pdfs/article-vitalsigns.pdf

Fornataro-Clerici, L., & Zajac, D. J. (1993). Aerodynamic characteristics of tracheostomy speaking valves. *Journal of Speech and Hearing Research, 36*, 529–532.

Gross, R. D., Atwood, C. W., Grayhack, J. P., & Shaiman, S. (2003). Lung volume effects on pharyngeal swallow physiology. *Journal of Applied Physiology, 95*, 2211–2217.

Hess, D. R. (2005). Facilitating speech in the patient with a tracheostomy. *Respiratory Care, 50*(4), 519–525.

Hoit, J. D., & Banzett, R. B. (1997). Simple adjustments can improve ventilator-supported speech. *American Journal of Speech Lang Pathology, 6*, 87–96.

Hoit, J. D., Banzett, R. B., Lohmeier, H. L., Hixon, T. J., & Brown, R. (2003). Clinical ventilator adjustments that improve speech. *Chest, 124*, 1512–1521.

Hoit, J. D., Shea, S. A., & Banzett, R. B. (1994). Speech production during mechanical ventilation in tracheostomized individuals. *Journal of Speech and Hearing Research, 37*, 53–63.

Holmberg, E. B., Hillman, R. E., & Perkell, J. S. (1988). Glottal airflow and transglottal air pressure measurements for male and female speakers in soft, normal, and loud voice. *Journal of the Acoustical Society of America, 84*(2), 511–529.

Kazandjian, M. S., & Dikeman, K. J. (2008). Communication options for tracheostomy and ventilator-dependent patients. In E. N. Myers & J. T. Johnson (Eds.), *Tracheostomy: Airway management, communication, and swallowing*. San Diego, CA: Plural Publishing.

Leder, S. B. (1990). Importance of verbal communication for the ventilator-dependent patient. *Chest, 96*(4), 792–3.

Leder, S. B., & Ross, D. A. (2000). Investigation of the causal relationship between tracheostomy and aspiration in the acute care setting. *Laryngoscope, 110,* 641–644.

Leder, S. B., & Traquina, D. N. (1989). Voice intensity of patients using a Communi-Trach I cuffed speaking tracheostomy tube. *Laryngoscope, 99,* 269–274.

Lichtman, S. W., Birnbaum, I. L., Sanfilippo, M. R., Pellicone, J. T., Damon, W. J., & King, M. L. (1995). Effect of a tracheostomy speaking valve on secretions, arterial oxygenation, and olfaction: A quantitative evaluation. *Journal of Speech and Hearing Research, 38*(3), 549–555.

MacBean, N., Ward, E., Murdoch, B., Cahill, L., Solley, M., Geraghty, T., et al. (2008, September). Optimizing speech production in the ventilator-assisted individual following cervical spinal cord injury: A preliminary investigation. *International Journal of Language and Communication Disorders,* 1–12.

Manzano, J. L., Lubillo, S., Henriquez, D., Martin, J. C., Perez, M. C., & Wilson, D. J. (1993). Verbal communication of ventilator-dependent patients. *Critical Care Medicine, 21*(4), 512–517.

Mozart, M. J., & Stuart, H. (2001). Subcutaneous emphysema caused by a fenestrated tracheostomy tube. *Anaesthesia, 56*(2), 191–192.

Nomori, H. (2004). Tracheostomy tube enabling speech during mechanical ventilation. *Chest, 125*(3), 1046–1051.

Orme, R. M., & Welham, K. L. (2006). Subcutaneous emphysema after percutaneous tracheostomy—time to dispense with fenestrated tubes? *Anaesthesia, 61*(9), 911–912.

Passy, V., Baydur, A., Prentice, W., & Darnell-Neal, R. (1993). Passy-Muir tracheostomy speaking valve on ventilator-dependent patients. *Laryngoscope, 102*(6), 653–658.

Saul, A., & Bergstrom, B. (1979). A new permanent tracheostomy tube-speech valve system. *Laryngoscope, 89*(6, Pt. 1), 980–983.

Shahvari, M.B.G., Kigin, C. M., & Zimmerman, J. E. (1977). Speaking tracheostomy tube modified for swallowing dysfunction and chronic aspiration. *Anesthesiology, 46*(4), 290–291.

Shea, S. A., Hoit, J. D., & Banzett, R. B. (1998). Competition between gas exchange and speech production in ventilated patients. *Biological Psychology, 49,* 9–27.

Shikani, A. H., French, J., & Sievens, A. A. (2000). New unidirectional airflow ball tracheostomy speaking valve. *Otolaryngology—Head and Neck Surgery, 123*(1), 103–107.

Suiter, D. M., McCullough, G. H., & Powell, P. W. (2003). Effects of cuff deflation and one-way tracheostomy speaking valve placement on swallow physiology. *Dysphagia, 18,* 284–292.

Tippett, D. C., & Siebens, A. A. (1995). Preserving oral communication in individuals with tracheostomy and ventilator dependency. *American Journal of Speech and Language Pathology, 4*(2), 55–61.

Tippett, D. C., & Vogelman, L. (2000). Communication, tracheostomy and ventilator dependency. In D. C. Tippett (Ed.), *Tracheostomy and ventilator dependency.* New York: Thieme.

Toremalm, N. G. (1968). A tracheotomy speech valve. *Laryngoscope, 78*(12), 2177–2182.

Zajac, D. J., Fornataro-Clerici, L., & Roop, T. A. (1999). Aerodynamic characteristics of speaking valves: An updated report. *Journal of Speech, Language, and Hearing Research, 42,* 92–100.

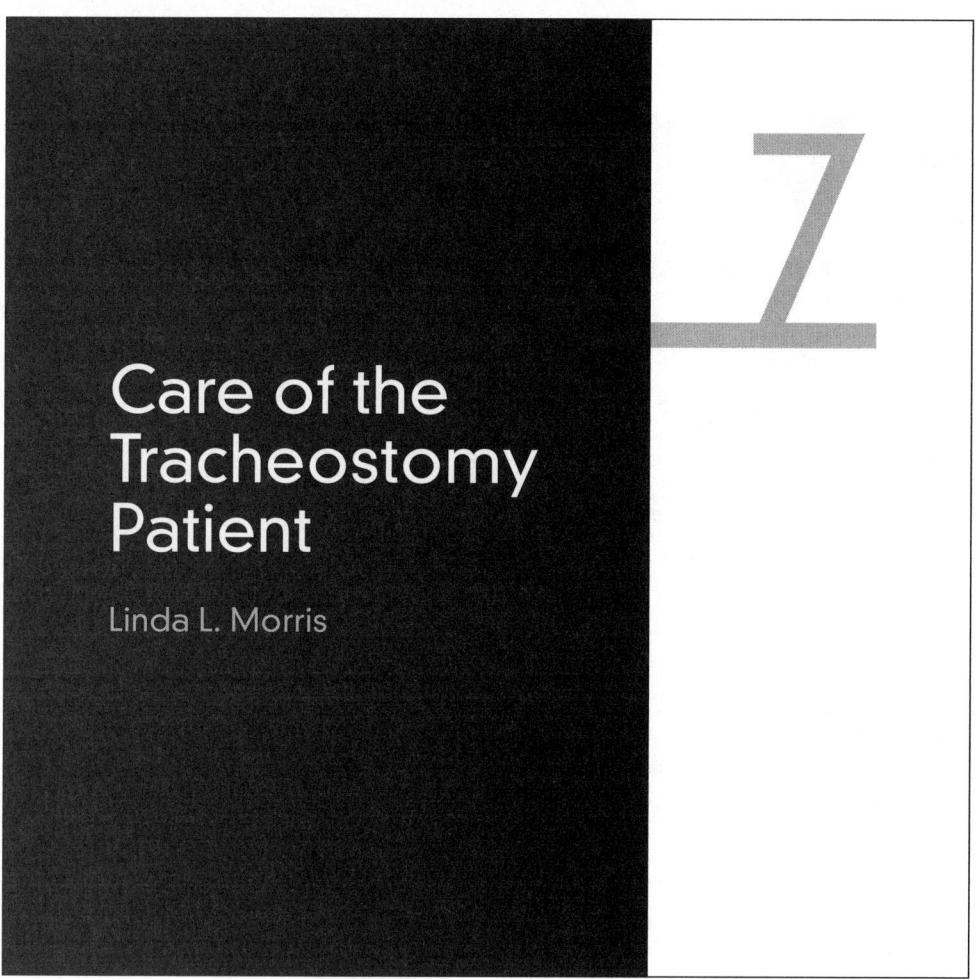

Care of the Tracheostomy Patient

Linda L. Morris

The tracheostomy patient requires vigilant care, especially in the first several postoperative days. Meticulous care and maintenance of the tracheostomy tube can prevent many complications. This chapter discusses the care required for the patient with a tracheostomy, including maintaining the tube, cleaning the inner cannula and stoma, caring for the cuff, mobilizing secretions, and caring for other tracheostomy appliances such as the T-tube. In addition, considerations for patients at home will also be reviewed, including managing home emergencies.

Maintenance of the Tracheostomy Tube

General care of the tracheostomy patient includes ensuring the presence of everyday and emergency supplies at all times, as well as complete familiarity with care of the tube. Bedside supplies, listed in Table 7.1, should include an extra tracheostomy tube of the same size and one size smaller, an obturator of appropriate size and type, a suction source and appropriately sized suction catheters, a

7.1 Contents of Emergency Kit

- Extra tracheostomy tube of same size
- Extra tracheostomy tube one size smaller
- Obturator
- Suction catheters
- Manual resuscitation bag
- Suction source, tubing
- Oxygen source
- Comparably sized endotracheal tube
- Tracheostomy dressings (drain sponges)
- Tracheostomy tube holders (or twill tape)
- Tracheostomy cleaning kits

manual resuscitation bag, an endotracheal tube of comparable size, and an oxygen source if needed (Seay & Gay, 2002). Additional supplies include dressings, tracheostomy tube holders or cotton twill tape, and tracheostomy cleaning kits.

Securing the Tracheostomy Tube

The first step in proper tracheostomy care is to ensure the security of the tube. After initial placement, most surgeons prefer to suture the tracheostomy tube in place (Hotter & Warfield, 1997). This is commonly done with a suture at each of the four corners of the neck flange in addition to snugly applied twill tape. This technique often makes care of the stoma challenging in the first postoperative week; however, the security of the tube during this time is a higher priority. Two groups have proposed more secure suturing techniques that differ from this conventional practice. Nouraie and others (2008) described a four-point technique done closer to the pivot point on the neck flange, while Liew, Gibbins, and Oyarzabal (2008) described securing the tracheostomy with two sutures through the central superior part of the neck flange. Both groups reported that their methods allow better care of the stoma, provide for easier replacement of stoma dressings, and function with different neck flange materials. Liew and coauthors reported that over the course of 10 years, their method has avoided tube dislodgements in the immediate postoperative period.

Most authors suggest that tracheostomy ties be secured snugly, allowing only one finger depth under the tracheostomy holder. Cotton twill tape is often used to secure the tracheostomy tube, especially in the early postoperative period. Twill tape does not slack when secured in place; however, over a longer period of time, it may cut into the neck of the wearer or fray at the ends (American Thoracic Society [ATS], 2000). A study of tracheostomy securing devices by Dixon and Wasson (1998) showed that Velcro holders were more comfortable, easier to use, and took significantly less time to apply; however, they may degrade over time, especially when washed in hot water (ATS, 2000). In fact, one manufacturer (Dale) specifically reported that their product should not be washed. While there is no consensus on the best device to use for anchoring the tracheostomy tube, it should be the priority in the early postoperative period. After the stoma and tract have matured, the clinician can consider comfort as well as tube security.

When the tracheostomy tube can move within the airway, the tip intermittently comes in contact with the trachea. Patient discomfort and coughing can result and are more pronounced with a rigid tube with a wider angle. The continued contact of the tube within the trachea may cause erosion of the trachea and the formation of granulation tissue within the airway. This granulation tissue can also occur in the suprastomal area, where the connection of the neck flange repeatedly comes in contact with the stoma. The resultant granulation tissue can fall back into the airway and create a partial obstruction (Yaremchuk, 2003).

Most authors state that the first tracheostomy tube change should be done at the end of the first postoperative week, which marks the transition from an immature to a mature tracheostomy. It usually takes 5–7 days for the tract to heal (Kost, 2008) and mature. If inadvertent decannulation were to occur during this time, the tissue planes would collapse, thus making simple reinsertion essentially impossible. It is inadvisable to attempt the reinsertion of a tube through an immature stoma because of the high likelihood of creating a false passage.

Care of the Inner Cannula

There is wide variation on the recommended frequency for cleaning or changing the inner cannula, but most authors suggest two to three times per day. Though cleaning may be required as often as every 2 hours, this frequency was challenged in one study, which suggested inner cannulas do not need to be changed often, if at all (Burns et al., 1998). Sixty patients were studied over 3 days to determine whether the interval of changing the inner cannula had an impact on tube obstruction or colonization. One group of patients had the inner cannula changed every 24 hours, while the other group did not have the inner cannula changed at all over a 3-day period. Surprisingly, the researchers found no difference on both outcome measures. The study had some limitations, however. All patients were suctioned in the hour before the inner cannula was examined, thus limiting the accurate interpretation of obstruction versus patency. Another limitation was the lack of defining the postoperative period in which the study took place. Results may differ between postoperative days 1–3 compared to postoperative days 10–12. Finally, the results could not be universally applied to all patients since the investigation was a small pilot study of only 60 patients in one surgical ICU. Comorbid conditions with large amounts of secretions—for example, pneumonia—might produce different results.

The inner cannula should be cleaned or changed when needed as long as it is inspected at least two to three times per day. Disposable inner cannulas are a convenience for the nursing staff; however, they can be a significant added expense for patients at home. Insurance coverage may be insufficient for home medical care and supplies such as disposable inner cannulas (Crimlisk, O'Donnell, & Grillone, 2006). Currently, the Medicare allowance is 30 inner cannulas per month and should be considered before discharging patients with

214 Tracheostomies

tracheostomies. Discharge and home care for the tracheostomy patient are covered in detail in chapter 12.

Procedure for Cleaning the Inner Cannula

The inner cannula must be regularly inspected and ideally cleaned using an aseptic technique. There are few studies that define the optimal frequency for cleaning or replacing the inner cannula. Cited frequency of cleaning has ranged from almost 16 times per day (Johnson, Wagner, & Sigler, 1988) to no cleaning at all (Burns et al., 1998). Most hospital policies recommend cleaning inner cannulas about 3 times per day.

Before beginning the procedure, supplies should be gathered and set up. Most tracheostomy cleaning kits (Figure 7.1) are sterile and contain all necessary supplies, including two small containers, stoma dressing (or drain sponge),

7.1

Contents of tracheostomy cleaning kit. Photo courtesy of Smiths Medical.

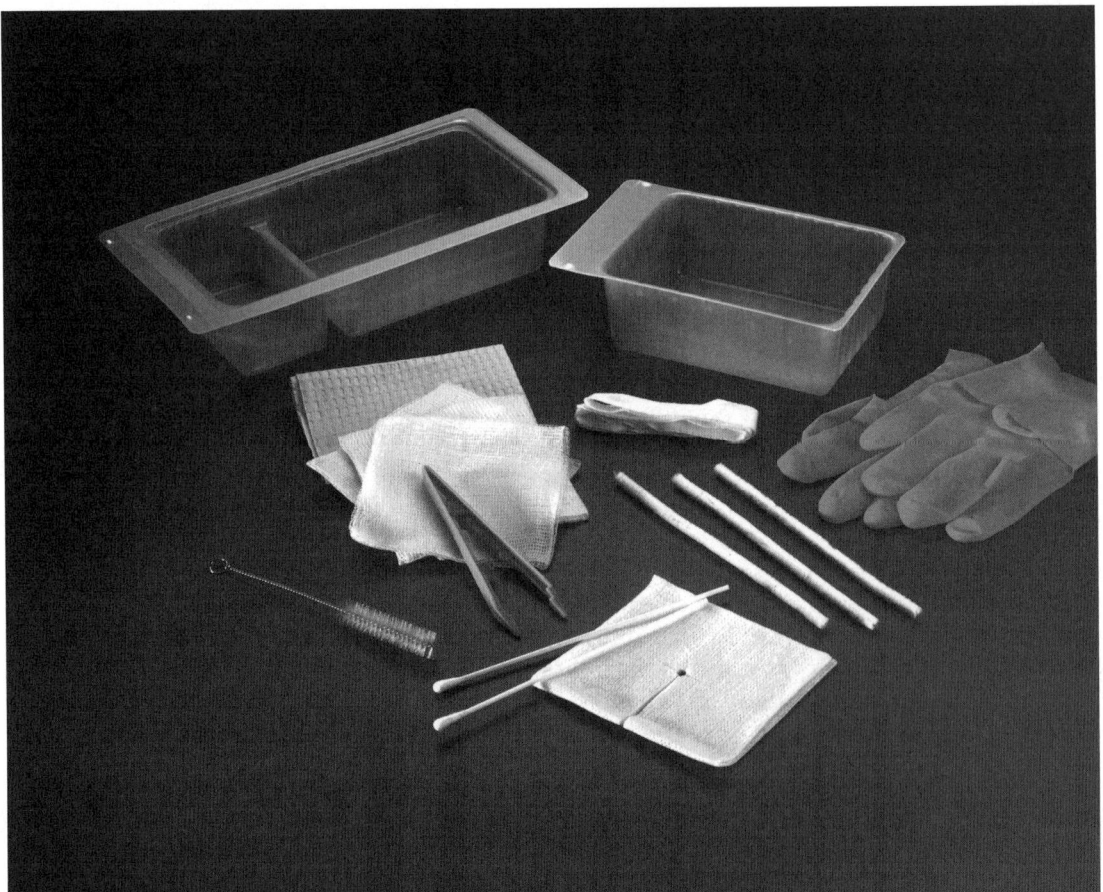

cotton twill tape, a small bottle brush, cotton-tipped swabs, pipe cleaners, a drape, and gloves. Hydrogen peroxide (3%) and sterile water are used for cleaning plastic tracheostomy tubes but should not be used for metal, silicone, or nylon tubes. Cleaning instructions for tubes of the latter materials are discussed in the following instructions for standard plastic tubes.

To clean plastic tubes, first fill one container with enough sterile water or saline to completely immerse the inner cannula. Fill the second container with the same amount of hydrogen peroxide. Some practitioners prefer to use hydrogen peroxide diluted to a 1:1 solution with sterile water (Hudak & Hickey, 2008). The solution will be used to soak the inner cannula, and the diluted hydrogen peroxide solution will take a longer time.

It is important to minimize the movement of the tracheostomy tube during manipulation in order to prevent discomfort and coughing. The tube should be steadied using the thumb and forefinger of one hand to stabilize the neck flange while the other hand removes the inner cannula. Small movements of the tube from the outside create large movements within the trachea, especially if the tube is rigid and has a wide angle. The inner cannula should be placed in the container of hydrogen peroxide solution and allowed to soak for 3–5 minutes in order to soften and dissolve the accumulated secretions. During this interval, the stoma can be cleaned with cotton swabs dipped in saline.

After the inner cannula has soaked in the peroxide bath, the secretions should be sufficiently loosened for cleaning. The small bottle brush can then be used to scrub the inside as well as the outside of the cannula. The point of contact of the 15-mm connector with the shaft of the cannula generally harbors secretions and should be scrubbed carefully. After all debris are removed, the inner cannula should be rinsed in sterile water and shaken free of water droplets. Alternatively, pipe cleaners can be used to dry the inside of the inner cannula. The inner cannula is then locked in place within the outer cannula while once again stabilizing the neck flange.

One Swedish study (Bjorling et al., 2007) demonstrated the superior efficacy of a cleaning method utilizing decontamination with chlorhexidine-alcohol followed by rinsing with sterile saline. The study was intended to create clinical evidence in support of a new national guideline compared to standard practice. In Sweden, common practice for cleaning the inner cannula utilized warm water with mild detergent. However, a national guideline recommended decontamination via an additional step of rinsing the inner cannula with chlorhexidine-alcohol followed by sterile saline. A study was undertaken to examine the difference in bacterial counts between the two methods. The authors studied 47 patients using a crossover design and cultured the inner cannulas before and after each cleaning procedure. Before the decontamination step, all but three samples had bacterial colonization. Median counts were 10,000 cfu/ml (colony-forming units per milliliter) for silver cannulas, 52,500 cfu/ml for Portex cannulas, 17,000 cfu/ml for Shiley cannulas, and 100,000 cfu/ml for TRACOE cannulas. Following decontamination using detergent and chlorhexidine-alcohol, 5 of 48 inner cannulas grew up to 160 cfu/ml; after using detergent alone, only 1 of 49 inner cannulas grew up to 10 cfu/ml. Furthermore, cleaning with both methods resulted in a near total elimination of all organisms. In view of the results of this study and considering the various materials used for tracheostomy tube components, the optimal approach for cleaning would be to follow the individual manufacturer's recommendations.

Tracheostomy tubes with disposable inner cannulas were developed in the late 1980s with the intent of saving significant nursing time. Johnson, Wagner, and Sigler (1988) compared the time to clean the inner cannula versus simply replacing it with a new one. They found that standard care of the inner cannula required over 5 minutes, while changing a disposable inner cannula took less than 1 minute. Even though disposable inner cannulas are popular in hospitals, the cost of supplies and insurance coverage may prohibit their use at home.

One of the primary benefits of plastic dual cannula tracheostomy tubes is that the inner cannula can be removed and cleaned while leaving the outer cannula in place within the airway. This may not be the case for tubes made of other materials.

Cleaning Metal Tracheostomy Tubes. Peroxide and enzyme cleaners should be avoided with sterling silver and stainless steel tubes. These solutions cause silver tubes to discolor, stain, and tarnish; in stainless steel, they cause the solder connection joints to weaken and the surface to pit and stain. Rather, the manufacturers recommend that metal tracheostomy tubes be removed and cleaned daily by soaking in mild dishwashing liquid for 1 hour to soften and loosen mucus. A flexible tracheal brush should be used to clean the inside of the tube; a soft toothbrush can be used to clean the outside of the tube and the neck flange. Dry heat sterilization is not recommended, and the tubes should not be exposed to temperatures above 204°C (400°F). The recommended use for patients at home is to place the tube in a pan of tap water and boil for 30 minutes, followed by wiping dry the cooled tube.

Cleaning Silicone Tracheostomy Tubes. The manufacturers' recommendations state that the Bivona and Arcadia lines of tracheostomy tubes (made of silicone) should be cleaned with a mild detergent. Because of its porous nature, silicone tends to absorb cleaning products, so they should not be used.

Cleaning Nylon Tracheostomy Tubes. The Air-Lon™ tracheostomy tube should be soaked in warm soapy water for a few minutes to loosen any dried mucus. A flexible tracheal brush can be used to clean the inside of the tube, and a soft toothbrush can be used to clean the outside of the tube and the neck flange. The Air-Lon™ tube can be autoclaved, boiled, gas sterilized, or soaked in a cold germicidal solution that does not contain phenol or formic acid as a base.

Care of the Tracheostomy Tube Cuff

It is important to minimize pressure from the air-inflated cuff against the trachea for several reasons. Proper inflation of the cuff can ensure an adequate delivery of tidal volume and prevent loss of air around the cuff, thus preventing hypoxemia. Inadequate cuff inflation has also been implicated in the development of ventilator-associated pneumonia. Alternatively, hyperinflation of the cuff can result in ischemia of the trachea, which can lead to tracheal necrosis, tracheomalacia, and tracheal stenosis. Cuff pressures above capillary perfusion pressure (25 cm H_2O or 20–30 mm Hg) for a prolonged time have been associated with ischemia and necrosis of the trachea (Bernhard, Yost, Joynes, Cothalis, & Turndorf, 1985; Hudak & Hickey, 2008). By contrast, cuff pressures below 20 cm H_2O have been associated with the leakage of oropharyngeal secretions around the cuff and are thought to contribute to ventilator-associated pneumonia (Rello et al., 1996; Sole et al., 2009).

There are three primary acceptable methods to ensure adequate cuff pressure: direct measurement of cuff pressure through manometry, minimal occlusive volume, and the minimal leak technique. Direct measurement of cuff pressure can be done intermittently with a manual pump manometer or continuously with an electronic manometer. The advantage of the electronic version is that it monitors cuff pressure as well as automatically regulates the pressure within the cuff and provides alarms to warn of leaks or overpressure. This electronic cuff-management device is not FDA approved as of this writing (personal communication, Boston Medical Products).

Several studies have considered palpation of the cuff as a technique to estimate pressure; however, its accuracy has been disappointing. Faris and colleagues (2007) asked experienced physicians and respiratory therapists to estimate cuff pressure by palpation and compared this value to a manometer measurement. Even the most experienced clinicians were accurate only 61% of the time. Stewart, Secrest, Norwood, and Zachary (2003) asked nurse anesthetists to use their usual cuff estimation techniques and compared these values with direct cuff manometry. They found that less than 31% of the nurse anesthetists inflated the cuff within the ideal range. Fernandez, Blanch, Mancebo, Bonsoms, and Artigas (1990) demonstrated that experienced physicians and nurses accurately estimated high cuff pressures only 69% of the time, normal cuff pressures 58% of the time, and low cuff pressures 73% of the time. Hoffman, Parwani, and Hahn (2006) showed that experienced faculty in emergency medicine were only 22% sensitive for detecting overinflation of the cuff. In that study, the average cuff pressure measured more than 93 cm H_2O (9.3 kPa), and 90% of the participants inflated the cuff to more than 120 cm H_2O (12 kPa). The investigators concluded that the inability to detect overinflated cuffs is not related to years of experience.

Morris, Zoumalan, Roccaforte, and Amin (2007) compared two hospitals using two different techniques for cuff inflation. One hospital used balloon palpation while the other used manometry. The study followed a total of 115 patients and found an overall overinflation rate of 38%, which, incidentally, was equal at both hospitals. They suggested the use of manometry alone did not prevent overinflation of the cuff and that more vigilant cuff monitoring practices were indicated.

Historically, high-pressure cuffs were exclusively found on tracheostomy tubes; and then routine cuff deflation was common practice to relieve pressure against the trachea. Intermittent cuff deflation provided an opportunity for reperfusion of the tracheal mucosa; however, there was no evidence that capillary blood flow was restored. In addition, routine cuff deflation was not well tolerated in hemodynamically unstable patients. Therefore, deep oropharyngeal suctioning should be done prior to cuff deflation to remove accumulated secretions above the cuff. Cuff deflation should also be timed with exhalation to prevent the aspiration of secretions above the cuff. A positive-pressure breath can also be used to blow secretions into the pharynx so they can be suctioned (Hudak & Hickey, 2008; Shapiro, Harrison, Kacmarek, & Cane, 1985).

Until recently, the potential role of continuous monitoring and adjustment of cuff pressure had not been studied. Sole and colleagues (2009) completed a pilot study of 10 patients in their ICU. Observational data coupled patient care activities with changes in cuff pressure. The pilot balloon was connected to a transducer, and cuff pressures were continuously monitored for 3.8 to 11.8 hours. The routine activities of suctioning, coughing, and patient-ventilator dyssynchrony increased cuff pressure an average of 20 cm H_2O. Other factors that increased cuff pressure included decreased pharmacologic sedation, turning in bed, and continuous lateral rotation therapy, whereas deeper positioning of the endotracheal tube, elevation of the head, and duration of intubation were associated with lower cuff pressures. The investigators concluded that intermittent monitoring of cuff pressures might give practitioners a false sense of security.

Duguet and colleagues (2007) studied nine mechanically ventilated patients to evaluate a prototype device that maintained constant pressure within endotracheal tube cuffs. Continuous measurements of cuff pressures were taken both when the cuffs were maintained by the device and when they were not. The investigators randomly ordered the sequence of measurements, varying days when the prototype device maintained constant pressure with days when constant cuff pressure was not maintained yet was continuously monitored. The target cuff pressure was set at 22–28 cm H_2O. On control days, cuff pressure ranged from 30–50 cm H_2O for 29% of the time and from 15–30 cm H_2O for 56% of the time. On prototype days, cuff pressure was maintained at 15–30 cm H_2O for 95% of the time. The study showed that cuff pressure was successfully controlled with minimal human intervention. Although cuff pressure maintenance devices are not yet widely available in the United States, clinical studies will determine their accuracy and clinical utility.

Accumulated secretions above the cuff have been implicated in the development of ventilator-associated pneumonia and, therefore, should be suctioned regularly in order to prevent seepage. Some tracheostomy and endotracheal tubes have a separate suction channel for this purpose.

Using intermittent and continuous suctioning schedules, Coffman, Rees, Sievers, and Belafsky (2008) compared the quantity of secretions removed from conventional tracheostomy tubes to those with a suction channel. The purpose of their benchtop study was to determine if an above-the-cuff suction channel could decrease tracheal aspiration. They compared standard Shiley tubes to Portex Blue Line Ultra Suctionaid tubes, which include a suction channel. Tubes of similar outer diameter were placed in a simulated tracheal model, and donor human saliva was used because of its unique rheology and viscoelastic properties. Each cuff was inflated to 30 cm H_2O, and 10 ml of human saliva was placed above the cuff. The amount of saliva that migrated past the Shiley tubes with no suction was approximately 8.5 ml. There was no difference in the amount of saliva that migrated past the cuff of the Portex tubes when no suction was applied.

Changing the Tracheostomy Tube

The entire tracheostomy tube should be changed on a regular basis in order to prevent infection, obstruction of the tube, and other complications associated with an indwelling airway device. An additional goal for this procedure in children is to keep up with their physical growth. Manufacturers' recommendations suggest entire tube changes every 1 to 2 months. However, one study (Yaremchuk, 2003) suggested that routine tracheostomy tube changes should take place more often. The author found that implementing a new policy of tracheostomy tube changes every 2 weeks decreased the number of surgical interventions required for the removal of granulation tissue. He further suggested that tracheostomy tubes should be changed as potential sources of infection when sepsis is present. Some patients have reported success with daily tracheostomy tube changes and cleaning while rotating the use of two primary tubes.

Most papers report the first tracheostomy tube change should take place on the seventh postoperative day. At this time, the tissue tract is considered mature. The first tube change is usually done by the surgeon who placed the tube, who typically signs off the case afterward (Yaremchuk, 2003). Ideally, care should then be transferred to another practitioner who will provide follow-up for the tracheostomy. There is anecdotal evidence that tracheostomy tube changes can be safely performed earlier than the fifth day; however, there are no randomized, controlled studies to identify the minimum safe interval following tracheostomy placement.

One of the biggest risks during the early postoperative period is inadvertent decannulation—an emergency requiring orotracheal intubation with an endotracheal tube. The rationale for orotracheal intubation is the lack of a mature tract and the collapse of tissue planes, which form an impediment to the emergency replacement of the tube. Refer to chapter 10 for a discussion of inadvertent decannulation.

Care of the Stoma

While the inner cannula is soaking in the peroxide bath, the stoma can be cleaned. A healthy stoma should be clean and dry with pink edges, though in the early postoperative period it is normal to see dried blood around the stoma. Any redness, swelling, or pus is abnormal. A small amount of blood should be expected with each tracheostomy tube change, especially when a cuffed tube is inserted or removed. However, if frank blood continues to be evident, the clinician may need to explore the wound to ligate or cauterize a leaking blood vessel or possibly apply packing.

The constant exposure of the stoma to secretions can be very irritating to the skin, much like diaper rash. Secretions left in place around the stoma become dried and encrusted quickly. In addition, moist secretions can act as irritants to the skin, so the stoma must be cleansed regularly and kept dry. A precut drain sponge should be applied around the stoma until secretions have significantly decreased. This dressing should be changed at least twice per day (Dennis-Rouse & Davidson, 2008; Wright & Van Dahm, 2003) or whenever secretions begin to collect. This can be challenging in the early postoperative period, as priority during that time is the security of the tube.

In the hospital, 3% hydrogen peroxide is often used to clean around the stoma and soften encrustations. It can be applied full or half strength to a cotton swab to cleanse the skin around the tracheostomy tube, underneath the neck flange along the entire circumference of the stoma, and particularly along the point of connection with the neck flange. For long-term use, however, saline-dipped cotton swabs are recommended. Patients at home are taught to use saline or tap water to gently cleanse the stoma. All excess moisture should be removed with another cotton-tipped applicator or gauze pad and additional tracheostomy dressing.

The stomal dressing has a dual purpose: to collect secretions and to cushion the neck flange from direct contact with the skin. There is no evidence of the optimal material for the stomal dressing, but the primary goal should be to keep the neck dry and free of secretions. Hydrophilic absorbent dressings can be used in patients with large amounts of secretions, but their effectiveness over gauze dressings has not been demonstrated in tracheostomy patients. One Japanese group used an absorbent dressing (Aquacel) on five patients and reported favorable results (Tsunezuka, Suzuki, Nitta, & Oda, 2005); however, there is a need for randomized studies comparing various methods of dressing the stoma. The major goal is timely replacement of the dressing when it becomes soiled or moist with secretions, which occasionally may necessitate several dressing changes per day.

Internal and external traction forces can create stomal erosion. The inward pressure of the neck flange against the skin can create erosion of the stoma from the outside. This is most often seen in tracheostomies with a rigid neck flange, as they tilt along one plane. This erosion can be exacerbated in patients with severe neck flexion, as in kyphosis. Excessive outward traction from ventilator tubing is also a significant problem because it can erode the stoma from the inside. Any additional rotational force, or torque, can also exacerbate this problem. Care must be taken to support ventilator tubing to prevent this outward traction and torque. There are also devices on the market, like the Shiley Stronghold (Figure 7.2), that support the connection of the ventilator tubing with the tracheostomy tube.

Shiley Stronghold connected to tracheostomy tube. Covidien.

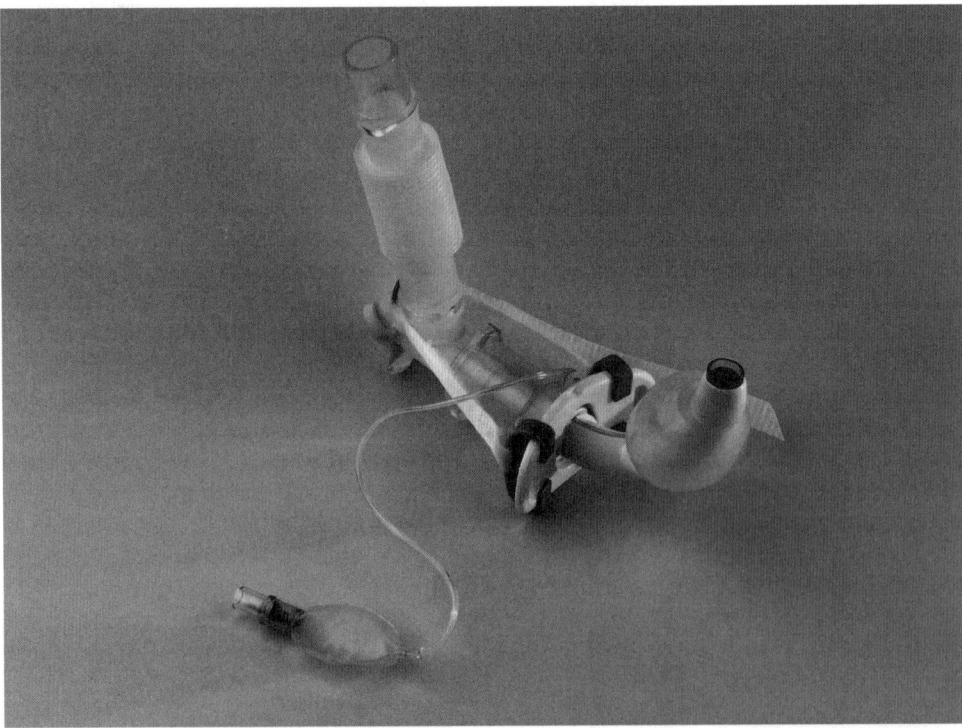

Occasionally, a large surgical incision is necessary, which can result in stomal discomfort and excessive drainage. One common option is to pack the wound with iodoform gauze. Hotter and Warfield (1997) recommended frequent wound packing with cloth ribbon impregnated with 15% sodium chloride (Mesalt). Surgicel can also be used to pack the wound. These approaches offer the advantages of absorbing secretions, keeping the wound dry, and providing a bacteriostatic/bacteriocidal medium.

Mobilization of Secretions

Airway mucus is a viscoelastic gel composed of water, carbohydrates, proteins, and lipids. It is a product of the goblet cells of the airway epithelium and submucosal glands. The volume of mucus secretion is between 10–100 ml per day in a healthy person. In instances of mucus hypersecretion or damage to the ciliary mechanism, cough is critical for effective bronchial hygiene (Rubin, 2002). Patients unable to cough effectively should be suctioned to prevent obstruction, decrease work of breathing, improve oxygenation and ventilation, and remove bacteria (Ireton, 2007; Lewis, 2002). Blackwood (1999) appropriately described the goal of suctioning as maximizing the removal of secretions and minimizing hazards. Two recent papers reviewed the evidence of secretion management for patients on mechanical ventilation (Branson, 2007; Pedersen, Rosendahl-Nielsen, Hjermind, & Egerod, 2008), although these studies involved patients intubated with endotracheal tubes. With the exception of one study in children (Ireton), the suctioning of secretions in tracheostomy patients has not been specifically studied. However, most studies' conclusions are likely applicable to any type of artificial airway, as the principles of secretion management apply no matter what type of appliance is in the airway.

Suctioning

The problem of secretion retention often begins in the ICU due to a confluence of additive factors. The patient is confined to bed and is relatively immobile. Atelectasis develops, and the coughing reflex is impaired and interfered with by endotracheal or tracheostomy tubes. Fluid restriction leads to thickened secretions. Finally, comorbid conditions compound the presence of secretions.

Suctioning is not without risk. Numerous complications may result from the suctioning procedure, including cardiac arrhythmias, hypoxemia, atelectasis, bleeding, and infection. Most of these complications can be prevented by meticulous attention to detail and technique.

There are no studies that identify whether the suctioning experience is different in tracheostomies versus endotracheal tubes, but numerous studies have discussed suctioning in general. An adequate explanation of the procedure is essential prior to suctioning. Patients report that suctioning is a painful procedure (Arroyo-Novoa et al., 2008; Pedersen et al., 2008; Puntillo et al., 2001), but it is essential to prevent the accumulation of secretions and promote adequate ventilation. Patients have described the suctioning procedure as "hell on earth" (Sawyer, 1997), a feeling of choking or breathlessness (Bergbom-Engberg & Halijamae, 1989), a "frightening and unpleasant experience" (Griggs, 1998), and "horrific" and "terrifying" (Sawyer). Peruzzi and Smith (1995) recommended that sedation and pain relief could lead to a reduction in stress, anxiety, and pain as well as increased effectiveness of the procedure itself.

Frequency of Suctioning. It is commonly held that suctioning should be done only as needed, rather than on a routine schedule. However, one small study of 14 patients showed no significant variation in complications between patients suctioned routinely and those suctioned as needed (Wood, 1998). Pedersen and colleagues (2008) reported that a number of studies have shown a decreased internal diameter to the airway because of the formation of a biofilm and the accumulation of secretions (Glass & Grap, 1995; Shah & Kollef, 2004; Tenaillon, 1990). Therefore, in order to prevent obstruction of the tube and the accumulation of secretions, the American Association of Respiratory Care recommends that patients may require suctioning at a minimum frequency (Branson, Campbell, Chatburn, & Covington, 1993). Pedersen and coauthors further defined a suctioning frequency of every 8 hours in order to reduce the accumulation of secretions and airway occlusion.

Kost (2008) described the clinical signs that indicate suctioning—visible secretions, audible gurgling, coarse or diminished breath sounds, dyspnea, increased airway pressures, and unexplained desaturation. Though the aforementioned list is intuitive, one must not overlook the importance of suctioning in order to check the patency of the tracheostomy tube, particularly in patients who do not produce secretions on their own due to inadequate physical strength or a neurological impairment of the normal cough reflex. These patients do not produce the usual cues of gurgling or visible secretions within the tube. Frequently, however, secretions are present deep within the airway of these patients, and they must be externally stimulated in order to produce secretions. External stimulation includes suctioning, turning, and regular physical mobility such as range-of-motion exercises. When used in combination on a regular basis, these maneuvers can effectively prevent inspissation of secretions and tube obstruction.

Size of Suction Catheter. The size of the suction catheter should be large enough to effectively remove secretions but small enough to prevent unnecessary obstruction. The effectiveness of the catheter is directly related to its size, with larger catheters being more effective. It is recommended that the catheter be no more than half the internal diameter of the endotracheal tube. This allows space around the outside of the suction catheter for air to pass to the lungs during suctioning (Pedersen, 2008). Odell and others (1993) introduced a formula for determining the appropriate size of a suction catheter:

$$(\text{Size of endotracheal tube or tracheostomy tube} - 2) \times 2$$
$$= \text{size of French catheter}$$

According to this formula, a patient with a size 8 tracheostomy tube should be suctioned with no greater than a 12 French suction catheter. This may be appropriate for some patients; however, one must also weigh the catheter's ability to remove the secretions effectively—especially when the tracheostomy tube is small in diameter.

Application of Suction. It must be remembered that when suction is applied, secretions as well as oxygen are removed from the tracheobronchial tree. The application of suction using high negative pressure for a prolonged period of time could result in trauma to the trachea in addition to hypoxemia and cardiac arrhythmias. These effects can be lessened by hyperoxygenation. It is recommended that suction be applied for less than 12 seconds, only upon withdrawal of the catheter, and with a suction pressure of less than −80 to −120 mm Hg (Kost, 2008; Oh & Seo, 2003). Studies of suctioning focus on defining the optimal pressure to remove secretions while reducing the risks of hypoxia, atelectasis, and tracheal damage (Pedersen et al., 2008; Wood, 1998). Most studies used a suction pressure of −80 to −120 mm Hg (Oh & Seo), and, in general, higher pressure more effectively removed secretions. The safety of higher suction pressures depends on appropriately sized suction catheters to avoid the aforementioned risks. Tenaillon (1990) recommended that a pressure of −200 to −300 mm Hg could be used safely with optimal-sized suction catheters; however, Pedersen and colleagues recommended a more cautious approach and advised −200 mm Hg as the acceptable upper limit. While higher suction pressures are tolerated in patients who have adequate oxygen reserves and hemodynamic profiles, a more cautious approach is advisable for those who do not.

The mobilization of secretions is not limited to suctioning alone but extends to methods for loosening, thinning, and facilitating the removal of secretions. The basis of mobilization begins with keeping the secretions thin, which is accomplished best with adequate fluid intake. Although a high-humidity tracheostomy collar is effective in providing humidity for comfort, it is not a substitute for adequate hydration. Strategies for the humidification of airways will be discussed in the following. Patients should be encouraged to drink plenty of fluids. If they are not able to take fluids orally, then additional fluids should be given enterally or parenterally unless otherwise contraindicated.

Oxygenation. Oxygenation is part of the suctioning procedure and is used to avoid hypoxia and its sequelae. Oxygenation can be accomplished prior to, during, and after the procedure even though it is usually referred to as preoxygenation. Preoxygenation is frequently used in the immediate postoperative period; however, its use tends to diminish over time. Most studies on preoxygenation were done on patients with endotracheal tubes; however, it is not known whether a tracheostomy tube would decrease preoxygenation requirements (St. John & Malen, 2004).

One source advises against using preoxygenation with manual resuscitation bags in patients with tracheostomies for head and neck cancer (Hudak & Hickey, 2008). The authors reported that although preoxygenation with the manual resuscitation bag helped increase inspiratory volume and mobilize secretions, it also placed stress on the anastomosis of the surgical wound. When patients were able to take deep breaths on their own through a tracheal mask, hyperventilation with a manual resuscitation bag was not necessary.

Hyperoxygenation is the delivery of oxygen at a greater concentration than the patient is already receiving, up to 100% concentration (Day, Farnell, & Wilson-Barnett, 2002; Glass & Grap, 1995; Swartz, Noonan, & Edwards-Beckett, 1996; Wood, 1998). Hyperoxygenation is advisable when the patient is critically ill and requires full ventilator support. The benefit from hyperoxygenation is not clear in patients who do not require ventilator support; therefore, its use is directed by clinical need.

Hyperinflation. Hyperinflation is the delivery of a tidal volume greater than that generated mechanically or spontaneously (Day et al., 2002; Wood, 1998). Hyperinflation can be accomplished by adjusting ventilator settings or with a manual resuscitation bag. A common method is the use of 150% of the preset tidal volume for at least three breaths (Oh & Seo, 2003; Swartz et al., 1996). Hyperinflation has been shown to decrease atelectasis and increase residual capacity, but the degree of hyperinflation necessary to prevent complications is not well defined (Day et al.).

Some studies separate hyperinflation from oxygenation, although, in practice, hyperinflation is usually used with hyperoxygenation. Stone, Preusser, Groch, Karl, and Gonyon (1991) studied the effects of hyperinflation delivered by a ventilator on oxygenation and hemodynamic values. The investigators delivered three consecutive hyperoxygenation/hyperinflation breaths with randomly selected tidal volumes (12, 14, 16, and 18 ml/kg of body weight). Significant increases in mean arterial pressure, pulmonary artery pressure, pulmonary airway pressure, and cardiac output were recorded during all hyperinflation/suctioning sequences and for all tidal volumes. No incidents of hypoxia were noted with any of the hyperinflation/suctioning sequences.

Depth of Suctioning. Depth of suctioning has also been studied, primarily in neonates and children, but there are a few adults studies. Shallow suctioning is placing the tip of the suction catheter no further than the depth of the airway, and deep suctioning is anything beyond that point. Numerous studies have recommended introducing the suction catheter to the level of the carina, and then withdrawing 1–2 cm before applying suction (Pedersen, 2008). In a national sample of pediatric centers, 71.2% of nurses reported inserting the catheter until it met resistance (Swartz et al., 1996). A Cochrane meta-analysis of deep versus shallow suctioning in infants and children examined the evidence but did not offer an evidence-based preference for one method over the other (Spence, Gillies, & Waterworth, 2003). However, in patients with large amounts of secretions, deep suctioning may be necessary (Van de Leur, Zwaveling, Loef, & Van der Shans, 2003).

Bleeding. Occasionally, mild bleeding occurs as a result of tracheal irritation and erosion during suctioning. This mild bleeding should not prevent suctioning but, rather, should be a cue to switch from standard suction catheters to soft rubber catheters to prevent continued irritation. Complete healing of tracheal lesions has been reported in as little as 24 hours when using softer suction catheters.

Open Versus Closed Suction Systems. There has been some debate about the use of open versus closed suction systems. Closed suction systems have gained popularity and are used frequently in the ICU while patients are on mechanical ventilation. Their widespread use has gained favor because of their convenience and containment of secretions. There is less concern for hypoxemia and desaturation because the ventilator tubing is not disconnected while suctioning takes place. One cautionary meta-analysis (Oh & Seo, 2003) showed that simultaneous insufflation of oxygen with suctioning in closed systems increased hypoxemia.

Most studies comparing open and closed suction systems show no difference in rates of ventilator-associated pneumonia (Niel-Weise, Snoeren, & van den Broek, 2007; Siempos, Vardakas, & Falagas, 2008; Vonberg, Eckmanns, Welte, & Gastmeier, 2006). One Turkish study (Topeli, Harmanci, Cetinkaya, Akdeniz, & Unal, 2004) found that closed suction systems resulted in a greater degree of colonization but did not have an effect on the development of ventilator-associated pneumonia.

A recent animal study compared the effectiveness of secretion removal between the two methods (Copnell et al., 2007). They found that open suction systems were more effective in removing thick as well as thin secretions no matter what type of ventilator mode was used. Combes, Fauvage, and Oleyer (2000) also investigated both infection and effectiveness and found that closed suction systems decreased the rate of ventilator-associated pneumonia but had a volume of tracheal aspirate similar to open systems.

In a review conducted by Maggiore and colleagues (2002), the most frequent complications with open and closed suctioning were related to desaturation and hemorrhagic secretions, and PEEP was the only independent risk factor for desaturation. They suggested that closed suction systems should not be considered routine but should only be used in those patients with higher oxygen requirements and levels of PEEP. Pedersen and others (2008) reviewed the evidence and did not find one method superior to the other.

Seymour, Cross, Cooke, Gallop, and Fuchs (2009) studied the recovery times of vital signs and hemodynamic parameters using the closed suction system on mechanically ventilated patients. Spontaneously breathing patients on pressure support mode were compared to those who were heavily sedated or paralyzed on volume-controlled continuous or intermittent mandatory ventilation. The median post-suctioning recovery time was greater than 5 minutes for minute volume, tidal volume, and respiratory rate. Heart rate, mean arterial pressure, and oxygen saturation increased after suctioning but were not clinically important. Furthermore, post-suctioning changes persisted longer in those breathing spontaneously on pressure support mode. The overall conclusion was that the timing of suctioning should be considered when assessing readiness to wean or extubate.

Although convenient, closed suction systems add a great deal of bulk, weight, and traction to the ventilator tubing (St. John & Malen, 2004). Traction or torque on the tracheostomy tube and stoma can have numerous deleterious effects. First, it can shift the position of the tracheostomy tube within the airway and create a positional leak of air around the cuff. This shifting can also move the tip of the tube in contact with the posterior wall of the trachea, resulting in erosion and stenosis. Second, the torque can twist the tube itself inside the trachea and create friction against the endotracheal wall. If these problems are not corrected early, they can create erosion and enlargement of the stoma from the inside. The entire tracheostomy tube, including the cuff, may be visible. It is advisable to eliminate the added traction whenever possible and reserve the use of closed suction systems to patients whose hemodynamic status cannot tolerate an open suction system.

Saline Instillation, or Lavage. The use of saline lavage with suctioning has been a topic of great debate for many years. The instillation of 2–10 ml of normal saline, followed by manual ventilation with a resuscitation bag, has been used for loosening and thinning secretions just prior to aggressive suctioning. It was also thought that saline lavage helped lubricate the suction catheter and dislodge bacteria from the biofilm inside the endotracheal tube (Blackwood, 1999; Hagler & Traver, 1994; O'Neal, Grap, Thompson, & Dudley, 2001; Pedersen et al., 2008). Numerous studies have been conducted over the years to evaluate the benefits of saline lavage and its effect on vital signs, oxygenation, airway pressures, infection, and amount of secretions.

Most studies do not favor the use of saline instillation; in fact, most have found detrimental effects (Raymond, 1995). Ackerman and Gugerty (1990) studied the effect of saline lavage on oxygen saturation and reported significant decreases after suctioning. Patients who received a prior bolus of saline had a much greater fall in saturation compared to those who did not receive a bolus. O'Neal and others (2001) used a crossover study design to quantify patients' perceptions of dyspnea with suctioning. Patients self-rated their level of dyspnea using a visual analog scale. They were randomized to two groups involving suctioning with or without saline. There was no difference in the level of dyspnea between the groups. However, the investigators found a significant correlation between age and level of dyspnea, with older patients experiencing higher levels of dyspnea with the use of saline.

No studies have been able to demonstrate that saline instillation actually loosens or thins secretions. Nevertheless, it has been shown to promote vigorous coughing (Branson, 2007; Pedersen, 2008). One study showed that less than 19% of the volume of saline was returned with suctioning (Hanley, Raud, & Butler, 1978). Perhaps the unfavorable effects of saline can be attributed to its characteristics. Blackwood (1999) reported that the earliest mention of the instillation of saline was questioned by Demers and Saklad (1973) "because mucus and water do not mix, even after vigorous shaking."

Gray, MacIntyre, and Kronenberger (1990) published one of the few studies to conclude that no apparent detrimental effects resulted from saline instillation. The investigators found that suctioning with and without instillation resulted in no differences in heart rate, respiratory rate, blood pressure, PaO_2, $PaCO_2$, or pH. In addition, there was no difference in peak airway pressure, minute ventilation, saturation, or forced vital capacity. Interestingly, the investigators noted that material suctioned after saline lavage weighed more than that suctioned without saline, and they concluded that the major effect of saline instillation was to stimulate a forceful cough.

Despite the lack of evidence showing its benefit, saline lavage is still widely practiced on a routine basis and is even advocated by some authors (Hudak & Hickey, 2008; Johnson, 2008; Walvekar & Myers, 2008). A national survey of pediatric centers in 1996 showed that 96.2% of nurses reported the use of an irrigant for suctioning, primarily normal saline (Swartz et al., 1996). Schwenker, Ferrin, and Gift (1998) reported the differences between nurses and respiratory therapists regarding the use of saline lavage: 64% of nurses rarely used saline, while 71% of respiratory therapists commonly used it. A more recent study published in 2003 surveying 27 centers across the United States reported that saline lavage was commonly practiced by 26% of nurses and 51% of respiratory therapists. One reason saline lavage is used frequently is because the technique is still taught in schools (Celik & Kanan, 2006). A study published in 2002 showed that 67% of respiratory therapists in a large acute-care hospital used saline lavage occasionally, and 24% used it routinely. There was no correlation between its use and the level of education or experience of the therapist. Sixty percent of therapists reported learning about the practice in school (French & Bauer, 2002).

One recent study (Caruso, Denari, Ruiz, Demarzo, & Deheinzelin, 2009) advocated the use of saline instillation as a means to decrease the incidence of ventilator-associated pneumonia. This was a blinded, controlled study where 262 patients were divided into two groups: a saline group that received 8 ml of saline before tracheal suctioning and a control group that did not. The authors found that the incidence of confirmed ventilator-associated pneumonia was significantly lower in the saline group, although clinical suspicion was the same in both groups. There was no difference between the groups in tube obstruction or atelectasis. The authors concluded that the decrease in ventilator-associated pneumonia could be a result of the improvement in secretion removal, which is primarily due to cough stimulation. They also suggested that frequently rinsing the tube with saline could have reduced biofilm. No apparent effect was noted on mortality, mechanical ventilation, or length of stay. The authors acknowledged the study's limitations, including single-center design and not blinding the respiratory therapists, who performed all of the suctioning.

Saline lavage has limited effectiveness in mobilizing, but not thinning, mucus plugs, especially when used in combination with hyperoxygenation, vigorous hyperinflation, and deep suctioning. Its use should be limited to cases in which standard methods have proven ineffective. Preventive measures such as hydration, humidification, and physical mobility should be provided to prevent mucus plugs from obstructing the airway.

Airway Humidification and Secretions

Mucous membranes often require added moisture because the tracheostomy tube bypasses the upper airway. Humidification can be provided by a tracheostomy collar, an HME, or atomized saline. Lack of adequate humidification can cause the trachea to develop squamous metaplasia, desiccation of the tracheal mucosa, and impaired ciliary function (Epstein, 2005). HMEs use moisture in exhaled air to humidify inspired air. There are models that connect within the ventilator circuit and those that attach directly to the tracheostomy tube.

Humidity prevents the drying of secretions, but a standard measure of optimal humidity is lacking. Proposed measures of optimal humidity include secretion volume and consistency, frequency of suctioning, changes in airway resistance, incidence of airway occlusion, and the need for lavage. Humidity is provided differently for patients on mechanical ventilation and those who are not. Patients on mechanical ventilation require either an in-line HME or heated humidifier. A meta-analysis comparing these two methods of providing humidity in over 1,000 mechanically ventilated patients demonstrated a fourfold increase in the risk of occlusion with an HME (Hess, 2002). Branson (2007) suggested HMEs should not be used in patients with retained secretions and their use should be limited to less than 5 days. There is no evidence to differentiate the effectiveness of humidity between heated humidified and nonheated tracheostomy collars.

In summary, the mainstay of secretion management rests on three primary interventions: suctioning, humidification, and physical mobility, which is discussed in the following section.

Mobility

Physical mobility is the third, but equally important, component of secretion mobilization. Physical movement of any kind helps mobilize secretions. Active or passive range-of-motion exercises for bedridden patients can be effective in mobilizing secretions, strengthening respiratory muscles, and improving cough ability. Although there have been no definitive studies to identify the optimal type or frequency of exercise, clinical experience has demonstrated that any type of movement is beneficial for the mobilization of secretions. Active or passive range of motion, frequent turning, and progressive ambulation are all recommended as early as possible. Many clinicians are reluctant to provide mobility to their patients because of a lack of time or a fear the patient's medical devices, including tracheostomy tube, will become dislodged.

One study recently published by Morris and others (2008) demonstrated benefit from initiating an early mobility program for patients with acute respiratory failure in the ICU. Their mobility therapy program was run by a dedicated team comprised of a critical care nurse, a nursing assistant, and a physical therapist. The protocol included four levels of activity. Level I consisted of passive range of motion administered three times per day to all joints except shoulder extension and hip flexion, which were limited by the patient's position in bed. In Level II, patients were sufficiently alert to participate in therapy and had progressed to active range of motion with assistance. In addition to passive range of motion, patients were placed in a sitting position for at least 20 minutes three times a day. In Level III, sitting at the edge of the bed was added to the previous regimen. In Level IV, patients also got out of bed and transferred to a chair for a minimum of 20 minutes per day.

The early mobility therapy program showed a significant decrease in the number of days patients were confined to bed rest, as well as length of stay in the ICU and the hospital. The number of bed rest days was 5 in the therapy group and 11 in the control group ($p \leq 0.0001$). The length of stay in the ICU was 5.5 days in the therapy group compared to 6.9 days in the control group ($p = 0.025$), whereas overall hospital length of stay was 11.2 days in the therapy group versus 14.5 days in the control group ($p = 0.006$). There was also a near-significant decrease in the incidence of ventilator-associated pneumonia in the therapy group (3%) compared to the control group (7.9%), ($p = 0.087$). Paradoxically, the rate of deep vein thrombosis was higher in the therapy group—5.4%, compared to 1.8% in the control group—although not significant ($p = 0.078$).

The results of this study showed that early mobility does no harm and can make a dramatic difference in length of stay. There were no incidents of cardiopulmonary compromise or inadvertent removal of any invasive device. This study did not report if this protocol made a difference in the numbers of tracheostomies performed or the time to tracheostomy. However, further research is needed to determine the optimal type of therapy, the frequency of therapy, and other outcomes that can be influenced by early mobility.

Oral Care

Poor oral hygiene has been implicated in the development of ventilator-associated pneumonia (VAP). Several factors are related to the development of VAP, and they include the colonization of dental plaque, bacterial colonization of the oropharynx, the development of biofilm around the walls of the tube, and accumulation of subglottic secretions around the inflated cuff.

Treatment for VAP is targeted antibiotic therapy in addition to bundled preventative steps as recommended by the Institute for Healthcare Improvement (IHI). Bundled care for mechanically ventilated patients includes elevating the head of the bed, daily sedation vacations, and prophylaxis for peptic ulcer disease and deep venous thrombosis. The elevation of the head of the bed to 30–45 degrees can prevent aspiration of gastrointestinal contents and/or oropharyngeal secretions. Daily ventilator weaning trials coupled with decreased sedation have been shown to lessen time on mechanical ventilation.

Currently, oral care is not included in the ventilator bundle, but it has been adopted in nursing practice as an effective quality measure for the prevention of VAP. Recommended oral care includes toothbrushing, chlorhexidine oral swabbing, and deep subglottic suctioning above the cuff. Several studies have shown that oral decontamination with chlorhexidine decreased rates of VAP with no effect on mortality or length of stay (Chan, Ruest, Meade, & Cook, 2007; Chlebicki & Safdar, 2007; Tantipong, Morkchareonpong, Jaiyindee, & Thamlikitkul, 2009; Wip & Napolitano, 2009). Sona and investigators (2009) demonstrated that toothbrushing every 12 hours decreased VAP rates by 46%. Fields (2008) demonstrated that toothbrushing every 8 hours eradicated VAP for the duration of the study. Bouza and colleagues (2008) showed that continuous aspiration of subglottic secretions decreased VAP in patients undergoing major heart surgery. Tsai, Lin, and Change (2008) found that intermittent suctioning of oral secretions prior to each position change decreased rates of VAP from 11% to 2.6% and decreased ICU length of stay from 27.6 to 20.3 days. Interestingly, there is no evidence to show an advantage of continuous over intermittent aspiration of secretions on the development of VAP. Thus, regular oral care and suctioning of subglottic secretions are recommended for patients with tracheostomies.

It is important to distinguish between infection and colonization. Brook (1979) reported that 100% of his pediatric patients with long-term tracheostomies were colonized with bacteria within the upper airway. Because most patients with chronic tracheostomies become colonized, it is usually not necessary to treat a positive culture unless there are other signs of active infection, such as leukocytosis, fever, or infiltrates on chest x-ray.

Other Tracheal Appliances

Care of the T-Tube

T-tubes are placed to support a weak or damaged trachea (Figure 7.3) caused by conditions such as tracheal stenosis, laryngotracheal injuries, tracheal reconstruction, or segmental resection. The T-tube consists of three lumens: the upper intraluminal limb, the lower intraluminal limb, and the external limb. In some cases, it may be necessary to shorten one or both of the intraluminal limbs

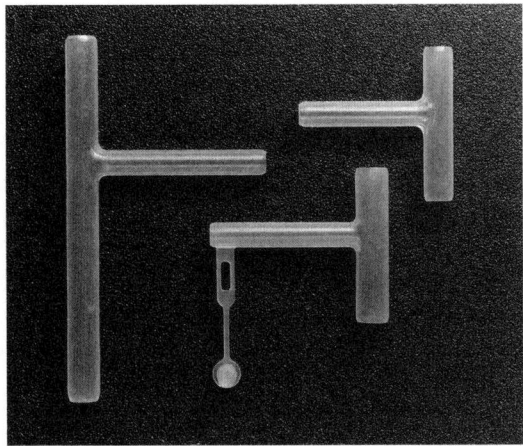

7.3

Hood T-tube.
Hood Labs
(Pembroke, MA).

in order to ensure a proper fit. If the required lengths are known prior to surgery, the manufacturer should be approached to customize the length. Customizing kits are also available to cut, taper, and smooth the internal limbs.

Generally, the T-tube should be plugged at all times to allow the natural humidification of the upper airway as well as normal phonation. Open T-tubes can promote dry secretions, which have a greater potential for obstruction. During the first few postoperative weeks, manufacturers recommend that 1 to 2 ml of saline be instilled into the lumen up to three times daily. The extraluminal limb should be cleaned with a hydrogen peroxide–soaked cotton-tipped swab.

Frequent suctioning several times a day is recommended during the early postoperative period after placement of a T-tube. One source stated that suctioning is not necessary after the initial postoperative period (Wahidi & Ernst, 2003); however, manufacturers recommend suctioning twice daily. The suction catheter should be small enough that it is easily inserted into the T-tube to traverse both the upper and lower limbs. To suction the lower limb, the extraluminal limb should be bent gently upward and the catheter should be directed caudad (Figure 7.4). To suction the upper limb, the extraluminal limb should be bent downward and the catheter should be directed cephalad. To avoid mucosal irritation, the suction catheter should not be advanced beyond the level of the intraluminal limbs.

A separate 15-mm adapter can be ordered for use when positive-pressure ventilation is needed with a T-tube (Jessup & Stephan, 1993). An alternative option is to replace the narrow lumen stent with a standard tracheostomy tube, but this approach should be considered carefully in terms of the patency of the airway. Wouters, Byreddy, Gleeson, and Morley (2008) presented a stimulating case discussion of the challenges presented by the T-tube when planning anesthetic management for a surgical procedure. Early removal of the T-tube may leave the tracheal graft unsupported. If positive-pressure ventilation is required, a simple solution recommended by the manufacturer is to occlude the upper limb of the T-tube with a small balloon catheter. It is necessary to first tilt the external limb downward and then insert the catheter cephalad and ensure the balloon remains within the T-tube. When the balloon is inflated, a closed

7.4

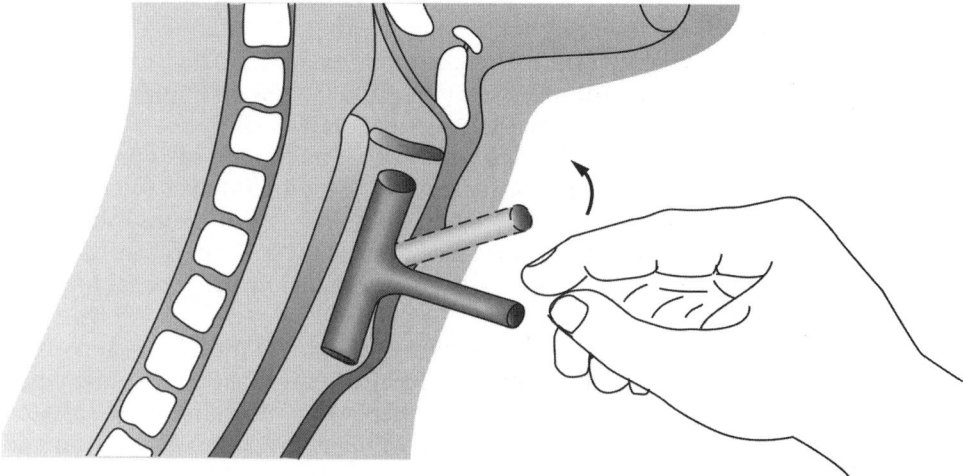

Suctioning T-tube. Note that the external limb is lifted up to straighten the tube and allow suctioning of the lower intraluminal limb. Alternatively, the external limb is pulled downward to suction the upper intraluminal limb.

system is achieved. Another option is to use a new T-tube device called the Hebeler tube, which has a built-in balloon around the upper intraluminal limb.

When a patient has a T-tube in place, emergency equipment, including a smaller cuffed tracheostomy tube and obturator, should be readily available. A curved hemostat should also be available to retrieve any pieces of the tube in case emergency removal is required. As the patient recovers from anesthesia, it is recommended to keep the external lumen plugged if possible. If plugging is not possible, then humidified air or oxygen should be used.

Postoperative care includes lavaging the tube and cleansing the stoma three times daily with a 1:1 solution of peroxide and saline. The stoma should also be inspected for redness or edema. The ring washer on the external limb should also be monitored for inward or outward movement. Any movement of this washer can indicate edema or posterior displacement.

Care of the Tracheal Cannula

A tracheal cannula is designed to provide a secondary airway instead of a standard tracheostomy tube. It fits within the stoma and against the anterior tracheal wall. It is effective for long-term use for up to 6 months, and then it should be replaced. However, the tracheal cannula cannot be used for positive-pressure ventilation or for patients at risk of aspiration.

After the surgical procedure to insert the cannula, it is recommended that the faceplate be left in place for up to 10 days or until the incision is healed. The skin under the faceplate or ring washer should be cleaned twice per day with cotton-tipped applicators soaked in a 1:1 solution of hydrogen peroxide and saline. When the cannula is not needed for access, it can be plugged.

Nutrition

Adequate nutrition is important to provide wound healing and the strength required to do the work of breathing. It is commonly held that "whenever the gut works, use it." Enteral feeding eliminates the problems, primarily infection, associated with parenteral nutrition. However, enteral feeding should be administered with caution in the patient with a tracheostomy.

The effectiveness of the swallowing reflex must be determined prior to beginning oral feeding. The prolonged presence of an artificial airway can interfere with glottic function by applying mechanical pressure against the vocal cords. Vocal cord edema, or temporary paresis, can result. Most often these issues resolve over time, but in a few cases, full function of the glottis does not return.

All patients should initially be considered at risk for aspiration when given enteral feedings. Patients should be placed with the head of their bed elevated at least 30 degrees or higher. The cuff of the tracheostomy tube should be inflated if there is a question of airway protection. A common practice has been to add blue food dye to enteral feedings to detect aspiration through the tube. However, several studies described severe consequences of prolonged use of blue dye, including enteral bacterial infections, diarrhea, systemic dye absorption, and death. The incidence of toxicity was higher in septic patients (Acheson, 2003; Bell & Fishman, 1990; Maloney & Metheny, 2002). Consequently, the American Association of Critical Care Nurses (AACN) has banned the use of blue dye mixed with enteral feedings (AACN Practice Alert, 2005), although blue dye is still commonly used as part of a test of swallowing function.

Continuous Versus Intermittent Feedings

Small-bore enteral feeding tubes are preferred over larger-bore nasogastric tubes. The smaller diameter reaches farther into the alimentary tract, making aspiration less risky as recently supported by guidelines (Martindale et al., 2009). An important consideration with enteral feedings should be the regular assessment of residual volumes. In contrast to previous practice, recent guidelines suggest that, in the absence of other signs of intolerance, one should provide enteral feeding unless the gastric residual volume is greater than 500 milliliters (Martindale et al.).

Enteral feedings should never be initiated until proper placement of the feeding tube has been confirmed. Local policies should govern the optimal method of assessing proper placement.

Care of the Patient at Home

Patients going home with a tracheostomy require much preplanning and at-home care. Family members must be taught the steps of care and strategies to prevent complications. Capable patients should learn how to care for themselves. The goal of this teaching is for the patients and caregivers to feel safe at home and in the community.

Patient and family teaching should begin with a review of the normal anatomy and physiology of the airway. Reviewing the location of the esophagus related to the trachea can sometimes help patients and family members understand the need for a cuff on the tracheostomy tube when the patient's swallowing mechanism is not optimal.

Patients and family members need to have a list of supplies so they can plan timely replenishment of inventory. All home caregivers need to know the location of emergency supplies so they can be reached immediately. They need to know what type of tracheostomy tube patients have in place and what size suction catheters to use. They should also have an extra tracheostomy tube of the same size and one size smaller to manage inadvertent decannulation if it occurs.

Patients need to know that tracheostomy care at home can be done as a clean procedure, rather than the sterile technique they saw in the hospital. All care of the tracheostomy begins with thorough hand washing. Patients and family members should be taught to wash their hands before touching the tracheostomy and again after care is complete. Gloves can and should also be used, but this is in addition to hand washing and not a substitute for it.

In addition to a review of anatomy and physiology, discharge teaching should also include care of the stoma, care of the inner cannula, suctioning, care of the cuff, and managing emergencies. The caregivers and patients should have a list of phone numbers to contact for support as well as general questions. These emergency phone numbers should include the primary care practitioner, the tracheostomy specialist, the home care company, and the number to summon emergency personnel (e.g., 911). Upon discharge, a phone call should be placed to alert the local fire department that the patient has a tracheostomy. This advance notification could facilitate the timely arrival of the paramedics in the event of an emergency when a tracheostomy patient in distress may not be able to speak.

It is best to conduct teaching sessions with the patient and all family members together so they can all hear the same information at the same time and discuss it among themselves and with the health professional. Supplemental written information should also accompany a demonstration of the techniques because patients and family members are usually overwhelmed with the amount of information provided. They will need reinforcement and repetition in order to feel competent.

Patients and family members should also be taught how to use the manual resuscitation bag. It can be used to give extra breaths with suctioning when needed, but it can also be used in an emergency to deliver air and facilitate a cough.

One of the most difficult procedures for family members to master is suctioning. The procedure itself is overtly unpleasant, and they do not want to harm their loved one and are usually reluctant to cause any discomfort. It is advisable to inform family members that inefficient suctioning is a disservice to their loved one. Each suctioning attempt should be with the goal of mobilizing as great a volume of secretions as possible, thereby minimizing multiple passes of the suction catheter. Useful advice to family members is to provide deep suctioning on the first attempt at minimum. Deep suctioning retrieves a large amount of secretions and also facilitates a deep cough—which, in turn, mobilizes more secretions. Subsequent passes of the suction catheter can be determined based on the yield of the previous pass. Three passes of the suction catheter is the usual maximum for each episode, but this depends on the results. The patient is usually aware of the need for suctioning by the time of hospital discharge. From the patient's perspective, optimal breathing is the anticipated result of suctioning.

In the home setting, Medicare and most insurance companies provide for 90 suction catheters per month, averaging 3 per day. This may not be enough to manage large volumes of secretions. In contrast to the hospital setting, suction catheters can be reused all day in the home. The catheter should be rinsed thoroughly to remove obvious secretions from the inside by filling a small disposable paper cup with tap water and flushing the catheter. In addition, the outside of the catheter should be wiped clean to remove secretions on the outside. Then the catheter can be laid on a paper towel and allowed to air dry in between uses. At the end of the day, the catheter and the paper cup can be discarded.

Patients need to be taught to observe the quality of their secretions. Changes in color, quantity, odor, or thickness should be watched closely and reported promptly to their health care professional.

Patients also need to cleanse the stoma to keep it dry and free of secretions. In the hospital, they may have seen the nurse use hydrogen peroxide; however, long-term use of peroxide on the skin can produce irritation. For this reason, the stoma should be cleansed with cotton-tipped swabs dipped in tap water or saline. Patients and family members should be told to examine the stoma area for redness, swelling, bleeding, or pus. Any of these signs should be reported to their health care provider.

In the early postoperative period, patients are encouraged to keep a drain sponge at the stoma site to protect the skin from constant exposure to secretions. Also, a drain sponge helps cushion the neck flange against the skin of the neck. Only presplit sponges should be used at the stoma site. Gauze dressings should not be cut because shreds may become embedded in the tissue and create inflammation.

Patients and family members should also be taught to clean the stoma and inner cannula on a regular basis. Depending on the patient's condition, a larger volume of secretions is often produced in the early postoperative period and tends to lessen over time. For this reason, care of the stoma and inner cannula is often done routinely up to three times per day in the hospital (and as needed) and can be decreased to twice per day when at home and secretions have diminished.

Managing Home Emergencies

Before emergency personnel are mobilized, patients and family members must begin efforts to manage an emergency (see Table 7.2). By far, most tracheostomy emergencies are the result of mucus plugs. Patients and family members should be aware that the best way to manage mucus plugs is to prevent them with adequate hydration to thin secretions and vigorous physical mobility to loosen secretions, strengthen respiratory muscles, and facilitate an effective cough to expel secretions.

7.2 Managing an Emergency

1. Remove inner cannula (clean if obstructed).
2. Suction deeply.
3. Use manual resuscitation bag to provide rescue breaths.
4. Change entire tracheostomy tube. (If tube is still obstructed and stoma is mature, remove tube and suction directly into stoma.)
5. Provide Heimlich maneuver.

The initial presenting symptom of a mucus plug is usually dyspnea or shortness of breath. The patient should first be taught to check his or her inner cannula. After it is removed, it will be obvious if it is clogged with secretions; if it is, it should be cleaned or replaced. If removal of the inner cannula is not successful in resolving the dyspnea, the problem is still likely to be a mucus plug further down in the tracheobronchial tree. If removal of the inner cannula does not relieve the shortness of breath, the patient should suction himself. If the patient is still short of breath after these two maneuvers, emergency help should be summoned. Meanwhile, there are other steps the patient can take. The manual resuscitation bag can be used to provide rescue breaths. Several small breaths can be delivered, followed by one or two large and forceful breaths. The purpose of the larger breaths is to promote a strong cough.

Patients and family members should be taught the Heimlich maneuver in order to help dislodge a mucus plug. If all of the aforementioned have not been successful, the entire tracheostomy tube should be changed. Often, a mucus plug is pulled out when the entire tracheostomy tube is changed.

Activities of Daily Living

At home, patients should be able to assimilate well into usual family life. Outside of the care required for the tracheostomy, there are few restrictions. A tracheostomy need not restrict activities, but a few simple precautions are necessary. Patients can shower and bathe normally as long as care is taken to avoid splashing or spraying water into the tracheostomy. Several devices such as shower collars can be used if there is concern about splashed water.

Tracheostomy patients may be more sensitive to odors and inhalants. Perfume and cologne use may need to be restricted. Of course, smoking should not be allowed in the home.

Pets may cause some concerns in terms of inhalation of stray hair. Pets that sleep next to, or in close proximity to, patients may need to be relocated to minimize the inhalation of pet hair or dander. A stoma grid or filter can be used if there are concerns about inhaled particulate matter.

Patients with tracheostomies need to minimize their exposure to dust and other allergens. If patients will be exposed to these environmental hazards, a filter or mask can be used to cover the tracheostomy.

Patients with tracheostomies who experience some discomfort with lack of humidity can use an HME. Misted saline (such as Ocean nasal spray) can be instilled into the tracheostomy and mucous membranes. Alternatively, patients can become comfortable simply by using a room humidifier.

Summary

Patients with tracheostomies require vigilant care in order to prevent complications. The most common complication is the development of mucus plugs resulting from thickened secretions. Routine care includes cleaning the stoma and inner cannula as well as regular tube changes to prevent infection. Colonization is common but does not require treatment unless there are outward signs of infection.

When discharged home, patients and their family members require extensive teaching in order to become comfortable with daily care and emergency procedures. It is essential for all caregivers to ensure supplies and emergency equipment are always available and functional. With attention to proper care, patients with tracheostomies can live long and productive lives.

Key Points

- During the first postoperative week, the security of the tracheostomy tube is a priority.
- The inner cannula, when present, should be cleaned regularly to prevent tube obstruction.
- Cuff pressures should be maintained at 20–25 cm H_2O to prevent overinflation or underinflation of the cuff.
- Routine tube changes should take place every 1–2 months.
- The mainstay of secretion management includes adequate hydration and humidity, suctioning, and physical mobility.

Available Resources for the Tracheostomy Patient

There are many resources available for patients with tracheostomies and many more for the health care professional.

Patient Resources

Devices for laryngectomy patients, including HMEs, shower collars, phonating devices such as electrolarynx, and reference books. Luminaud, Inc. Retrieved October 26, 2009, from http://www.luminaud.com

Discussion forums for tracheostomy patients and caregivers. Tracheotomy.info: A community for tracheotomy wearers and the people who love them. Retrieved October 26, 2009, from http://www.tracheotomy.info/index.php

Information about oral cancer, American Head and Neck Society. Retrieved October 26, 2009, from http://www.headandneckcancer.org/patienteducation/docs/oralcavity.php

Pediatric tracheostomy information, advice for parents, and listserv. Aaron's Tracheostomy Page. Retrieved October 26, 2009, from http://www.tracheostomy.com

Tracheostomy products, featuring TRACOE and Moore tracheostomy tubes, Montgomery buttons and valves, and Singer and TRACOE laryngectomy tubes. Also features protective neckwear, shower protection, cleaning supplies, and accessories. Boston Medical Products, Inc. Retrieved October 26, 2009, from http://www.trachs.com

Professional Resources

Devices for laryngectomy patients. Atos Medical. Retrieved October 26, 2009, from http://www.atosmedical.com

Education and research forum for healthcare professionals regarding care of the tracheostomy patient, TrachResource.com, www.TrachResource.com

Passy-Muir speaking valves and educational materials. Passy-Muir, Inc. Retrieved October 26, 2009, from http://www.passy-muir.com/

Pilling products catalog 2007. Teleflex Medical. 2917 Weck Drive, Research Triangle Park, NC 27709.

Portex and Bivona tracheostomy products. Smiths Medical. Retrieved October 26, 2009, from http://www.smiths-medical.com/products/tracheostomy/

Shiley tracheostomy products. Nellcor Tyco Healthcare. Retrieved October 26, 2009, from http://www.nellcor.com/prod/List.aspx?S1=AIR

Tracheostomy and airway products, featuring TRACOE and Moore tracheostomy tubes, Montgomery and Dumont stents, and Singer and TRACOE laryngectomy tubes. Boston Medical Products. Retrieved October 26, 2009, from http://www.bosmed.com

References

Acheson, D. (2003). FDA Public Health Advisory. *Reports of blue discoloration and death in patients receiving enteral feedings tinted with the dye, FD&C Blue No. 1.* Retrieved September 23, 2008, from http://www.cfsan.fda.gov/~dms/col-ltr2.html

Ackerman, M., & Gugerty, B. P. (1990, Spring). The effect of normal saline bolus instillation in artificial airways. *Journal of the Society of Otorhinolaryngology and Head-Neck Nursing*, 14–17.

American Association of Critical Care Nurses. (2005). AACN Practice Alert: Dye in enteral feeding. Retrieved from http://www.aacn.org/WD/Practice/Docs/Dye_in_Enteral_Feeding_4-2005.pdf

American Thoracic Society. (2000). Care of the child with a chronic tracheostomy. *American Journal of Respiratory Critical Care Medicine, 161,* 297–308.

Arroyo-Novoa, C. M., Figueroa-Ramos, M. I., Puntillo, K. A., Stanik-Hutt, J., Thompson, C. L., White, C., et al. (2008). Pain related to tracheal suctioning in awake acutely and critically ill adults: A descriptive study. *Intensive and Critical Care Nursing, 24,* 20–27.

Bell, R., & Fishman, S. (1990). Eosinophilia from food dye added to enteral feedings [Letter]. *New England Journal of Medicine, 322,* 1822.

Bergbom-Engberg, I., & Halijamae, H. (1989). A retrospective study of patients' recall of respiratory treatment: Nursing care factors and feelings of security/insecurity. *Intensive Care Nursing, 4*(3), 95–101.

Bernhard, W. N., Yost, L., Joynes, D., Cothalis, S., & Turndorf, H. (1985). Cuff pressures in endotracheal and tracheostomy tubes. Related cuff physical characteristics. *Chest, 87,* 720–725.

Bjorling, G., Belin, A., Hellstrom, C., Schedin, U., Ransjo, U., Alenius, M., et al. (2007). Tracheostomy inner cannula care: A randomized crossover study of two decannulation procedures. *American Journal of Infection Control, 35,* 600–605.

Blackwood, B. (1999). Normal saline instillation with endotracheal suctioning: Primum non nocere (first do no harm). *Journal of Advanced Nursing, 29*(4), 928–934.

Bouza, E., Perez, M. J., Munoz, P., Rincon, C., Barrio, J. M., & Hortal, J. (2008). Continuous aspiration of subglottic secretions in the prevention of ventilator-associated pneumonia in the postoperative period of major heart surgery. *Chest, 134*(5), 938–946.

Branson, R. D. (2007). Secretion management in the mechanically ventilated patient. *Respiratory Care, 52*(10), 1328–1347.

Branson, R. D., Campbell, R. S., Chatburn, R. L., & Covington, J. (1993). Endotracheal suctioning of mechanically ventilated adults and children with artificial airways. *Respiratory Care, 38*(5), 500–504.

Brook, I. (1979). Bacterial colonization, tracheobronchitis, and pneumonia following tracheostomy and long-term intubation in pediatric patients. *Chest, 76*(4), 420–424.

Burns, S. M., Spilman, M., Wilmoth, D., Carpenter, R., Turrentine, B., Wiley, B., et al. (1998). Are frequent inner cannula changes necessary? A pilot study. *Heart and Lung, 27*(1), 58–62.

Caruso, P., Denari, S., Ruiz, S.A.L., Demarzo, S. E., & Deheinzelin, D. (2009). Saline instillation before tracheal suctioning decreases the incidence of ventilator-associated pneumonia. *Critical Care Medicine, 37*(1), 32–38.

Celik, S. A., & Kanan, N. (2006). A current conflict: Use of isotonic sodium chloride solution on endotracheal suctioning in critically ill patients. *Dimensions in Critical Care Nursing, 25*(1), 11–14.

Chan, E. Y., Ruest, A., Meade, M. O., & Cook, D. J. (2007). Oral decontamination for prevention of pneumonia in mechanically ventilated adults: Systematic review and meta-analysis. *BMJ, 334*(7599), 1–11.

Chlebicki, M. P., & Safdar, N. (2007). Topical chlorhexidine for prevention of ventilator-associated pneumonia: A meta-analysis. *Critical Care Medicine, 35*(2), 595–602.

Coffman, H.M.S., Rees, C. J., Sievers, A.E.F., & Belafsky, P. C. (2008). Proximal suction tracheotomy tube reduces aspiration volume. *Otolaryngology—Head and Neck Surgery, 138*(4), 441–445.

Combes, P., Fauvage, B., & Oleyer, C. (2000). Nosocomial pneumonia in mechanically ventilated patients, a prospective randomized evaluation of the Stericath closed suctioning system. *Intensive Care Medicine, 26*(7), 878–882.

Copnell, B., Tingay, D. G., Kiraly, N. J., Sourial, M., Gordon, M. J., Mills, J. F., et al. (2007). A comparison of the effectiveness of open and closed endotracheal suction. *Intensive Care Medicine, 33,* 1655–1662.

Crimlisk, J. T., O'Donnell, C., & Grillone, G. A. (2006). Standardizing adult tracheostomy tube styles: What is the clinical and cost-effective impact? *Dimensions in Critical Care Nursing, 25*(1), 35–43.

Day, T., Farnell, S., & Wilson-Barnett, J. (2002). Suctioning: A review of current research recommendations. *Intensive and Critical Care Nursing, 18*(2), 79–89.

Demers, R. R., & Saklad, M. (1973). Minimizing the harmful effects of mechanical aspiration. *Heart and Lung, 2*(4), 542–545.

Dennis-Rouse, M. D., & Davidson, J. E. (2008). An evidence-based evaluation of tracheostomy care practices. *Critical Care Nursing Quarterly, 31*(2), 150–160.

Dixon, L., & Wasson, D. (1998). Comparing use and cost effectiveness of tracheostomy tube securing devices. *Medsurg Nursing, 7*(5), 270–274.

Duguet, A., D'Amico, L., Biondi, G., Prodanovic, H., Gonzalez-Bermejo, J., & Similowski, T. (2007). Control of tracheal cuff pressure: A pilot study using a pneumatic device. *Intensive Care Medicine, 33,* 128–132.

Epstein, S. K. (2005). Late complications of tracheostomy. *Respiratory Care, 50*(4), 542–549.

Faris, C., Koury, E., Philpott, J., Sharma, S., Tolley, N., & Narula, A. (2007). Estimation of tracheostomy tube cuff pressure by pilot balloon palpation. *Journal of Laryngology and Otology, 121*(9), 869–871.

Fernandez, R., Blanch, L., Mancebo, J., Bonsoms, N., & Artigas, A. (1990). Endotracheal tube cuff pressure assessment: Pitfalls of finger estimation and need for objective measurement. *Critical Care Medicine, 18*(12), 1423–1426.

Fields, L. B. (2008). Oral care intervention to reduce incidence of ventilator-associated pneumonia in the neurologic intensive care unit. *Journal of Neuroscience Nursing, 40*(5), 291–298.

French, B. A., & Bauer, B. S. (2002). Incidence of normal saline lavage by RTs in a large acute care hospital. *Respiratory Care,* 2002 Open Forum Abstracts.

Glass, C. A., & Grap, M. J. (1995). Ten tips for safer suctioning. *American Journal of Nursing, 95*(5), 51–53.

Gray, J. E., MacIntyre, N. R., & Kronenberger, W. G. (1990). The effects of bolus normal-saline instillation in conjunction with endotracheal suctioning. *Respiratory Care, 35*(8), 785–790.

Griggs, A. (1998). Tracheostomy: Suctioning and humidification. *Nursing Standard, 13*(2), 49–53.

Hagler, D. A., & Traver, G. A. (1994). Endotracheal saline and suction catheters: Sources of lower airway contamination. *American Journal of Critical Care, 3*(6), 444–447.

Hanley, M. V., Raud, T., & Butler, J. (1978). What happens to endotracheal instillations? [Abstract]. *American Review of Respiratory Disease, 117*(4, Pt. 2), 124.

Hess, D. R. (2002). And now for the rest of the story [Letter]. *Respiratory Care, 47*(6), 696–699.

Hoffman, R. J., Parwani, V., & Hahn, I. (2006). Experienced emergency medicine physicians cannot safely inflate or estimate endotracheal tube cuff pressure using standard techniques. *American Journal of Emergency Medicine, 24,* 139–143.

Hotter, A. N., & Warfield, K. (1997). Technique for promoting healing of complex tracheostomy wounds. *Otolaryngology—Head and Neck Surgery, 11*(6), 693–695.

Hudak, M., & Hickey, M. M. (2008). Nursing management of the patient with a tracheostomy. In E. M. Myers & J. T. Johnson (Eds.), *Tracheotomy: Airway management, communication, and swallowing.* San Diego, CA: Plural Publishing.

Ireton, J. (2007). Tracheostomy suction: A protocol for practice. *Paediatric Nursing, 19*(10), 14–18.

Jessup, B., & Stephan, N. (1993). What nurses need to know and teach their patients about the care and maintenance of the Montgomery Safe-T-Tube. *ORL Head and Neck Nursing, 11*(3), 23–27.

Johnson, J. T. (2008). Tracheostomy in patients with the obstructive sleep apnea syndrome. In E. N. Myers & J. T. Johnson (Eds.), *Tracheotomy: Airway management, communication, and swallowing* (pp. 141–146). San Diego, CA: Plural Publishing.

Johnson, J. T., Wagner, R. L., & Sigler, B. A. (1988). Disposable inner cannula tracheostomy tube: A prospective clinical trial. *Otolaryngology—Head and Neck Surgery, 99*(1), 83–84.

Kost, K. M. (2008). Tracheostomy in the intensive care unit setting. In E. N. Myers & J. T. Johnson (Eds.), *Tracheotomy: Airway management, communication, and swallowing* (pp. 83–116). San Diego, CA: Plural Publishing.

Lewis, R. M. (2002). Airway clearance techniques for the patient with an artificial airway. *Respiratory Care, 47*(7), 808–817.

Liew, L., Gibbins, N., & Oyarzabal, M. (2008). How I do it: Securing tracheostomy tubes. *European Archives of Otorhinolaryngology, 265*(5), 607, 608.

Maggiore, S. M., Jacobone, E., Zito, G., Conti, G., Antonelli, M., & Proietti, R. (2002). Closed versus open suctioning techniques. *Minerva Anestesiologica, 68,* 360–364.

Maloney, J., & Metheny, N. (2002). Controversy in using blue dye in enteral feedings as a method for detecting pulmonary aspiration. *Critical Care Nurse, 22,* 84–86.

Martindale, R. G., McClave, S. A., Vanek, V. W., McCarthy, M., Roberts, P., Taylor, B., et al. American College of Critical Care Medicine, ASPEN Board of Directors (2009). Guidelines for the provision and assessment of nutrition support therapy in the adult critically ill patient: Society of Critical Care Medicine and American Society for Parenteral and Enteral Nutrition: Executive summary. *Critical Care Medicine, 37*(5), 1757–1761.

Morris, L. G., Zoumalan, R. A., Roccaforte, J. D., & Amin, M. R. (2007). Monitoring tracheal tube cuff pressures in the intensive care unit: A comparison of digital palpation and manometry. *Annals of Otology, Rhinology, and Laryngology, 116*(9), 639–642.

Morris, P. E., Goad, A., Thompson, C., Taylor, K., Harry, B., Passmore, L., et al. (2008). Early intensive care unit mobility therapy in the treatment of acute respiratory failure. *Critical Care Medicine, 36*(8), 2238–2243.

Niel-Weise, B. S., Snoeren, R. L., & van den Broek, P. J. (20007). Policies for endotracheal suctioning of patients receiving mechanical ventilation: A systematic review of randomized controlled trials. *Infection Control and Hospital Epidemiology, 28*(5), 531–536.

Nouraei, S. A., Nouraei, S. M., Upile, T., Taylor, M., Patel, A., & Sandhu, G. S. (2008). A four-point suture fixation technique for securing surgical tracheostomies. *Clinical Otolaryngology, 33,* 196–199.

Odell, A., Allder, A., Bayne, R., Everett, C., Scott, S., Still, B., et al. (1993). Endotracheal suction for adult non-head injured patients. A review of the literature. *Intensive & Critical Care Nursing, 9*(4), 274–278.

Oh, H., & Seo, W. (2003). A meta-analysis of the effects of various interventions in preventing endotracheal suction-induced hypoxemia. *Journal of Clinical Nursing, 12,* 912–924.

O'Neal, P. V., Grap, M. V., Thompson, C., & Dudley, W. (2001). Level of dyspnoea experienced in mechanically ventilated adults with and without saline instillation prior to endotracheal suctioning. *Intensive & Critical Care Nursing, 17,* 356–363.

Pedersen, C. M., Rosendahl-Nielsen, M., Hjermind, J., & Egerod, I. (2008). Endotracheal suctioning of the adult intubated patient: What is the evidence? *Intensive & Critical Care Nursing, 25*(1), 21–30.

Peruzzi, W. T., & Smith, B. (1995). Bronchial hygiene therapy. *Critical Care Clinics, 11*(1), 716–720.

Puntillo, K. A., White, C., Morris, A. B., Perdue, S. T., Stanik-Hutt, J., Thompson, C. L., et al. (2001). Patients' perceptions and responses to procedural pain: Results from Thunder Project II. *American Journal of Critical Care, 10,* 238–251.

Raymond, S. J. (1995). Normal saline instillation before suctioning: Helpful or harmful? A review of the literature. *American Journal of Critical Care, 4*(4), 267–271.

Rello, J., Sonora, R., Jubert, P., Artigas, A., Rue, M., & Valles, J. (1996). Pneumonia in intubated patients: Role of respiratory airway care. *American Journal of Respiratory Critical Care Medicine, 154*(1), 111–115.

Rubin, B. K. (2002). Physiology of airway mucus clearance. *Respiratory Care, 47*(7), 761.

St. John, R. E., & Malen, J. F. (2004). Contemporary issues in adult tracheostomy management. *Critical Care Nursing Clinics of North America, 16*(3), 413–430.

Sawyer, N. (1997). Back from the twilight zone. *Nursing Times, 93*(7), 28–29.

Schwenker, D., Ferrin, M., & Gift, A. G. (1998). A survey of endotracheal suctioning with instillation of normal saline. *American Journal of Critical Care, 7*(4), 255–260.

Seay, S. J., & Gay, S. L. (2002). Tracheostomy emergencies: Correcting accidental decannulation or displaced tracheostomy tube. *American Journal of Nursing, 102*(3), 59–63.

Seymour, C. W., Cross, B. J., Cooke, C. R., Gallop, R. L., & Fuchs, B. D. (2009). Physiologic impact of closed-suction endotracheal suctioning in spontaneously breathing patients receiving mechanical ventilation. *Respiratory Care, 54*(3), 367–374.

Shah, C., & Kollef, M. H. (2004). Endotracheal tube intraluminal volume loss among mechanically ventilated patients. *Critical Care Medicine, 32*(1), 120–125.

Shapiro, B. A., Harrison, R. A., Kacmarek, R. M., & Cane, R. D. (1985). *Clinical application of respiratory care* (3rd ed.). Chicago: Yearbook Medical Publishers.

Siempos, I. I., Vardakas, K. Z., & Falagas, M. E. (2008). Closed tracheal suction systems for prevention of ventilator-associated pneumonia. *British Journal of Anaesthesia, 100*(3), 299–306.

Sole, M. L., Penoyer, D. A., Su, X., Jimenez, E., Kalita, S. J., Poallilo, E., et al. (2009). Assessment of endotracheal cuff pressure by continuous monitoring: A pilot study. *American Journal of Critical Care, 18*(2), 133–143.

Sona, C. S., Zack, J. E., Schallom, M. E., McSweeney, M., McMullen, K., Thomas, J., et al. (2009). The impact of a simple, low-cost oral care protocol on ventilator-associated pneumonia in a surgical intensive care unit. *Journal of Intensive Care Medicine, 24*(1), 54–62.

Spence, K., Gillies, D., & Waterworth, L. (2003). Deep versus shallow suction of endotracheal tubes in ventilated neonates and young infants. *Cochrane Database of Systematic Reviews, 3,* CD003309.

Stewart, S. L., Secrest, J. A., Norwood, B. R., & Zachary, R. (2003). A comparison of endotracheal tube cuff pressures using estimation techniques and direct intracuff measurement. *AANA Journal, 71*(6), 443–7.

Stone, K. S., Preusser, B. A., Groch, K. F., Karl, J. I., & Gonyon, D. S. (1991). The effect of lung hyperinflation and endotracheal suctioning on cardiopulmonary hemodynamics. *Nursing Research, 40*(2), 76–80.

Swartz, K., Noonan, D. M., & Edwards-Beckett, J. (1996). A national survey of endotracheal suctioning techniques in the pediatric population. *Heart and Lung, 25*(1), 52–60.

Tantipong, H., Morkchareonpong, C., Jaiyindee, S., & Thamlikitkul, V. (2009). Randomized controlled trial and meta-analysis of oral decontamination with 2% chlorhexidine solution for the prevention of ventilator-associated pneumonia. *Infection Control and Hospital Epidemiology, 29*(2), 131–136.

Tenaillon, A. (1990). Tracheobronchial suctions during mechanical ventilation. *Update in Intensive Care Emergency Medicine, 10,* 196–200.

Topeli, A., Harmanci, A., Cetinkaya, Y., Akdeniz, S., & Unal, S. (2004). Comparison of the effect of closed versus open endotracheal suction systems on the development of ventilator-associated pneumonia. *Journal of Hospital Infection, 58*(1), 14–19.

Tsai, H., Lin, F., & Change, S. (2008). Intermittent suction of oral secretions before each position change may reduce ventilator-associated pneumonia: A pilot study. *American Journal of Medical Science, 336*(5), 397–401.

Tsunezuka, Y., Suzuki, M., Nitta, K., & Oda, M. (2005). The use of fibrous wound dressing sheets made of carboxymethylcellulose natrium in the postoperative management of tracheostomy. *Kyobu Geka, 58*(12), 1063–1067.

Van de Leur, J. P., Zwaveling, J. H., Loef, B. G., & Van der Shans, C. P. (2003). Endotracheal suctioning versus minimally invasive airway suctioning in intubated patients: A prospective randomized controlled trial. *Intensive Care Medicine, 29*(3), 426–432.

Vonberg, R. P., Eckmanns, T., Welte, T., & Gastmeier, P. (2006). Impact of the suctioning system (open vs. closed) on the incidence of ventilation-associated pneumonia: Meta-analysis of randomized controlled trials. *Intensive Care Medicine, 32*(9), 1329–1335.

Wahidi, M. M., & Ernst A. (2003). The Montgomery T-tube tracheal stent. *Clinics in Chest Medicine, 24,* 437–443.

Walvekar, R. R., & Myers, E. N. (2008). Technique and complications of tracheostomy in adults. In E. N. Myers & J. T. Johnson (Eds.), *Tracheotomy: Airway management, communication, and swallowing.* San Diego, CA: Plural Publishing.

Wip, C., & Napolitano, L. (2009). Bundles to prevent ventilator-associated pneumonia: How valuable are they? *Current Opinion in Infectious Disease, 22*(2), 159–166.

Wood, C. J. (1998). Can nurses safely assess the need for endotracheal suction in short-term ventilated patients, instead of using routine techniques? *Intensive Critical Care Nursing, 14*(4), 170–178.

Wouters, K.M.A., Byreddy, R., Gleeson, J., & Morley, A. P. (2008). New approach to anaesthetizing a patient at risk of pulmonary aspiration with a Montgomery T-tube in situ. *British Journal of Anaesthesia, 101,* 354–357.

Wright, S. E., & Van Dahm, K. (2003). Long term care of the tracheostomy patient. *Clinics in Chest Medicine, 24,* 473–487.

Yaremchuk, K. (2003). Regular tracheostomy tube changes to prevent formation of granulation tissue. *Laryngoscope, 113,* 1–10.

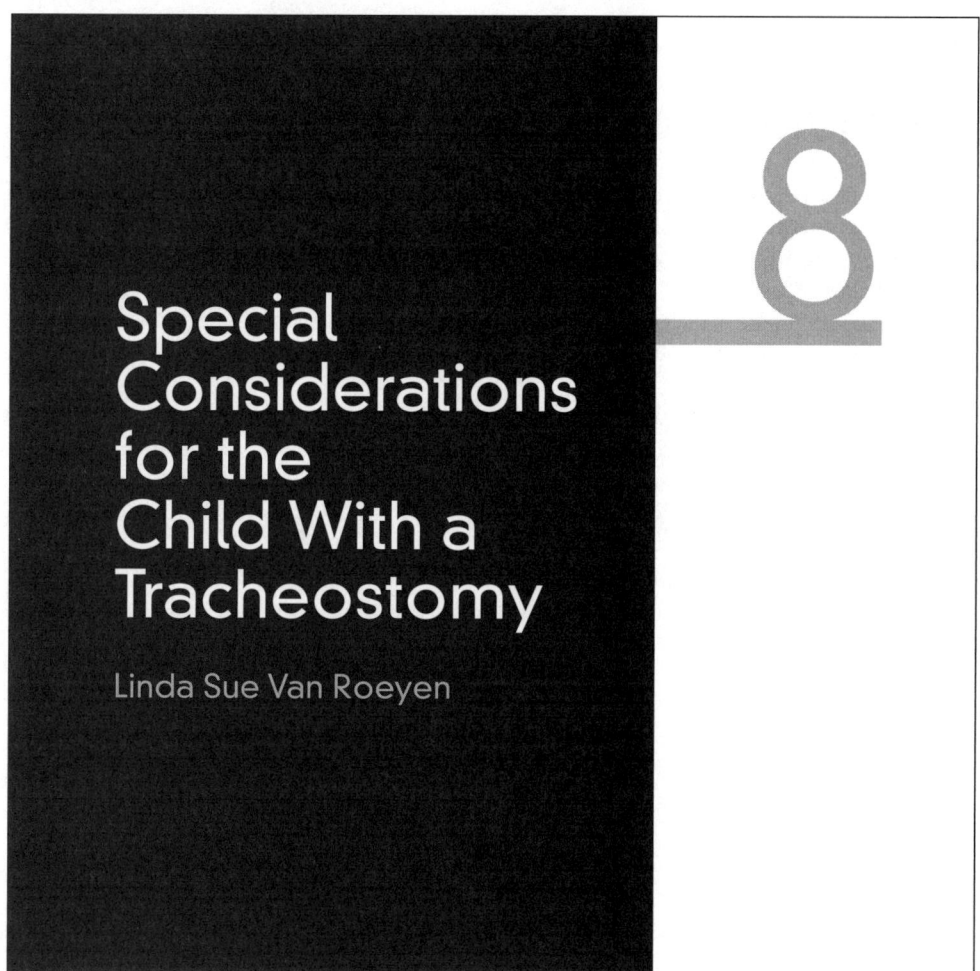

Special Considerations for the Child With a Tracheostomy

Linda Sue Van Roeyen

Advances in technology have brought about new developments in noninvasive ventilatory support, and increasing numbers of premature infants and children with tracheostomies require home care. Additionally, home ventilation with a tracheostomy is becoming an increasingly available alternative to prolonged intubation and hospitalization.

Changing trends in pediatric care have become apparent over the past 30 years. The numbers of tracheotomies for upper airway obstruction have decreased while the need for prolonged mechanical ventilation has increased. More tracheotomies are performed during the first year of life than any other pediatric age group (Wooten et al., 2006). Feudtner and others (2005) found that 20% of children discharged from children's hospitals were dependent on a medical device. Lewis, Carron, Perkins, Sie, and Feudtner (2003) found significant regional variation in the discharge disposition of children with tracheostomies. A notable finding was that children from the northeastern or Midwestern United States were more likely to be discharged to long-term health facilities, with the exception of children admitted to children's hospitals or teaching institutions, where they were less likely to be discharged to long-term care facilities.

Indications for Tracheostomy in Children

The decision to provide a tracheostomy for a child is made on an individual basis and is based on family dynamics, individual patient factors, and the initial process that led to prolonged intubation. The patient's underlying disease process dictates whether the child is a candidate for a tracheostomy and/or long-term ventilation. Ventilator-dependent children must repeatedly demonstrate their inability to maintain independent oxygenation and ventilation prior to the initiation of a tracheostomy.

Indications for tracheostomy in children fall into several categories: pulmonary and airway disorders, neuromuscular conditions (including diaphragm and chest wall), central nervous system disorders, and acquired conditions such as trauma and smoke inhalation. See Table 8.1 for a list of indications for tracheostomy in children.

Patient prognosis depends on the underlying medical condition. In many neonatal units, the complications of long-term intubation have become one of the most important indicators for tracheostomy. Parilla, Scarano, Guidi, Galli, and Paludetti (2007) reviewed current trends in pediatric tracheostomies. In a study of 38 patients given tracheostomies for respiratory failure and upper airway obstruction, the complication rate of long-term intubation in children less than 1 year of age was 42.1% compared to 26.3% for those over 1 year of age. The change in indication also showed a decrease in the average age of children who required tracheostomies.

Patients with chronic lung and diaphragm problems can become candidates for weaning from ventilator support. As diaphragm strength increases and new lung tissue continues to develop until approximately age 2, children are more likely to tolerate decreasing ventilator support. Growth and development issues are carefully monitored from infancy to early childhood to ensure calories are used for normal growth and development. Children with neuromuscular disease require supportive care over a lifetime, while those with central nervous system conditions may only need ventilator support during sleep.

Outcome of Children With Tracheostomies

There are few studies related to the outcome of children with tracheostomies. One retrospective survey examined home mechanical ventilation in 20 Italian children (Otonello et al., 2007). Their diagnoses included myopathic disorder, congenital central hypoventilation syndrome, chest wall disorder, cystic fibrosis, pulmonary hypertension, and diaphragmatic paralysis. The goals for optimal ventilation included maintaining normal oxygenation and ventilation, minimizing work of breathing, and supporting normal growth and development. Unfortunately, the children with tracheostomies had frequent elective hospital admissions, an increased number of emergency admissions, longer inpatient stays, and many readmissions within a short time from discharge.

A recent retrospective study at Baylor College of Medicine reviewed 70 children and adolescents who underwent tracheostomy placement over a 24-month period. Median hospital stay was 46 days. Within a 6-month period, 63% of children were readmitted, and there was a mortality rate of 13%. None

8.1 Indications for Tracheostomy in a Child

General Condition	Indication
Pulmonary disorders	■ Chronic lung disease ■ Bronchopulmonary dysplasia ■ Meconium aspiration ■ Congestive heart failure ■ Respiratory distress syndrome ■ Chronic aspiration ■ Airway disease ■ Stenosis ■ Malacia ■ Congenital malformation of the chest wall or diaphragm ■ Diaphragmatic hernia ■ Omphalocele ■ Phrenic nerve injury
Neuromuscular disorders	■ Spinal muscular atrophy ■ Degeneration of the anterior horn cells ■ Muscular atrophy ■ Fatty infiltration of muscle ■ Spinal cord injury
Central nervous system disorders	■ Central hypoventilation ■ Central sleep apnea
Acquired conditions	■ Trauma ■ Smoke inhalation ■ Foreign body aspiration
Other	■ Infection ■ Neoplasms ■ Respiratory papillomatosis ■ Respiratory hemangiomas ■ Obstructive sleep apnea ■ Aspiration due to neurologic lesions ■ Pulmonary toilet for chronic aspiration ■ Tracheoesophageal fistula ■ Cleft larynx

of the deaths, however, were related to the tracheostomy (Graf, Montagnino, Hueckel, & McPherson, 2008a).

A German retrospective study of 85 children in a pediatric ICU reviewed the experience of tracheostomies over an 8-year period. Indications for tracheostomy included upper airway obstruction, craniofacial syndromes, long-term mechanical ventilation, neurological deficits, trauma and sequelae, and bilateral vocal cord paralysis. Successful decannulation occurred in 50.6% of patients, with a mean cannulation time of 21.6 months (Zenk et al., 2009).

Procedural Steps in the Care of the Child With a Tracheostomy

Tube Selection

Performing a tracheostomy in children can be more difficult than in adults. (See chapter 2 for discussion of a pediatric tracheotomy.) The trachea is more pliable, making it difficult to palpate, and the operative area is smaller, requiring an otolaryngologist skilled with pediatric patients. There are many types of neonatal and pediatric tracheostomy tubes available (Figure 8.1, Figure 8.2, Table 4.3). Like adult tubes, materials include polyvinyl chloride, polyurethane, silicone, and metal. Cuffed tubes are rarely used with neonatal and pediatric patients but can improve the delivery of tidal volume when the patient is ventilator dependent. When a tube with extended length is required, a pediatric tube should still be chosen over an adult tube because they are significantly shorter. Inner cannulas are never used because of the very narrow inner diameter of neonatal and pediatric tubes.

8.1

Shiley pediatric tracheostomy.

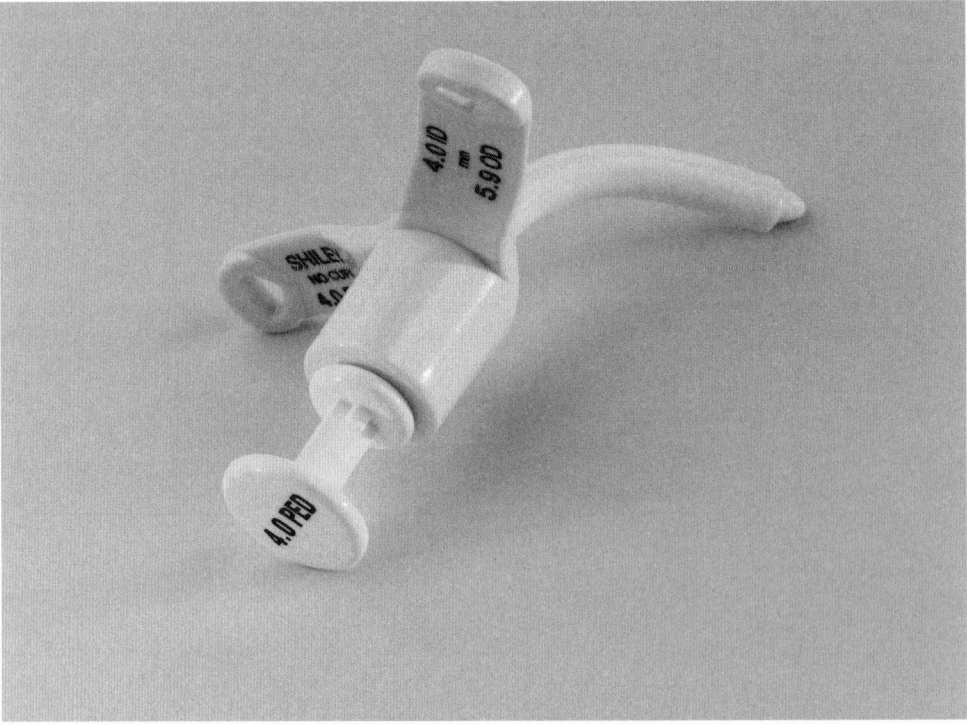

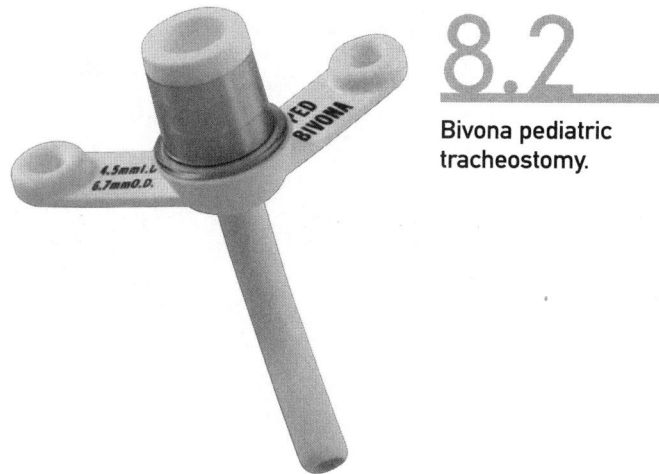

8.2

Bivona pediatric tracheostomy.

The type of tracheostomy tube is also selected based on the shape and length of the airway to prevent pressure on any portion of the neck or trachea. The flexibility of the tube is also taken into consideration. For example, tubes made of silicone are generally more flexible than those made from polyvinyl chloride (PVC) or plastic. Tubes made from PVC may become stiffened after 3 to 4 months of use and cleaning, while tubes made from silicone remain flexible. Metal tubes, which can be reused indefinitely, are generally not used in pediatrics due to their inflexibility (ATS, 2000).

The clinician must also evaluate the need for a cuffed versus an uncuffed tube. If the patient is mechanically ventilated, a cuffed tube may be preferable to decrease the possibility of a leak during ventilation and the risk of aspiration. The cuff provides the ability to adjust the fit of the tube within the airway (ATS, 2000). Considerations for tube selection should exclude the presence of tracheomalacia. If tracheomalacia is present, the tube should be long enough to ventilate past that area. Occasionally, children have areas of granulation tissue within their airway, which must also be considered in determining the length of the tube. Finally, it is important to select a tube that does not cause pressure or erosion on sensitive areas within the trachea.

The difference between the internal and external diameter may not be significant until the child begins to speak. At that time, the child may not be able to get enough air around the tube to enable vocalization. If this is the case, the tracheostomy tube should be downsized until a leak occurs. If the patient is mechanically ventilated, monitoring the return of tidal volume is helpful to ensure the leak is not too large.

The neck flanges of the tracheostomy tube are shaped like wings, remain on the outside of the neck, and are used to attach tracheostomy ties to secure the tube around the neck. A v-neck flange is often preferable with children's neck anatomy to allow for better placement against the neck (Figure 8.3). A soft Velcro tracheostomy holder is used predominantly in pediatrics. Other tracheostomy holders include a chain tracheostomy holder, utilized frequently in preteens, or the Snappy tracheostomy holder, which uses an elastic material that snaps onto the flanges. The Velcro tracheostomy holder is secured behind

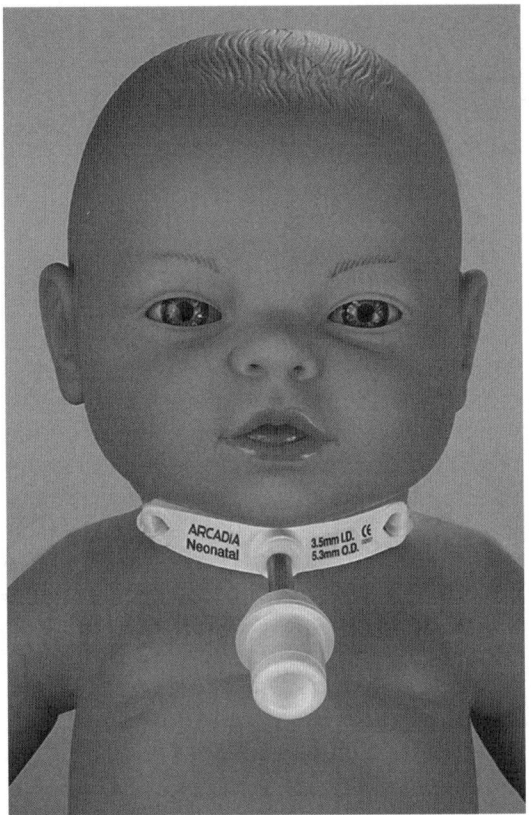

8.3 Tracheostomy in situ.

the patient's neck and at the flanges. If the patient is mechanically ventilated, the ventilator tubing is secured with cotton twill tracheostomy ties to the swivel adapter.

General Care of the Tracheostomy

During the first postoperative week, the stomal area should be cleansed with a solution of hydrogen peroxide and sterile water. Using a sterile gauze pad, a 1:1 concentration of hydrogen peroxide and sterile water should be used to cleanse the stoma, wiping in a semicircular motion around the top half of the stoma and repeating with another pad along the inferior portion of the stoma. After the first postoperative week, individual soap cleansing pads (e.g., Castille soap) or plain soap and water may be used to clean around the tracheostomy tube. The dressing should be changed at least three times per day, and skin care of the stoma should be performed daily. Gauze dressings should not be cut to fit around the tube, as loose fibers can work their way into the tracheostomy.

Precautions While Bathing

A child with a tracheostomy should never be submerged in water without covering the tube, either with an artificial nose or the ventilator tubing. When bathing a toddler with a tracheostomy, the water level should not be higher than the child's waist. This prevents water from entering the tracheostomy, with subsequent risk for aspiration pneumonia.

Changing the Tracheostomy Tube

After the initial tracheotomy, a tube change should be avoided for at least 5–7 days to allow the tract time to become well established (Wilson, 2005). The first tube change should be done by the surgeon to allow for evaluation of the stoma and confirmation it has healed enough for other professionals and family members to safely change the tube. The tracheostomy tube of a child should be changed weekly and at a time when the child is awake and least irritable. This will improve cooperation for a successful outcome.

The tracheostomy tube should be changed by two people whenever possible. The goal is to change the tracheostomy in a calm manner, without fear on the part of the child or caregiver. Depending on the age of the child, it is best if a pattern is established. Small children should be instructed to keep their hands at their sides each time the procedure is begun. The two-person method is used so that one person does the work of the tracheostomy tube change while the other person provides a distraction. In this way, the tube change can be done without traumatizing the child or increasing the anxiety of the child or caregiver.

Prior to the tube change, it is wise to organize the necessary equipment and plan to ventilate the child if required. This involves inserting the obturator into the new tube, lubricating the tip, and attaching the Velcro ties, which should be cut to fit the child's neck. The caregiver should inflate the cuff and inspect it prior to insertion. An infant or small child should have his or her tracheostomy tube changed while lying down in bed, while an older child may sit in a chair or stand. If the supine position is used, a rolled blanket should be placed under the patient's neck so his or her chin is pointing to the ceiling and his or her head is tilted back to a neutral position. The child's head should not be tilted too far back because this will make it more difficult to insert the tube. To prevent the child from coughing out the tube, one person should secure the neck flange while the other is undoing the ties. The tracheostomy tube should be removed and a new one reinserted with the curve of the tube pointing downward into the trachea. Contrary to the adult insertion procedure, in children it is not necessary to make a significant caudal turn when inserting the tracheostomy tube. This is because the anatomy of the child is much smaller; therefore, the angle of the caudal turn does not need to be accentuated. After insertion, the obturator should be removed while holding the tracheostomy tube in place. The tracheostomy holder should be secured, allowing for only one finger width under it. The tube should not be released until the ties are secure. If the tracheostomy leans to the left or right, the ties may be too tight (Downs, Beland, Reamer, & Hird, 2008).

Suctioning

Suctioning of the tracheostomy occurs only when needed. The risks associated with suctioning include trauma, atelectasis, hypoxemia, laryngospasm, bronchospasm, infection, and increased mucus production (Ireton, 2007). Suctioning should occur after waking, before meals, before leaving home, before bedtime, and as needed during the day or night. Children, especially those with neurological impairment, require frequent assessments for suctioning. Suctioning is an opportune time to evaluate secretions for color, odor, and consistency. When possible, encourage coughing to enhance airway clearance with suctioning. Surveillance cultures should be obtained weekly on all hospitalized patients with tracheostomies. Many patients are colonized with specific types of organisms, and this information is helpful to identify organisms that respond to treatment.

Suctioning pressures recommended for children are detailed as follows. Adolescents require pressures of 80–120 mm Hg (10–16 kPa), children require 80–100 mm Hg (10–13 kPa), and neonates, 60–80 mm Hg (8–10 kPa). Three-holed suction catheters are recommended, and they should be no larger than half the internal diameter of the child's tracheostomy (Ireton, 2007). To determine the length of the suction catheter, the tracheostomy tube should be measured and 1.5 cm added for suctioning purposes. Measurement is especially important with customized tubes. It is helpful to leave a catheter at the bedside as an example of how deep the suction catheter should be when entering the tracheostomy tube. In neonates, the length of the suction catheter introduction may be shorter due to their smaller anatomy.

During suctioning, it is important to avoid contact with the carina because of the high potential for trauma and scarring. Scarring can interfere with later decannulation. The catheter should remain in the airway for 5–10 seconds. Some authors (Hooper, 1996) recommend twisting the suction catheter upon withdrawal from the airway to avoid adherence to the tracheal mucosa. In a review of tracheostomy care in children, isotonic sodium chloride should not be routinely instilled for suctioning. Routine instillation of saline may dislodge bacteria, cause infection, and be detrimental to oxygenation (ATS, 2000; Neill, 2001).

Humidification

Humidification is extremely important to maintain airway patency and prevent the destruction of epithelium, ciliary function, and atelectasis (Wissing, 2004). If the airway is dry, there may be increased incidence of mucus plugs. Mucus plugs occur when secretions become thick and block the tracheostomy tube. When the patient is ventilated, the in-line humidifier should be set at 37°C. An artificial nose or high-humidity tracheostomy collar may be used while the patient is awake to filter and humidify the air. Nebulized saline treatments have been shown to thin secretions with uniform distribution and may be helpful when secretions are too thick (Klockare et al., 2006).

Medications

Common issues related to children with tracheostomies include excessive oral and tracheal secretions and the inability to manage them. Occasionally, it can be helpful to use ammonium glycopyrrolate (Robinul) to dry secretions slightly. It is important to start with a very low dose in order to prevent drying secretions too much, thereby causing a mucus plug. The dosing range for Robinul is 40–100 mcg/kg up to four times per day. It is preferable to start with a 40-mcg/kg dose three to four times per day and increase as needed. If copious secretions continue to be an issue, surgical removal of the salivary glands has been helpful in some cases. Laryngeal tracheal separation reconstruction is sometimes done to alleviate excessive oral/tracheal secretions preventing aspiration. An intraglandulary injection of Botulinum toxin-A (BTX-A) may be used to block the release of acetylcholine from motor and autonomic nerve terminals and decrease saliva production (Svetel et al., 2009).

Pulmonary Medications. The administration of respiratory medications for tracheostomy patients is accomplished via in-line or manual devices. Children with tracheostomies utilize a spacer for metered dose inhalation (MDI) administration. For children on ventilator support, an in-line device is placed in the ventilator circuit proximal to the patient's airway. With a dual limb circuit, the placement of the spacer should be on the inspiratory side to ensure better absorption of the medication into the airway. Aerosols can be delivered through hand bag-in methods, which do not disturb the integrity of the circuit. If given into the circuit, medications pass through the exhalation valve and cause the valve to stick over time, causing nuisance alarms.

Management of the Child With a Tracheostomy in the Community

Resources for Home Care

The prevalence of children in the United States under 18 years of age with special health care needs is high—approaching 14% (U.S. Department of Health and Human Services, Health Resources and Services Administration, 2009). In 2008, Baylor College of Medicine studied 70 children and adolescents undergoing tracheostomy over a 24-month period. Their objective was to describe an educational program and timeline for the discharge of children with new tracheostomies and to identify common impediments to education and the discharge process. Multiple medical and social factors can impede the child's transition to the outpatient setting. These include regional variations in rates of tracheostomy throughout the United States as well as variations in discharge disposition (home versus chronic care facilities). In addition, technology-dependent children require frequent readmission. Implementing a structured education and discharge program resulted in shorter hospitalization and more successful discharge to home (Graf et al., 2008b).

The stress of having a child with a tracheostomy has not been quantified; however, several studies have attempted to identify the challenges to parents and families with children with tracheostomies or on ventilators. In a study from the United Kingdom, the effects on the quality of life of both the patient and caregiver were evaluated. Questionnaires were received from 26 caregivers who reported adverse effects on all aspects of their quality of life, including sleep, relationships, social life, and ability to work. This study identified the need for improved preoperative care and increased community support for families of children with tracheostomies or on mechanical ventilation (Hopkins, Whetston, Foster, Blaney, & Morrison, 2009).

A review of children with tracheostomies and gastrostomies evaluated parental stress and coping mechanisms (Montagnino & Mauricio, 2004). A convenience sample of 50 families with children who had tracheostomies or gastrostomies over the prior 2 years was included in the study. Questionnaires included the Impact on Family Scale (Stein & Reissman, 1980) and the Family Crisis Oriented Personal Evaluation Scale (McCubbin, Olsen, & Larsen, 1981). The data demonstrated that caregivers believed there was a disruption of social interactions within and outside the family because of the child's condition. The study suggested that respite services might be helpful in supporting the families (Montagnino & Mauricio).

A multidisciplinary team approach is best for supporting and facilitating the outpatient needs of these medically complex children. In a recent study of children with new tracheostomies, the inpatient stay was typically 3 weeks (Graf et al., 2008b). During this time, nursing resources were identified and caregivers were given a cardiopulmonary resuscitation (CPR) class and demonstrated proficient care following a 24-hour stay with the child.

In addition to the great need for social/emotional support in families caring for children with tracheostomies, the health insurance coverage for home care is variable. The availability of home care nursing varies from state to state; however, resources are limited even in the best circumstances. The cost of the tracheostomy tubes, suction catheters, suction equipment, and other supplies is high, and families without insurance frequently rely on Medicaid, the state-supported health insurance for low-income and disabled patients. However, Medicaid resources are decreasing, which places a difficult burden on the families of children with special needs. Benefits vary between state Medicaid providers and private insurers, resulting in significant differences in degree of nursing services (Graf et al., 2008b). Title V federal funding, enacted by Congress in 1935, authorized funding for maternal and child health programs. Individual states determine how to apply the funds for these medically complex patients (U.S. Department of Health and Human Services, 2009). Some states provide a waiver system for the medical expenses of these children until they are 21 years of age. New resources must be identified to support these children and young adults, as their needs continue well beyond 21 years of age. The needs of medically complex children are many, and they continue to require much support in the outpatient setting.

Goldson, Louch, Washington, and Scheu (2006) described the concept of multidisciplinary medical home care as an approach to the needs of children with multiple medical problems. They identified the common experiences, special needs, and financial burden of families with children with multiple medical problems. The study highlighted common experiences in children with tracheostomies and multiple medical problems, including variable funding resources (which differed from state to state), lack of home nursing support, and developmental speech challenges. Furthermore, children with progressive deterioration requiring chronic mechanical ventilation encountered related ethical issues.

Physiologic Monitoring of Children With Tracheostomies at Home

During the child's hospitalization, the parent or primary guardian for the child with a tracheostomy must identify a primary and secondary caregiver. Identification of the secondary caregiver can be problematic in single parent or nontraditional families. Children with a tracheostomy need 24-hour observation and frequent assessment throughout the day. The home monitoring of children with tracheostomies is facilitated with pulse oximeters and capnography devices. Many children, due to age or disability, are unable to communicate their needs; therefore, the caregiver must be extremely perceptive in recognizing and anticipating the child's needs. Before discharge from the hospital, families must be instructed on suctioning, changing tubes, and general care of the tracheostomy tube and stoma. Families must also be trained in using the ventilator and basic life support. They should be supervised during a 24-hour stay while the child is an inpatient to demonstrate their ability to meet the comprehensive needs of the child prior to discharge.

Emergency Care

Identification of Respiratory Distress. All caregivers should be well trained in resuscitation. It is important they understand the principles of a manual resuscitation bag as well as mouth-to-tracheostomy ventilation. The caregiver must remember to close the child's mouth and nose while ventilating through either the stoma or the tracheostomy tube. Symptoms of respiratory distress include restlessness, rapid breathing, retractions, cyanosis, an inability to pass the suction catheter into the tube, and occasionally a whistling sound from the tracheostomy tube. Mucus plugs can be difficult to remove and put the patient at risk for obstruction. Although saline lavage for suctioning is not generally recommended on a routine basis, 5 ml of saline instilled in the tube may assist in loosening a mucus plug, enabling the caregiver to suction it out. Care should be taken to avoid pushing the plug further down into the airway. If this maneuver is ineffective, the tube should be replaced. If a new tube is difficult to insert, make sure the patient's head is in the correct (neutral) position. If insertion is still difficult, the caregiver may attempt to use the old tube or a tube one-half size smaller. If insertion of the tube is unsuccessful, a suction catheter can be inserted into the stoma to allow some passage of air while additional help is summoned. If it is suspected the new tracheostomy tube is displaced, ventilation through the tube should not be attempted. In this case, the use of a manual resuscitation bag will push air into the subcutaneous space, leading to subcutaneous emphysema, pneumothorax, or pneumomediastinum. This is a life-threatening emergency that interferes with the ability to safely ventilate the child. (See chapter 10 for further discussion on emergency management of a displaced tracheostomy.)

Infection

Because the tracheostomy is a foreign object and the stoma is an additional orifice, children with tracheostomies are more prone to respiratory infections. The stoma itself can occasionally develop a buildup of granulation tissue or a keloid formation. Granulation tissue lesions should be monitored by an otolaryngologist, who will generally perform annual bronchoscopies. Superficial granulation tissue can be removed with silver nitrate. In other cases, the granulation tissue can be excised under bronchoscopic guidance in the operating room. Skin infections are fairly common around the tracheostomy stoma. Fungal infections may appear as bright red, irritated, or scaly rashes with softening and breakdown of the skin. Some fungal skin infections appear with a central pallor. The edges of the lesion may present with tiny pustules. For example, *Candida* is a yeast infection that generally occurs in moist areas of the skin, typically in skin folds. Unless a child is mechanically ventilated, humidified tracheostomy collars are generally used. The constant humidity provides an excellent growth medium for *Candida*. For fungal skin infections, an antifungal such as Nystatin can be applied three times per day to the exterior portion of the stoma until the infection is resolved.

In addition, skin lesions often appear under the tube ties. When the skin appears broken down under the ties, Bacitracin can be an effective first-line treatment, followed by a 1% hydrocortisone cream or other topical anti-inflammatory agent as needed. Depending on the severity, location, and underlying cause of the skin irritation, a barrier method such as Duoderm may be used. Duoderm is a latex-free hydrocolloid adhesive occlusive material used for exudative wounds that provides a moist environment for wound healing. It can be used for areas of irritation under the tracheostomy ties but not over the stoma itself. If redness does not improve after 1–2 days, the patient should be referred to an otolaryngologist for further evaluation. Other possible causes of skin irritation can be due to trauma from the tracheostomy ties or infections that are fungal, bacterial, or viral in origin. Many superficial skin infections are caused by *Staphylococcus aureus* on the surface of the skin. Left untreated, an abscess might develop near the stoma that could threaten the patency of the airway. Bacterial infections may require topical or systemic antibiotics, and viral infections may require antiviral medications.

Shape of Stoma

A healthy stoma should appear round in shape, without redness or drainage. If the stoma appears to be changed in shape or color, the otolaryngologist should be contacted. This may indicate an underlying skin infection, which needs to be addressed quickly to prevent airway obstruction.

Bleeding

If the child is bleeding from the stoma, the health care professional should assess the respiratory status of the child. Questions to explore include the following: Is the child on supplemental oxygen? Are the oxygen demands of the child increasing? Has recent suctioning been traumatic? Has changing the tracheostomy tube been difficult? Aggressive suctioning can cause bleeding due to trauma; over time, it can also create an obstruction through the development of granulation tissue. If changing the tracheostomy tube is difficult, the caregiver should place a one-half size smaller tube until the child can be examined by the otolaryngologist, where a bedside dilatation with laryngobronchoscopy may be required.

One or more episodes of pink-tinged secretions should be taken seriously, as they may represent an emerging tracheitis. Families should ideally have a culture trap at home for the collection of a culture specimen. The culture can be delivered to the nearest laboratory or pediatrician's office with a prescription from the medical provider. It is also helpful to examine the organisms obtained from previous tracheostomy cultures. Many children with tracheostomies are colonized with specific organisms. Most commonly, patients may be colonized with *Pseudomonas aeruginosa,* which is not generally treated unless the child is symptomatic. The culture should be followed for specificity of organism to ensure adequate antibiotic coverage. Ideally, daily telephone contact by the health care provider should be made to ensure the child is responding to treatment. If the child is not responding, he or she should be seen in the office for assessment and possible hospitalization. Rarely, bright red, brisk bleeding can be due to artery rupture or vascular wall erosion, which constitute an immediate life-threatening emergency. See chapter 10 for further discussion of bleeding emergencies.

Developmental Issues

Activity and Behavioral Issues

As children become more developmentally aware of their world, they explore everything, including their ventilator and tracheostomy tube. Frequently, families with children aged 15–30 months experience disruptive, stubborn, and attention-seeking behavior. For this reason, changing the tracheostomy tube must always be approached as a serious event. As children become more mobile, the ventilator tubing may become somewhat encumbering. Children who have never been without their ventilator may not even notice their tubing becoming tangled; however, the caregiver must be vigilant in order to prevent disconnection from the ventilator or possible decannulation. Additionally, some children become aware of the attention they receive when the ventilator alarms and begin a cycle of purposefully disconnecting the ventilator in order to see the caregiver run to their assistance. Some children have not only intentionally disconnected but have also pulled their tracheostomy tube out of their neck in an effort to get attention. It is not uncommon to hear a family member complain about the child disconnecting from the ventilator and running in the opposite direction in a playful "chase me" action. It is important for the caregiver to remain calm. Even if the child loses consciousness, the caregiver can quickly replace and secure the tracheostomy tube.

These instances must be approached in a consistent pattern of behavior modification to avoid a poor outcome from decannulation. A serious tone of voice, saying no, and time-outs on a consistent basis seems to be the most effective series of responses to this attention-seeking behavior. As a result, the importance of CPR training in maintaining the safety of a child with a tracheostomy grows. Children with tracheostomies should also be monitored while playing. As children without tracheostomies explore their environment and themselves freely, so will the child with a tracheostomy. Many children present to the emergency room with foreign body aspiration simply because they were exploring toys or other objects by placing them in their mouths. Furthermore, an occasional toddler will insert an object into his or her tracheostomy tube or stoma only to realize it is uncomfortable when inhaled into the lungs. In 2006, a total of 4,100 deaths (1.4 deaths per 100,000 population) from the unintentional ingestion or inhalation of food or other objects resulting in airway obstruction were reported (National Safety Council, Research and Statistics Department, 2008).

Language Development

Toddlers with early tracheostomy placement do not experience the progression of early vocalization that is critical for speech development and communication. Studies have documented that tracheostomy placement negatively affects the development of expressive language skills—including phonation, vocal quality, and articulation—in children (Hull, Dumas, Crowley, & Kharasch, 2005).

Children 0–3 Months. Children from 0–3 months of age begin to develop different levels of social/emotional self-awareness, with subsequent problem-solving abilities. These abilities are demonstrated through play by imitation, spatial and sensory integration, and the development of language comprehension through auditory processing. Through imitation, the infant learns by repeating nonspecific vocalizations. Language production begins with vocalization through a nasalized cry and the production of nasalized vocal sounds. Infants demonstrate self-control by stopping crying when comforted. On a cognitive level, crying is used as a signal, and infants progress to seeking sound/vision relationships. In the area of language, infants learn through imitation by smiling in response to the adult smile and imitating vocalizations.

The newborn displays a sensitive gag reflex, and at 1 month of age practices the suck-swallow pattern with some liquid loss. At this time, a sequence of moving the tongue forward and backward occurs. At age 3–6 months, vocalization occurs with prolonged coos and goos. The infant begins to produce throaty sounds when supine, labial sounds when prone, and tongue sounds when sitting. All these developmental steps are greatly affected when a child has a tracheostomy (Illinois State Board of Education, 2009).

Central control of vocalization becomes differentiated during the first months of life. Laryngeal functions expand from protective reflexes to intentional vocalizations for communication (Kelchner & Miller, 2008). It is well-known that earlier phonation encourages phonation in the young infant, providing improved outcomes later. It also improves long-term speech and language development. In normal growth and development, the child develops expressive language as receptive language is taken in. The reinforcement of hearing one's own voice and the experience of social interaction improves language development (Kertoy, Guest, Quart, & Lieh-Lai, 1999).

Children 3–6 Months. The infant aged 3–6 months continues to develop gross motor skills. The child begins to bear weight on his elbows, pushes his chest up off a flat surface, begins to arch his back, holds his head up, and rotates in a prone position. At approximately 4 months, he rolls side to side when in a prone position. The infant with a tracheostomy must also have "tummy time" and the opportunity to develop abdominal muscles when in the supine position. As children begin to hold things in their hands and use a palmar grasp, they begin to bring objects to their mouth. Children with cuffed tracheostomy tubes frequently find the pilot balloon and may begin to pull on it or explore it with their mouth. Many children are fascinated with the pilot balloon; this needs to be discouraged gently by tucking the inflated portion under their clothing or behind their neck.

Infants who are orally intubated for prolonged periods of time have an uncoordinated suck/swallow. They may initially require a nasogastric tube for enteral feedings due to dysphagia. Subsequently, infants with tracheostomy tubes may require a gastrostomy tube until they are developmentally able to coordinate their suck/swallow without aspiration. A nasogastric feeding tube may also be used; however, this presents skin breakdown issues and interferes with parent bonding. It is preferable for the parent to be able to view the child's entire face, smile, and oromotor skills without the interference of a nasogastric tube. In some cases, such as in children with diaphragmatic hernia repair, a gastrostomy tube is contraindicated, and the only initial option is a nasogastric tube until the child is able to manage oral foods/fluids. Infants begin solid foods between 4–6 months, starting with cereal and followed by vegetables, meats, and fruits. Infants with tracheostomies must have a swallow study to determine their ability to manage the introduction of foods without aspiration. During the swallow study, a blue dye is introduced by way of a thickened formula offered by the speech therapist to determine the infant's ability to swallow without aspiration.

Children 6–9 Months. The 6- to 9-month-old infant begins to develop more interest in touch, taste, smell, and investigation of objects. Infants with tracheostomies frequently develop communication through sign language, as simple gestures develop naturally to meet their needs. Imitating social games begins at this time, including the imitation of behavior that cannot be seen by oneself when performed—for example, the tongue click. At this age, many children begin to drink from a cup with assistance (Illinois State Board of Education, 2009). Children with tracheostomies may be delayed in feeding if they are unable to manage their oral secretions. The age at which a child receives a tracheostomy is critical in terms of how it affects growth and development. Children who receive a tracheostomy during early infancy may not have as much difficulty adjusting as an older child, who quickly recognizes the difference between their abilities pre- and post-tracheostomy.

Children 9–12 Months. The 9- to 12-month-old is developing a sense of humor, follows simple commands, and imitates adult vocalizations. The child develops problem-solving abilities and notices changes in predictable patterns. The 9- to 12-month-old pushes away an unwanted hand and begins to coordinate actions with people and objects. As children become more able to communicate their needs, they naturally become less frustrated with social interactions. At this age, they easily cruise around furniture while holding on with two hands and walk with both hands held. Fine motor skills are developing, enabling the child to pick up small objects with a pincer grasp, and they begin to fling objects in play. Hearing develops as demonstrated by the ability to localize voices, singing, and environmental sounds. Chewing using vertical, nonrhythmical movement develops, and the infant begins to close his or her lips around the edge of a cup (Illinois State Board of Education, 2009).

Children 12–15 Months. The child aged 12–15 months begins to identify body parts and resists adult control but also needs and expects rituals and routines. In social play, the child enjoys imitating adult behavior and taking the lead in social games. His or her cognitive ability to problem solve initiates a whole new world of exploring cabinets and drawers and using trial-and-error problem-solving strategies. At this time, the child begins to imitate the vocal intonation patterns of others and imitates some animal sounds and familiar words. Children in this age group may recognize the differences between themselves and other children who do not have tracheostomies (Illinois State Board of Education, 2009).

Children 15–36 Months. During the 15- to 18-month period, the child imitates sounds and words more clearly. The child engages in parallel play and develops adaptive behaviors such as indicating when he or she is wet or soiled. The concept of object permanence develops during this time, and the child may use echolalia—the repetition of sounds. Language comprehension is increasing at this point, and the child can identify at least three body parts and understands at least 50 words. At 15–18 months, the suck-swallow sequences are well coordinated. There is more defined tongue tip elevation for swallowing with chewing, and the child uses active lip movement in cup drinking with control at the lip corners. The child's appetite may lessen due to decreased metabolic demands in conjunction with decreased growth needs. The average child at this age consumes 1,000–1,300 calories per day (Illinois State Board of Education, 2009).

In the 18–24 month period, the child develops a strong sense of self-importance and often does the opposite of what is asked. Parallel play is common, and the child may use some pronouns. The child uses 50–200 words by 24 months of age. Nutritionally, children become more selective in what they eat and have strong food preferences. They require less milk intake; 24–32 ounces per day at 24 months is appropriate.

During the 24–30 month period, children exhibit more tantrum behavior, which may be difficult in children with tracheostomies. Firm, consistent behavioral modification techniques should be used to enable the caregiver to remain in control. By 30 months, the child performs more adaptive behaviors, such as putting on shoes and demonstrating improved toileting. The child generally is able to suck through a straw and drink from a cup with coordination of sip-swallow breathing. Children with tracheostomies may take a little longer to coordinate this effort. The 36-month-old shows increasing independence and may experience difficulty with transitions. Children this age begin more abstract thinking and use logic to relate experiences. Imitating peers is commonplace, and children may repeat two to three elements in a series. At this time, they produce intelligible speech 90% of the time with a vocabulary of 400–800 words (Illinois State Board of Education, 2009).

Preschool and Elementary Years. As children enter their preschool years, they are able to tell a story, using 4–5 word sentences with about 1,000 words in their vocabulary. They can recite several nursery rhymes. It is helpful to know normal milestones in child development to enable early identification of speech and language issues (University of Michigan Health System, 2009).

Healthy children are screened during preschool years for hearing and vision. It is extremely important to identify hearing and vision loss as early as possible. Premature infants can have developmental delays, including speech and hearing problems. Some children may have hearing loss, but identify visual clues to enable them to understand what is being said. Children who have tracheostomies and a ventilator must be checked regularly for hearing impairment. Due to the noise of the ventilator, children may have hearing deficits that might be overlooked unless they undergo a yearly hearing evaluation. At this age, if a child is neurologically appropriate, children may have behavioral hearing tests performed to assess hearing and the ability to understand spoken words.

Kindergarten-age children increase the size of their vocabulary and begin to use the past tense. At this age, they are able to identify colors, shapes, and begin to ask how and why questions. At ages 5 and 6 years, the vocabulary increases, and children begin to understand spatial relationships, such as in, on, over, under, and so forth.

Elementary-age children are able to understand stories that contain a theme or logical chain of events. Their oral language and word order is more adult-like, and they begin to discuss abstract concepts that are not of their own experience (State Education Resource Center, 2009).

Middle and Preteen Years. Children in the middle and preteen years may be more concerned about what their peers think about their tracheostomy than the importance of why they have it. These children may be able to participate in sports and other activities with their peers; however, an emergency bag with suctioning must be available at all times. There may be frequent discussions with the pulmonologist about the possibility of removing the tracheostomy to enable the child to appear more like everyone else. Specifically, children with central hypoventilation, who may only require ventilator support at night, may not fully appreciate the significance of their condition. They may request to have their tracheostomy removed in an effort to be more similar to their peers but may not be ventilating enough, causing significant cognitive impairment. Preteen to teenage children with their tracheostomy tubes capped during daytime hours may attempt to camouflage the tracheostomy with scarves or other clothing. Medical personnel must be sensitive to the concerns of the adolescent with a tracheostomy to encourage him or her to maintain compliance with the treatment plan.

After a tracheotomy, some children develop the ability to speak on their own after their airway opens enough for air to flow around the tube and reach their vocal cords. Others may require help in the form of a speaking valve. Hull and others (2005) reviewed 12 children age 8 months to 21 years. This study documented that supervision and training with speaking valves can enhance communication options for children with tracheostomies and ventilator dependence. Speaking can also occur by covering the tracheostomy tube with finger or chin. As children develop and explore, they may discover on their own that they have the ability to tuck their chin for phonation. However, this is not desirable and can contribute to suprastomal collapse (ATS, 2000).

Use of the Speaking Valve

An otolaryngologist must evaluate the child for medical clearance before they use a speaking valve. Medical clearance involves the exclusion of stenosis or malacia above the area of the tracheostomy. If the airway above the tracheostomy is patent, the child is ready for a speech therapy consult to determine whether a speaking valve is a safe option. Contraindications to the use of the speaking valve are listed in Table 8.2. In the pediatric setting, the respiratory therapist and primary health care provider should also be present when a speaking valve trial is first initiated. If the child is on a ventilator, alarm adjustments should be made while trying the speaking valve. When using the speaking valve in conjunction with the ventilator, the child should be monitored for carbon dioxide retention with a transcutaneous capnograph to ensure adequate ventilation. See chapter 6 for proper placement of the speaking valve within the ventilator circuit.

The speaking valve works by allowing inhalation through the tracheostomy tube and exhalation through the upper airway. Because of their smaller anatomy, children may have less tolerance for speaking valves. In addition to phonation, however, speaking valves may assist in weaning from the ventilator and improving swallow function. This is because patients with speaking valves can close their vocal cords through increased subglottic pressure and protect their airway during swallowing.

The speaking valve has been shown to facilitate upper airway breathing; decrease oral-nasal secretions; and improve expectoration, olfaction, appetite, swallowing, voice quality, intensity, pitch, and intonation. It also allows for vocalization, babbling, or speech production; encourages communication; eliminates finger occlusion; and decreases the child's frustration with communication. The speaking valve increases subglottic pressure to approximate the vocal cords, improve cough response, and provide airway clearance. Because children move air through their mouth and nose with a speaking valve, the sensations of taste and smell are enhanced. Tracheomalacia interferes with tolerance of the speaking

---

8.2 Contraindications for the Use of a Speaking Valve

- Severe tracheal or laryngeal obstruction
- Laryngectomy
- Excessive secretions that cannot be adequately managed
- Gross aspiration
- Bilateral adductor vocal cord paralysis
- Serious illness
- Upper airway stenosis with no voice
- Craniofacial anomalies that prevent oral or pharyngeal air flow
- No voice with tracheal occlusion
- Use of a cuffed or tight-fitting tube
- Reactive airway disease requiring treatments more than every 3 hours
- Chronic aspiration
- Absence of a swallow reflex
- Unconsciousness
- Medical instability

From "Assessing and Managing Medically Fragile Children: Tracheostomy and Ventilator Support," by G. Woodnorth, 2004. *Language, Speech, and Hearing Services in Schools, 35,* 363–372.

valve. Children with anatomic abnormalities or malacia of the upper airway may have difficulty with exhalation while the speaking valve is in place.

Attending School With a Tracheostomy Tube

Children who have tracheostomies as well as those who are ventilator dependent should be encouraged to attend school. They require the assistance of a home health nurse to provide suctioning and other necessary care. Many children attend mainstream classes depending on their limitations and comorbidities. Patel and colleagues (2009) studied a cohort of 38 school-aged children with tracheostomies and reviewed their experiences in the school system. The study revealed that 53% of children with tracheostomies with long-term ventilator dependency attended mainstream schools. The child should be accompanied with an emergency bag containing a manual resuscitation bag, a portable suction machine, an adequate amount of properly sized suction catheters, saline for lavage, an HME, spare identical and smaller-sized tracheostomy tubes, extra tube ties, lubricant, dry and wet tissues or hand sanitizer, and oxygen if needed. The emergency bag must be restocked daily by the parent or guardian. In a pilot study investigating the school experiences of 11 children with tracheostomies, it was determined that children with tracheostomies can successfully and safely achieve full-time education in both mainstream and special schools (Smith, Williams, & Gibbin, 2003).

The inability to communicate effectively is a common concern in children with tracheostomies. The lack of trained personnel caring for these children in the school system creates undue anxiety for families. Much organizational work is required for schools to coordinate the availability of special resources to manage these children with special needs.

Decannulation

Once the child has been successfully weaned from mechanical ventilator support, a plan for decannulation ensues. The patient must meet two specific criteria in order to be considered for decannulation: the original need for the tracheostomy tube must no longer be present, and the patient must be able to maintain a safe and adequate airway independent of the tracheostomy tube (ATS, 2000). Leung and Berkowitz (2005) found that the ongoing need for tracheostomy and the patient diagnosis were significant variables predicting early decannulation in pediatrics. For example, if the initial reason for the tracheostomy was malacia that has subsequently resolved, decannulation may be considered. If granulation tissue is removed at the time of the endoscopic exam, swelling of the airway may delay decannulation for up to 2–3 weeks.

Decannulation can be done in an inpatient or outpatient setting. In the inpatient setting, the child may be admitted to progressively downsize the tracheostomy tube. Downsizing the tracheostomy tube in small children causes a proportionately larger increase in airway resistance compared with a larger child. It also creates an increased risk of a mucus plug. If this technique fails, it is important to evaluate the patient's airway endoscopically to ascertain the reason for failure (ATS, 2000). After the endoscopic exam, the smaller tube may be left in place for 24 hours and then capped. While the tube is capped, the child should be observed overnight in the inpatient setting and monitored with a pulse oximeter. If no airway obstruction occurs overnight, the tube may be removed in the morning and a dressing placed over the stoma. Patients are preferably monitored in the hospital for 24–48 hours after decannulation (ATS, 2000).

For outpatient decannulation, the tracheostomy tube should be downsized to the smallest size tube through which the child can breathe comfortably. If the child tolerates the downsized tube, it should be capped to determine whether the child is able to breathe without discomfort through the upper airway. The family should be reminded that the caps are not sterile. If the child coughs or pulls the cap off, it can be washed in warm soapy water, rinsed and dried thoroughly, and reattached to the tracheostomy tube. During this trial period, the tube should be capped only while the child is awake. If the child shows any signs of difficulty breathing, the cap should be removed immediately. The child must be monitored with a pulse oximeter at all times during the initial capping trial to determine the level of oxygenation. Once a child can tolerate capping all day, capping trials can begin at night. The child should be monitored by a nighttime attendant for the first week to ensure he or she can tolerate capping while sleeping. When the child can tolerate continuous capping for at least 7 days, an appointment for decannulation should be scheduled.

After decannulation, all tracheostomy equipment for the child should be kept in the home for 2 weeks. After the child's follow-up visit with the otolaryngologist, the equipment and nursing support can be discontinued. This follow-up appointment will allow the otolaryngologist to evaluate the closure of the stoma. Most stomas will close on their own; however, they can be surgically closed if necessary.

Summary

As children grow and develop, their needs change. Fitting a tracheostomy tube to accommodate growth and prevent pressure against the trachea is especially important, as granulation tissue and malacia can interfere with the downsizing and decannulation process. Children with tracheostomies can attend mainstream schools but should have emergency and suction equipment with them at all times. Speaking valves are especially important for children with tracheostomies because of the developmental issues related to delayed speech.

The care of children with tracheostomies can be extremely complicated and requires frequent interaction with pediatricians, nurse practitioners, otolaryngologists, speech therapists, physical therapists, occupational therapists, respiratory care practitioners, and other health care specialists. Health care professionals play an important role in supporting the families of children with tracheostomies by providing medical knowledge and psychosocial support to allow the child and family to lead as normal a life as possible.

Key Points

- Contrary to adults, prolonged endotracheal intubation is common in children.
- Because of the narrow inner diameter of pediatric tracheostomy tubes, inner cannulas are never used, and cuffed tubes are rarely used.

- The sizing of tracheostomy tubes must keep up with the child's normal growth and development.
- Tracheostomy placement early in life negatively affects the development of expressive language skills, including phonation, vocal quality, and articulation.
- The decannulation process takes longer in children than in adults and generally includes at least 7 days of continuous capping.

Acknowledgments

Special thanks to Linda Downs, RN; Sylvia Finley, RRT; and Susie Willette, MS, CCC-SLP, for their contributions to this chapter.

References

American Thoracic Society. (2000). Care of the child with a chronic tracheostomy. *American Journal of Respiratory Critical Care Medicine, 161*(1), 297–308.

Downs, L., Beland, A., Reamer, P., & Hird, L. (2008). Tracheostomy care at home. *Children's Memorial Hospital* (patient education manual), 2–19.

Feudtner, C., Villareale, N. L., Morray, B., Sharp, V., Hays, R. M., & Neff, J. M. (2005). Technology dependency among patients discharged from a children's hospital: A retrospective cohort study. *BMC Pediatrics, 5,* 8.

Goldson, E., Louch, G., Washington, K., & Scheu, H. (2006). Guidelines for the care of the child with special health care needs. *Advances in Pediatrics, 54,* 165–182.

Graf, J. M., Montagnino, M. S., Hueckel, R., & McPherson, M. (2008a). Pediatric tracheostomies: A recent experience from one academic center. *Pediatric Critical Care Medicine, 9,* 96–100.

Graf, J. M., Montagnino, B. A., Hueckel, R., & McPherson, M. L. (2008b). Children with new tracheostomies: Planning for family education and common impediments to discharge. *Pediatric Pulmonology, 43*(8), 788–794.

Hooper, M. (1996). Nursing care of the patient with a tracheostomy. *Nursing Stand, 15*(10), 40–43.

Hopkins, C., Whetston, S., Foster, T., Blaney, S., & Morrison, G. (2009). The impact of paediatric tracheostomy on both patient and parent. *International Journal of Pediatric Otorhinolaryngology, 73*(1), 15–20.

Hull, E. M., Dumas, H. M., Crowley, R., & Kharasch, V. S. (2005). Tracheostomy speaking valves for children: Tolerance and clinical benefits. *Pediatric Rehabilitation, 8*(3), 214–219.

Illinois State Board of Education. (2009). *Family Enrichment Program, ECHO Joint Agreement.* Retrieved October 23, 2009, from http://www.FePecho.com

Ireton, J. (2007). Tracheostomy suction: A protocol for practice. *Paediatric Nursing, 19*(10), 18.

Kelchner, L. N., & Miller, C. K. (2008). Current research in voice and swallowing outcomes following pediatric airway reconstruction. *Current Opinion in Otolaryngology—Head and Neck Surgery, 16*(3), 221–225.

Kertoy, M. K., Guest, C. M., Quart, C. M, & Lieh-Lai, M. (1999). Speech and phonological characteristics of individual children with history of tracheostomy. *Journal of Speech Language and Hearing Research, 42*(3), 621–635.

Klockare, M., Dufva, A., Danielsson, A. M., Hatherly, R., Larsson, S., Jacobsson, H., et al. (2006). Comparison between direct humidification and nebulization of the respiratory tract at mechanical ventilation: Distribution of saline solution studies by gamma camera. *Journal of Clinical Nursing, 15*(3), 301–307.

Leung, R., & Berkowitz, R. G. (2005). Decannulation and outcome following pediatric tracheostomy. *Annals of Otology, Rhinology, and Laryngology, 114*(10), 743–748.

Lewis, C. W., Carron, J. D., Perkins, J. A., Sie, K. C., & Feudtner, C. (2003). Tracheotomy in pediatric patients: A national perspective. *Archives in Otolaryngology—Head and Neck Surgery, 129,* 523–529.

McCubbin, H. I., Olsen, D. H., & Larsen, A. S. (1981). Family crisis oriented personal scales (F-COPES). In H. I. McCubbin, A. I. Thompson, & M. A. McCubbin (Eds.), *Family assessment:*

Resiliency, coping, and adaptation—Inventories for research and practice (pp. 455–507). Madison: University of Wisconsin System.

Montagnino, B. A., & Mauricio, R. V. (2004). The child with a tracheostomy and gastrostomy: Parental stress and coping in the home—A pilot study. *Pediatric Nursing, 30*(5), 373–380, 389–390, 401.

National Safety Council, Research and Statistics Department. (2008). *Injury Facts 2008 Edition* (Vol. 8, pp. 14–15). Itasca, IL: Author.

Neill, K. (2001). Normal saline instillation prior to endotracheal suction: A literature review. *Nursing Critical Care, 6*(1), 34–39.

Otonello, G., Ferrari, L., Pirroddi, J. M., Diana, M. C., Villa, G., Nahum, L., et al. (2007). Home mechanical ventilation in children: Retrospective survey of a pediatric population. *Pediatrics International, 49*(6), 801–805.

Parilla, C., Scarano, E., Guidi, M. L., Galli, J., & Paludetti, G. (2007). Current trends in paediatric tracheostomies. *International Journal of Pediatric Otorhinolaryngology, 71*(10), 1563–1567.

Patel, M., Zdanski, C., Abode, K., Reilly, C., Malinzak, E., Stein, J., et al. (2009). Experience of the school-aged child with tracheostomy. *International Journal of Pediatric Otorhinolaryngology, 73*(7), 975–980.

Smith, J. C., Williams, J., & Gibbin, K. P. (2003). Children with a tracheostomy: Experience of their careers in school. *Childcare Health Development, 29*(4), 291–296. Nottingham, England: Blackwell Publishing.

State Education Resource Center. (2009). Typical speech and language development for school-age children: A checklist for school nurses. Retrieved October 29, 2009, from http://www.ctserc.org/s/index.php?option=com_content&view=article&id=373:typical-speech-and-language-development-for-school-age-children&catid=33:relevant&Itemid=140

Stein, R. E., & Reissman, C. K. (1980). The development of an impact-on-family scale: Preliminary findings. *Medical Care, 18*(4), 465–472.

Svetel, M., Vasić, M., Dragasević, N., Pekmezović, T., Petrović, I., & Kostić, V. (2009, January). Botulinum toxin in the treatment of sialorrhea. *Vojnosanitetski Pregled, 66*(1), 9–12. Clinical Centre of Serbia, Institute of Neurology, Belgrade, Serbia.

University of Michigan Health System. (2009). *Your child development and behavior resources: A guide to information and support for parents.* Retrieved October 29, 2009, from http://www.med.umich.edu/yourchild/topics/speech.htm

U.S. Department of Health and Human Services. (2009). *Title V history.* Retrieved October 23, 2009, from https://perfdata.hrsa.gov/mchb/mchreports/LEARN_More/Title_V_History/title_v_history.asp

U.S. Department of Health and Human Services, Health Resources and Services Administration. (2009). *The National Survey of Children With Special Health Care Needs.* Retrieved October 23, 2009, from http://mchb.hrsa.gov/cshcn05

Wilson, M. (2005). Tracheostomy management. *Pediatric Nursing, 17*(3), 38–43.

Wissing, D. R. (2004). Humidity and aerosol therapy. In J. M. Cairo & S. P. Pilbeam (Eds.), *Mosby's respiratory equipment* (7th ed., pp. 87–129). St. Louis, MO: Elsevier.

Woodnorth, G. (2004). Assessing and managing medically fragile children: Tracheostomy and ventilator support. *Language, Speech and Hearing Services in Schools, 35,* 363–372.

Wooten, C. T., French, L. C., Thomas, R. G., Neblett, W. W., Werkhaven, J. A., & Cofer, S. A. (2006). Tracheotomy in the first year of life: Outcome in term infants, the Vanderbilt experience. *Otolaryngology—Head and Neck Surgery, 134,* 365–369.

Zenk, J., Fyrmpas, G., Zimmerman, T., Kosh, M., Constandinidis, J., & Iro, H. (2009). Tracheostomy in young patients: Indications and long-term outcome. *European Archives of Otorhinolarngology, 266*(5), 705–711.

9

Special Considerations for the Patient With a Laryngectomy

Jeri A. Logemann

The patient who undergoes a laryngectomy poses a clinical challenge because of the varied nature of the procedure, which is based on the extent of disease. These patients are without a voice in the literal and figurative senses of the word. Laryngeal cancer seems to be a forgotten cancer, as other cancers attract more attention for research and funding (Dobbins et al., 2005). Laryngeal cancer accounts for half of all head and neck cancers, which together account for about 3% of all of cancers. In 2009, the American Cancer Society estimated about 12,290 new cases of laryngeal cancer and 3,660 deaths (2,250 men and 600 women; American Cancer Society, 2009). Squamous cell carcinoma accounts for the majority of cases and the 5-year survival rate is 65%. Laryngeal cancer is most frequently diagnosed in a 60- to 70-year-old with a long history of smoking and, frequently, alcohol abuse. However, it is beginning to be apparent in younger people without these risk factors (Scheich, 2007). Malnutrition due to chronic dysphagia has been identified as an impediment in the care of these patients (Iseli, Agar, Dunemann, & Lyons, 2007).

The presenting symptoms of laryngeal cancer include hoarseness, persistent ear pain, sore throat or coughing, painful swallowing, difficulty breathing, or a mass in the neck (Scheich, 2007). Head and neck cancers and their treatment can affect the patient's upper airway and generally require the introduction of a tube to maintain patency. Treatments may include surgical removal of the tumor with or without a particular reconstruction, radiation therapy, and/or chemotherapy. The clinician's first step is to define the nature of the tumor treatment and how it may affect the airway. Generally, it is a good idea to do pretreatment counseling with the patient to help him or her understand the nature of the treatment and his or her own role in recovery and rehabilitation. Often patients require therapy to strengthen the muscles affected by their treatment, particularly after surgery or radiotherapy. In order to be successful during rehabilitation, the patient should become comfortable with post-treatment changes, including the presence of a tracheostomy or laryngectomy tube. Patient questions should also be answered during the pretreatment counseling session. Generally, a speech pathologist, working with the physician, nurse, and respiratory care practitioner, should be involved in the rehabilitation.

The upper digestive and respiratory tracts perform three critical and often interrelated functions: (a) maintenance of respiration, (b) facilitation of swallowing, and (c) production of speech and voice. The most critical of these biologic functions is respiration. When any medical device or respiratory tube is introduced into the upper airway, all three functions must be considered; however, respiration is always primary as it supports life.

Types of Laryngectomy

There are three primary types of laryngectomy that require a tracheostomy or laryngectomy tube, whether temporarily or permanently. Refer to Figure 1.1 to identify the structure of the larynx affected by surgical resection.

Supraglottic Laryngectomy

The supraglottic laryngectomy is used to remove small tumors at the tongue base or aryepiglottic folds, and it includes the resection of the epiglottis, the hyoid bone, a portion of the tongue base and valleculae, and the aryepiglottic folds. The amount of tissue removed from each structure will depend upon the exact size and location of the tumor. The surgical procedure is usually called a supraglottic laryngectomy, but the extent can vary between patients. The procedure should be clearly documented in the patient's medical record. Generally, recovery from supraglottic surgery takes 5–7 days (Rademaker et al., 1993). The recovery of swallowing generally involves learning to use the tongue base region to facilitate airway protection at the valleculae (Logemann et al., 1994), which is accomplished by pulling the tongue base backward to touch the anteriorly tilting arytenoids. The recovery of the swallow function will depend upon the patient's ability to achieve airway entrance closure. In the supraglottic laryngectomy, the respiratory tract is usually maintained with a standard tracheostomy tube (generally adult size 8). The size of the tracheostomy tube will vary, however, depending upon the size of the patient's trachea.

Hemilaryngectomy

A hemilaryngectomy involves the resection of one vertical half of the larynx—including the false vocal folds, the true vocal folds, and the aryepiglottic folds—but excluding the epiglottis. Usually the epiglottis is left intact as are both arytenoid cartilages. Depending on the exact location of the tumor, the surgical resection may include parts of the tongue base or vocal fold on the contralateral side. Generally, the tracheostomy tube is the same size as the patient's trachea, usually an adult size 8. The recovery of the airway and normal swallowing occur rapidly after a hemilaryngectomy, usually within 5–7 days (Rademaker et al., 1993).

Total Laryngectomy

A total laryngectomy typically involves removing the laryngeal cartilage, the true and false vocal folds, the epiglottis, the most inferior portion of the tongue base, and a portion of the trachea, depending upon the exact location of the tumor. At the end of the surgical resection, the tracheal stump is angled forward and sewn into an incision in the anterior neck at approximately the fifth cervical vertebra, forming a permanent stoma. The construction of the stoma is often difficult and may need to be modified later as the tissue at the edge of the stoma heals, thus narrowing the airway entrance. The tube worn in the stoma typically is designed to maintain the opening and reduce the risk that the skin at the top of the stoma will contract, making breathing more difficult. After several years, many laryngectomized patients need a revision of their stoma due to the shrinkage and narrowing of the tissues at the stoma entrance. This is generally a simple procedure, but many patients find it upsetting because it involves their airway entrance. As with other respiratory tubes, the diameter and length of the tube and the duration of cannulation will vary between patients. Some patients need to wear a short tube for several years until the stoma entry stabilizes in size.

Postoperative Care After Laryngectomy

Postoperative care after total laryngectomy includes the inspection and care of the drains on either side of the neck and frequent assessment of the airway. The patient should have nothing by mouth for the first postoperative week but should receive enteral nutrition to promote wound healing. The patient should be suctioned and the laryngectomy tube cleaned regularly to prevent obstruction. The surgical site should be examined frequently to assess for hematoma formation. The patient should also be monitored for withdrawal from tobacco and alcohol, as these are frequently associated with this type of cancer. Patients who have also had a total thyroidectomy are at risk for hypocalcemia, so they should be counseled to report numbness and tingling around the mouth, fingers, and toes; muscle cramps or spasms; irritable mood; or personality changes. These patients will also require physical therapy, as neck dissection also affects the arm and shoulder muscles (Scheich, 2007). The speech language pathologist should also be seeing the patient to discuss and practice communication options.

Swallowing After Laryngectomy

The patient who has undergone a supraglottic laryngectomy must learn how to swallow differently by closing the reconstructed airway entrance—the arytenoid cartilage to the base of tongue. It takes about a month (Logemann et al., 1994) of therapy from a speech language pathologist to relearn to swallow. Patients are given exercises to increase the movement of the base of their tongue and arytenoid cartilages so they can contact each other and cause airway entrance closure. Approximately 30% of patients will not need to have any therapy, as they achieve closure of their new airway entrance spontaneously in the first postoperative month. Before beginning any swallowing (with or without therapy), the patient should receive a modified barium swallow to define his or her ability to protect the airway and determine which muscles need strengthening.

In contrast to the supraglottic laryngectomy, hemilaryngectomy patients generally achieve glottic closure spontaneously in the first few postoperative weeks. If the patient's x-ray study does not show good airway closure at that point, exercises to improve the range of motion of the remaining vocal fold should be initiated by a speech language pathologist (Logemann, 1998).

Total laryngectomy patients generally do not require swallowing therapy, as they do not have significant difficulty swallowing or protecting their airway. Their airway is surgically separated from their digestive tract such that they cannot aspirate. However, they may need to learn to squeeze a bit harder when swallowing in order to efficiently swallow.

When conducting a bedside clinical or radiographic study of swallowing, the clinician should examine the tracheostomy tube to determine the presence and status of the cuff (inflated or deflated), the size of the tracheostomy tube, and the presence or absence of a fenestration. The clinician should also review the patient's medical record to determine the length of time the tracheostomy has been in place. If the tracheostomy tube has been in place more than 6 months, scar tissue may have formed, which can restrict laryngeal elevation. A tracheostomy tube in place for more than 6 months also results in reduced airflow and stimulation to subglottic sensory receptors that play a role in vocal fold closure. These patients may have reduced vocal fold closure for swallowing and vocalization. When the tube has been in place for a shorter time, it may have little effect on laryngeal elevation when the cuff is deflated. *If medically feasible,* the tracheostomy cuff should be deflated during the bedside or radiographic study because an inflated cuff can reduce laryngeal elevation by creating friction against the tracheal wall. However, the tracheostomy cuff should not be deflated until medical clearance is given. If the tracheostomy cuff is inflated during the bedside or radiographic study, the clinician should note this in the report. Prior to cuff deflation, it is important to suction deeply in the posterior oropharynx to remove any secretions that have accumulated above the cuff. Ideally, cuff deflation should be timed to occur upon expiration.

If the radiographic study of the swallow confirms benefit, the patient may be taught to lightly cover the external end of the tracheostomy tube with a gauze pad or gloved finger during the moment of the swallow and for several seconds after the swallow. In this way, increased airflow is directed through the larynx, which stimulates subglottic sensory receptors before the swallow and may improve vocal fold closure. Most swallows occur during the expiratory phase of the respiratory cycle, when expiration is temporarily stopped by the swallow (Martin, Logemann, Shaker, & Dodds, 1994). Expiration usually resumes after the swallow. Thus, if the patient's tracheostomy is occluded during and immediately after the swallow, this exhaled airflow may clear residual food away from the top of the airway, lessening the chance of aspiration. It is also thought that covering the tracheostomy tube helps restore more normal subglottic pressures during swallowing and, thus, helps improve closure of the vocal folds during the swallow (Shin, Maeyama, Morikawa, & Umezaki, 1988). Several reports indicate reduction or elimination of aspiration with the tube covered (Muz, Hamlet, Mathog, & Farris, 1994; Muz, Mathog, Nelson, & Jones, 1989). Other studies and personal experience indicate variable or less consistently positive results from tube occlusion (Leder, Tarro, & Burrell, 1996). A study completed in our laboratory found that digital tube occlusion does not negatively affect swallowing and, in fact, may improve laryngeal elevation (Logemann, Pauloski, & Colangelo, 1998). However, such effects are not universal and must be examined during the radiographic study.

The use of a one-way valve may be helpful in place of light digital occlusion if the patient's respiratory status is stable and he or she can tolerate the valve comfortably. In addition to facilitating speech production, it also can produce swallowing benefits. The one-way valve is open at rest and closes when expiration pressure increases for speech. When the valve is closed, air is directed up and around the tracheostomy tube. The patient's tolerance for a valve should be determined by the respiratory care practitioner in conjunction with the swallowing therapist, usually the speech language pathologist. Like digital occlusion, the effects of the valve on the patient's swallow should be examined radiographically. Although one report (Dettelbach, Gross, Mahlmann, & Eibling, 1995) indicated uniformly positive effects of one-way valves with dysphagic, tracheostomized patients, personal experience demonstrates variable effects, making it necessary for the clinician to define the effects for each patient radiographically.

Maclean, Cotton, and Perry (2009) used a questionnaire with 120 members of the Laryngectomy Association of New South Wales, Australia. Dysphagia was reported by 71.8%, and their symptoms included increased time required to swallow, the need for fluids to wash down a bolus, and avoidance of certain food consistencies. Higher levels of depression, anxiety, and stress were also reported by those patients who reported dysphagia. Social activities, such as eating with friends at their homes or at restaurants, were curtailed in 57% of patients.

Swallowing Assessment and Therapy After Tracheostomy

In general, tracheostomy and enteral feeding tubes are left in place during swallowing assessment and therapy, as no studies have indicated these tubes significantly deter swallowing rehabilitation. However, the cuff of the tracheostomy tube should be deflated if medically feasible during assessment and therapy. An inflated cuff can restrict laryngeal elevation and cricopharyngeal opening during the swallow, as discussed previously. An inflated tracheostomy cuff can also cause tracheal irritation by rubbing on the tracheal walls as the larynx elevates during each swallow. Therefore, it is inappropriate to feed a patient with an inflated tracheostomy cuff. If the patient is aspirating, he or she should not be fed orally. On occasion, it may be absolutely necessary to leave the cuff inflated, such as when the patient is ventilator dependent, because most patients require cuff inflation while ventilated.

Cavalot and others (2009) found that preoperative swallowing therapy influenced the duration of nasogastric feedings. They studied 43 patients who underwent subtotal laryngectomy from 1990 to 2000. Prior to 1997, patients received swallowing therapy only after surgery. From 1997 on, patients scheduled for subtotal laryngectomy also received some swallowing therapy prior to surgery. The authors discovered that the average time to resumption of swallowing was 28 days for the patients who received only postoperative swallowing therapy and 16 days for those who experienced both pre- and postoperative therapy. The investigators concluded that preoperative swallowing therapy enhances earlier resumption of normal deglutition and quicker discontinuation of nasogastric tube feedings.

Speech After Laryngectomy

Patients who have undergone hemilaryngectomy and supraglottic laryngectomy will have natural voice production because part of their larynx has been retained. However, they generally need to work on quality of voice, which is rough and uneven. This generally involves an exercise in prolonging voice at various pitch and volume levels to create a smoother voice quality. To facilitate more consistent loudness and voice quality, patients are usually seen weekly for vocal exercises and are encouraged to complete daily exercises for a few weeks. Generally, this type of exercise begins several weeks after surgery. Some patients feel their voice is adequate and are not interested in improving, even though their voice may be rough or husky.

Surgical-Prosthetic Voice Restoration After Total Laryngectomy

Speech language pathologists generally begin discussing communication options with the total laryngectomized patient within the first few days after surgery. Options include artificial larynges, esophageal voice, and surgical prosthetic voice restoration. In the late 1970s, surgical prosthetic voice restoration techniques were developed and became more common. These techniques involve placing a surgical needle puncture (size 18) at the 12-o'clock position in the back of the stoma and fitting the resultant puncture with a small prosthesis, enabling airflow through the stoma and into the pharyngoesophagus. A prosthesis is worn in the puncture to keep it open such that airflow through the stoma passes through the puncture and into the pharyngoesophagus, vibrating whatever tissue is flaccid enough to respond to the airflow.

Tracheoesophageal puncture (TEP) is a procedure used only for total laryngectomy. Patients may choose to get a TEP at the time of primary laryngectomy or later. Some laryngectomized patients, by their own choice, prefer to use esophageal voice or an artificial larynx. The prosthesis is washed daily, and sometimes more often; generally, patients are taught to place and replace it themselves.

In a total laryngectomy, the stomal tube is generally short and is intended only to maintain an adequate stomal opening. Once the tube is placed into the stoma, the tracheal cartilage maintains the opening. It is only the entrance of the stoma that can become a problem. However, when a laryngectomy patient is interested in receiving a TEP for voice rehabilitation, an immediate factor is how to introduce the airflow below the vibratory segment and within the reconstructed laryngopharynx. In general, there is great anatomic variability in the laryngopharynx after total laryngectomies. Diedrich and Youngstrom (1966) described this variability in the location and size of the tissue serving as the vibratory element in total laryngectomees. The key to successful surgical prosthetic voice restoration is to introduce the airflow below the tissues that will vibrate. The patient wears a small prosthesis in the surgical puncture within the stoma. In order to speak, the patient must inspire, drawing air in through the stoma, and then cover the stoma with a gloved finger or second prosthesis and exhale, thus directing the airflow into the stomal prosthesis. As the patient exhales through the puncture prosthesis into the pharyngoesophagus, the tissue above the prosthesis begins to vibrate. A second small prosthesis placed at the stomal entrance, in lieu of the patient's finger, redirects air from the stoma through the prosthesis and into the pharyngoesophagus.

A similar problem is found in mechanically ventilated patients with normal laryngeal anatomy who use leak speech to exhale air through their pharynx to produce voice. Most ventilators are positive-pressure devices in which delivered airflow facilitates the vibration of the vocal folds to produce voicing. The patient on a ventilator has different dynamics in generating voice than the total laryngectomee. The removal of the vocal folds with a total laryngectomy necessitates the presence of adequate airflow through the pharyngoesophagus to guarantee vibration, yet the pharyngoesophageal tissue must be flaccid enough for the pharyngoesophagus to respond to airflow.

Deschler, Bunting, Lin, Emerick, and Rocco (2009) explored the value of early (primary) TEP and tracheoesophageal prosthesis with total laryngectomy. The investigators found that 29 of 30 patients had initial success with tracheoesophageal voice production. After 1 year, 23 of 30 (77%) had successful voice restoration. Five patients failed because of recurrent disease, one patient never achieved successful voice, and one patient wanted the prosthesis removed although successful voice was achieved. Overall, 92% of disease-free patients had functional voice restoration at 1 year.

Woodard, Oplatek, and Petruzzelli (2007) found that patients who had primary placement of TEP had statistically better outcomes with eating and overall functioning compared with those who had later placement of TEP. Furthermore, patients with primary TEP had higher speech scores and less social disruption. The authors reasoned that these patients were more motivated to learn how to speak with the prosthesis because they had no other means to communicate vocally, whereas patients who had TEP placed after their laryngectomy had time to learn other methods of vocal communication.

Patients should be counseled that TEP is an imperfect method of speech production and usually involves some speech therapy in order to achieve optimal voice restoration. A physician, Brook (2009), provides a discussion of his own experience as a patient with a total laryngectomy undergoing voice rehabilitation with a TEP. He reported the following experience:

> The task of talking again was most challenging and frustrating. I was unable to speak for over 2 months and later wished I had used an electrolarynx during that period.... I... realized that this field was not only a science, but also an art.... I soon realized that this process was going to be a long process of trial and error, repeated TEP failures due to leaks, and learning how to master the art of sealing the housing of the heat-moisture exchanging filter.... Fortunately, things improved significantly with the passage of time and the reduction of the neck edema.

Patients who are about to undergo a total laryngectomy have a number of choices, only one of which is a puncture procedure. The speech-language pathologist will provide advice to the patient and family as they proceed through the process.

Ventilator-Dependent Tracheostomized Patients

The newest airway, developed by Dr. Eric Blom, enables a ventilator-dependent patient with a larynx to maintain positive-pressure ventilation while still diverting some airflow into the larynx and creating voice. This new device facilitates airflow around the tube and into the patient's larynx, vibrating the vocal folds. In all cases where the tube is used to facilitate speech as well as respiration, the patient's respiratory airflow must be adequate to move through the prosthesis and vibrate whatever tissues produce voice. If airflow is low or the patient has poor respiratory strength, these prostheses will provide suboptimal results. Similarly, the patient's articulatory ability must be adequate to shape the vibratory airflow into speech sounds and words.

Balancing Breathing, Speech, and Swallowing

There are many conditions that may affect the patient's ability to produce speech or breathe with the respiratory tube in place, and the clinician who introduces these tubes or airflow devices must be able to identify the precipitating condition (Hess, 2005a, 2005b). The patient's airflow may be inadequate or the device may be clogged with mucous or other secretions.

The upper aerodigestive tract is important in respiration, swallowing, and speech and voice production. The trachea's role in respiration is obvious, as it delivers air to the lungs. Its role in swallowing, while critical, is often not entirely recognized.

The upper aerodigestive tract delivers airflow stimulation to the larynx and other structures of the upper airway. This stimulation contributes to vocal fold closure. Patients who are mechanically ventilated for even a short period of time often lose their vocal fold closure when they attempt to vocalize. This problem often requires speech therapy to stimulate vocal fold movement. Airway closure during swallow is necessary to protect the airway from food or liquid. The prevention of aspiration is essential to reduce the risk of pneumonia due to food entering the lungs. Again, patients may need intensive therapy to facilitate or improve airway closure during swallow. Maintaining upper airway function is critical to successful swallowing and speaking as well as respiration.

Swallowing Function With Ventilator-Dependent Patients

Swallowing and respiration are reciprocal processes. Swallowing normally occurs toward the beginning of exhalation; thus, it is usually helpful to present food to the patient at that time. Since a mechanical ventilator controls the respiratory cycle, the patient cannot fully coordinate exhalation time with swallowing. If the patient has slow oral or pharyngeal stages of swallowing that cannot be completed during the time allocated for exhalation by the ventilator, the swallow may be disrupted by the next inspiration. If the patient restarts inspiration early, any residual food may be directed into the airway. The inflated cuff of the tracheostomy tube in a ventilator-dependent patient interferes with laryngeal elevation and, thus, reduces closure of the entrance of the airway. In turn, food or liquid may enter the airway and be aspirated after the swallow.

The blue dye test may be used at the bedside for a tracheostomized patient (Thompson-Henry & Braddock, 1995; Tippett & Siebens, 1996). This test screens for the presence of aspiration. The patient is given measured amounts of blue-dyed foods, and the tracheostomy is suctioned immediately after the swallow for the presence of the blue-dyed foods, which would indicate aspiration. The test does not reveal the anatomic or physiologic cause(s) of aspiration, however, which is critical information. If the result is clearly positive (i.e., blue-dyed material is coughed or suctioned from the tracheostomy), the clinician should recommend a modified barium swallow to determine the cause of the aspiration and define the type of therapy needed. If blue-tinged secretions are later suctioned from the tracheostomy tube, the conclusion should not necessarily be that the patient is aspirating. The normal flow of secretions is downward from the mouth and pharynx, and it is quite normal for blue dye to mix with secretions and gradually coat the trachea. Also, the patient may aspirate on certain food consistencies and not on others.

Quality of Life

Because of the life-changing nature of the procedure and its sequelae, there are numerous studies assessing quality of life in the patient who has undergone a laryngectomy. Van den Brink and investigators (2006) studied 90 patients in the first 3 months following discharge after surgery for head and neck cancer. They found three factors that strongly associated with poorer quality of life: laryngectomy, lower levels of education, and being single. They also found that the dimensions of loss of control and physical self-efficacy worsened during this time period.

Lennie, Christman, and Jadack (2001) studied the eating-related experiences and educational needs of people following total laryngectomy. Most participants were not satisfied with the information they received from health care professionals and were unprepared for the potential alterations in eating following total laryngectomy. Ninety percent of the participants experienced a change in one or more aspects of eating. The most prominent changes were decreased sense of smell, decreased taste, decreased enjoyment of eating, and increased time required to eat meals. The investigators concluded that total laryngectomy produced significant changes in factors related to eating that could affect nutritional intake and quality of life.

Terrell and others (2004) studied a sample of 570 patients with upper aerodigestive cancers. The presence of a feeding tube had the most negative impact on quality of life, followed by medical comorbidities, the presence of a tracheostomy tube, chemotherapy, and neck dissection. They found that those patients who took the survey more than 1 year after their diagnosis had improved quality of life in the domains of physical health and more favorable scores for pain, social functioning, speech, and emotion. Furthermore, factors such as age, education level, sex, race, and marital status were significant predictors of quality of life. The authors postulated that the feeding tube and the process of tube feeding were constant reminders of the patients' disease in spite of the completion of therapy and/or eradication of the cancer. They also suggested that patients were less likely to enjoy the social aspects of eating due to their dysphagia. Limitations on activities such as going out to dinner may explain the decrements in social functioning and emotion for patients with feeding tubes.

Hanna and colleagues (2004) studied the differences in quality of life for patients who underwent total laryngectomy with radiation therapy compared to those who underwent chemo-radiation (chemotherapy and radiation therapy) for laryngeal preservation. They found no significant differences in demographics and overall quality of life scores; however, they found some differences in the subscales. Patients in the surgery and radiation therapy group experienced greater difficulties in social functioning, sensory disturbances (e.g., taste and smell), coughing, and greater use of pain medication compared to the chemo-radiation group. By comparison, chemo-radiation patients reported problems with dry mouth.

Eadie and Doyle (2005) compared quality of life in two male patient populations in two different hospital systems; the patients studied underwent total laryngectomy and used tracheoesophageal speech as their primary method of communication. One group of patients had higher quality of life measures in the domains of communication, eating, pain, and emotion. The authors reasoned that the better scores were due to a higher level of education and membership in a support group.

Su, Xian, Chai, Jiang, and Luo (2004) compared quality of life scores in patients who underwent a partial laryngectomy to those with a total laryngectomy and found significantly higher composite quality of life scores in the first group. They also found significant enhancements in physical function, laryngeal function, psychological state, and the ability to live independently in the partial laryngectomy group.

Quality of life seems to be affected by both treatment courses and social factors. In general, there is a trend toward improved quality of life and improved physical functioning with the following conditions: less invasive forms of laryngectomy, higher education, and the presence of a supportive environment.

Summary

There are three types of surgical laryngectomy procedures: the supraglottic laryngectomy, the hemilaryngectomy, and the total laryngectomy. The supraglottic and hemilaryngectomy are procedures that retain parts of the larynx, and recovery is relatively rapid. The severity of swallowing difficulties varies based on the extent of the surgical resection involved. In contrast, a total laryngectomy involves the removal of the entire laryngeal apparatus, and the stump of the trachea is pulled forward to form a stoma. Because there is no longer a connection between the trachea and the digestive tract, there is no risk of aspiration, although these patients may experience problems with dysphagia.

The restoration of voice also depends on the type of surgery involved. Supraglottic and hemilaryngectomy patients can benefit from exercises to strengthen the voice and swallowing. TEP can be used in patients with total laryngectomies to create esophageal speech by vibrating tissue in the pharyngoesophagus.

In summary, the successful use of laryngectomy and/or tracheostomy tubes and the management of respiratory function depend on a multidisciplinary approach and careful assessment by all team members. Generally, this team includes the speech-language pathologist, the nurse, the respiratory therapist, the patient's physician, and others involved in assessment and treatment of the patient.

Key Points

- Patients who undergo supraglottic and hemilaryngectomy may require speech therapy, but they reestablish functional swallowing and retain the ability to use their natural voice; however, the patient with a total laryngectomy must learn new methods of phonation.
- Patients may have difficulty swallowing after laryngectomy, particularly with an inflated cuff on the tracheostomy tube.
- TEP, used only with total laryngectomy patients, creates a passageway between the trachea and esophagus and uses airflow to vibrate the tissue of the pharyngoesophagus.
- The quality of life following total laryngectomy can be characterized by changes in self-image perception as well as social factors and may encompass affective disorders.

References

American Cancer Society. (2009). *All about laryngeal and hypopharyngeal cancer.* Retrieved July 4, 2009, from http://www.cancer.org/docroot/CRI/content/CRI_2_4_1X_What_are_the_key_statistics_for_Laryngeal_and_Hypopharyngeal_cancer_23.asp?rnav=cri

Brook, I. (2009). A physician's experience as a cancer of the neck patient. *Surgical Oncology,* doi:10.1016/j.suronc.2009.05.005.

Cavalot, A. L., Ricci, E., Schindler, A., Roggero, N., Albera, R., Utari, C., et al. (2009). The importance of preoperative swallowing therapy in subtotal laryngectomies. *Otolaryngology—Head and Neck Surgery, 140*(6), 822–825.

Deschler, D. G., Bunting, G. W., Lin, D. T., Emerick, K., & Rocco, J. (2009). Evaluation of voice prosthesis placement at the time of primary tracheoesophageal puncture with total laryngectomy. *Laryngoscope, 119*(7), 1353–1357.

Dettelbach, M. A., Gross, R. D., Mahlmann, J., & Eibling, D. E. (1995). Effect of the Passy-Muir valve on aspiration in patients with tracheostomy. *Head and Neck, 17*(4), 297–302.

Diedrich, W. M., & Youngstrom, K. A. (1966). *Alaryngeal speech.* Springfield, IL: Thomas.

Dobbins, M., Gunson, J., Bale, S., Neary, M., Ingrams, D., & Brown, M. (2005). Improving patient care and quality of life after laryngectomy/glossectomy. *British Journal of Nursing, 14*(12), 634–640.

Eadie, T. L., & Doyle, P. C. (2005). Quality of life in male tracheoesophageal (TE) speakers. *Journal of Rehabilitation Research and Development, 42*(1), 115–124.

Hanna, E., Sherman, A., Cash, D., Adams, D., Vural, E., Fan, C. Y., et al. (2004). Quality of life for patients following total laryngectomy vs. chemoradiation for laryngeal preservation. *Arch Otolaryngology—Head and Neck Surgery, 130*(7), 875–879.

Hess, D. R. (2005a). Facilitating speech in the patient with a tracheostomy. *Respiratory Care, 50*(4), 519–525.

Hess, D. R. (2005b). Tracheostomy tubes and related appliances. *Respiratory Care, 50*(4), 497–510.

Iseli, T. A., Agar, N.J.M., Dunemann, C., & Lyons, B. M. (2007). Functional outcomes following total laryngecopharyngectomy. *ANZ Journal of Surgery, 77*(11), 954–957.

Leder, S. B., Tarro, J. M., & Burrell, M. I. (1996). Effect of occlusion of a tracheotomy tube on aspiration. *Dysphagia, 11*(4), 254–258.

Lennie, T. A., Christman, S. K., & Jadack, R. A. (2001). Educational needs and altered eating habits following a total laryngectomy. *Oncology Nursing Forum, 28*(4), 667–674.

Logemann, J. A. (1998). *Evaluation and treatment of swallowing disorders* (2nd ed.). Austin, TX: Pro-Ed.

Logemann, J. A., Gibbons, P., Rademaker, A. W., Pauloski, B. R., Kahrilas, P. J., Bacon, M., et al. (1994). Mechanisms of recovery of swallow after supraglottic laryngectomy. *Journal of Speech and Hearing Research, 37*(5), 965–974.

Logemann, J. A., Pauloski, B. R., & Colangelo, L. (1998). Light digital occlusion of the tracheostomy tube: A pilot study of effects on aspiration and biomechanics of the swallow. *Head and Neck, 20*(1), 52–57.

Maclean, J., Cotton, S., & Perry, S. (2009). Dysphagia following a total laryngectomy: The effect on quality of life, functioning, and psychological well-being. *Dysphagia,* doi 10.1007/s00455–009–9209–0.

Martin, B.J.W., Logemann, J.A., Shaker, R., & Dodds, W.J. (1994). Coordination between respiration and swallowing: Respiratory phase relationships and temporal integration. *Journal of Applied Physiology, 76*(2), 714–723.

Muz, J., Hamlet, S., Mathog, R., & Farris, R. (1994). Scintigraphic assessment of aspiration in head and neck cancer patients with tracheostomy. *Head and Neck, 16*(1), 17–20.

Muz, J., Mathog, R. H., Nelson, R., & Jones, L. A., Jr. (1989). Aspiration in patients with head and neck cancer and tracheostomy. *American Journal of Otolaryngology, 10*(4), 282–286.

Rademaker, A. W., Logemann, J. A., Pauloski, B. R., Bowman, J. B., Lazarus, C. L., Sisson, G. A., et al. (1993). Recovery of postoperative swallowing in patients undergoing partial laryngectomy. *Head and Neck, 15*(4), 325–334.

Scheich, L. (2007). Looking at laryngeal cancer. *Nursing2007, 37*(5), 50–55.

Shin, T., Maeyama, T., Morikawa, I., & Umezaki, T. (1988). Laryngeal reflex mechanism during deglutition—observation of subglottal pressure and afferent discharge. *Otolaryngology—Head and Neck Surgery, 99*(5), 465–471.

Su, Z. Z., Xian, Z. X., Chai, L. P., Jiang, A. Y., & Luo, F. T. (2004). Investigation and analysis of quality of life for patients after laryngectomy. *Zhonghua Er Bi Yan Hou Ke Za Zhi, 39*(6), 364–367.

Terrell, J. E., Ronis, D. L., Fowler, K. E., Bradford, C. R., Chepeha, D. B., Prince, M. E., et al. (2004). Clinical predictors of quality of life in patients with head and neck cancer. *Arch Otolaryngology—Head and Neck Surgery, 130*(4), 401–408.

Thompson-Henry, S., & Braddock, B. (1995). The modified Evan's blue dye procedure fails to detect aspiration in the tracheostomized patient: Five case reports. *Dysphagia, 10*(3), 172–174.

Tippett, D. C., & Siebens, A. A. (1996). Reconsidering the value of the modified Evan's blue dye test: A comment on Thompson-Henry and Braddock. *Dysphagia, 11*(1), 78–79.

van den Brink, J. L., de Boer, M. F., Pruyn, J. F., Hop, W. C., Verwoerd, C. D., & Moorman, P. W. (2006). Quality of life during the first 3 months following discharge after surgery for head and neck cancer: Prospective evaluation. *Journal of Otolaryngology, 35*(6), 395–403.

Woodard, T. D., Oplatek, A., & Petruzzelli, G. J. (2007). Life after total laryngectomy: A measure of long-term survival, function, and quality of life. *Archives of Otolaryngology—Head and Neck Surgery, 133,* 526–532.

Complications and Emergency Procedures

Michiel J. Bové and
Linda L. Morris

Complications related to tracheostomies can be classified into immediate, early, and late (Table 10.1). Immediate complications occur during or immediately after the tracheotomy procedure and include hemorrhage and pneumothorax. Early complications often happen within the first postoperative week and include pneumonia, stomal infection, pneumomediastinum, pneumopericardium, obstruction, subcutaneous emphysema, and inadvertent decannulation, which can result in the creation of a false passage or complete loss of the airway. Later complications include the development of mucus plugs, pneumonia or stoma infection, tracheoinnominate hemorrhage, tracheoinnominate fistula, tracheoesophageal fistula, tracheocutaneous fistula, stomal stenosis, stomal granulation tissue, tracheomalacia, tracheal stenosis, mediastinitis, mediastinal fistula, and tracheocele (DeLeyn et al., 2007; Heffner, 2005; Henderson, Harrington, Izenberg, Dyess, & Silver, 1995; Neema & Manikandan, 2005; Singh, Fung, & Cole, 2007; St. John & Malen, 2004; Watanakunakorn, 1989; Wright & Van Dahm, 2003; Yaremchuk, 2003). It should be noted that there may be an overlap in the time frame in which early, intermediate, and late complications present.

10.1 Complications of Tracheostomy

Immediate	Early	Late
■ Hemorrhage ■ Pneumothorax ■ Intra-operative fire ■ Air embolism	■ Pneumonia ■ Stoma infection ■ Pneumomediastinum ■ Pneumopericardium ■ Obstruction ■ Subcutaneous emphysema (crepitus) ■ Inadvertent decannulation, loss of airway ■ False passage ■ Mucus plugs	■ Mucus plugs ■ Pneumonia ■ Stoma infection ■ Tracheitis ■ Tracheomalacia ■ Tracheoinnominate hemorrhage ■ Tracheoinnominate fistula ■ Tracheoesophageal fistula ■ Tracheocutaneous fistula (persistent stoma) ■ Stomal stenosis ■ Stomal granulation tissue ■ Tracheal stenosis ■ Mediastinitis ■ Mediastinal fistula ■ Tracheocele

The rate of complications has been shown to be significantly elevated in specific patient populations, such as in the pediatric, post–head trauma, obese, burn, or seriously debilitated groups (Goldenberg et al., 2000). Published rates of tracheotomy-related complications vary greatly (5%–65%) and depend on study design, length of follow-up, and definition of complications (Francois et al., 2003; Waldron, Padgham, & Hurley, 1990).

The first study to prospectively quantify complications from tracheostomy was by Dane and King (1975), who observed 40 patients after tracheostomies were placed. Their study did not involve intraoperative complications. Five percent of patients (2 patients) had significant bleeding from the wound. Another 2 patients had bleeding from stomal granulation tissue. One patient bled upon decannulation, and another patient bled endotracheally as a result of granulation tissue extending from the stoma to the tracheal lumen. These 2 patients later developed stomal stenosis. One patient developed tube obstruction, 2 developed bilateral tension pneumothorax during the first tube change, and 4 developed severe necrotizing pneumonia. The investigators followed up all patients with a bronchoscopic exam. Fifteen patients died while still receiving mechanical ventilation, all of whom had severe tracheitis. All 25 patients who were successfully decannulated survived. Of these survivors, 60% had "minimal deformity" of the trachea, 32% had moderate deformity, and 8% had symptomatic tracheal stenosis.

Francois and others (2003) reported a 2-year prospective trial of the complications following tracheostomy performed in the ICU. Out of their group of 118 patients, 86 patients underwent conventional subthyroid tracheotomy, while 32 underwent surgical cricothyroidotomy. Overall, complications occurred in 36 patients (30%), with 4 patients developing two complications. The incidence of complications was similar between conventional tracheotomy and cricothyroidotomy. There were 6 patients with serious complications (5%), and minor complications occurred in 30 patients (25%). The two most common complications during the immediate period were pneumothorax and minor bleeding. One minor episode of bleeding occurred in a patient with a cricothyroidotomy. In the patients with standard tracheotomies, there was one case of pneumothorax, four episodes of minor bleeding, and one episode of difficult cannulation.

For the early postoperative period, the researchers found 25 early complications, of which 5 were considered major and 20 were considered minor. Major complications included subglottic stenosis, accidental decannulation causing acute respiratory failure, tracheal fistula, and chronic vocal cord dysfunction. Minor complications included accidental decannulation, laryngeal edema, stomal granulations, and temporary vocal cord dysfunction. There were 8 minor complications in the late postoperative phase. These included tracheal granulations, persistent wound, and scar formation. No deaths were attributable to surgical tracheostomy in this study.

This study had an unusually high percentage of cricothyroidotomies (27%), and it was reported that this procedure was done mainly in older patients. Overall mortality rates tended to be higher in these patients, although their APACHE II scores were not significantly different from those undergoing the standard tracheotomy procedure. At the end of the 6-month follow-up period, 32 patients (35%) still had a tracheostomy in place, with a similar proportion in both groups.

A retrospective 10-year study in Israel reviewed 1,130 tracheostomies performed in one hospital from January 1987 through December 1996. None were percutaneous tracheostomies. Indications included prolonged mechanical ventilation, adjunct to head or neck or chest surgery in which prolonged mechanical ventilation was anticipated; extensive maxillofacial trauma; or upper airway obstruction. Only three tracheotomies were performed as emergencies; however, none of these three developed any postoperative complications. In this study, major complications occurred in 49 cases (4.3%) and included subglottic or tracheal stenosis (21), hemorrhage (9), severe postoperative hemorrhage (7), massive hemorrhage due to tracheoinnominate fistula (2), tracheocutaneous fistula (also called persistent fistula or persistent stoma; 6), severe infection (5), decannulation or tube obstruction (4), subcutaneous emphysema or pneumomediastinum (3), and tracheoesophageal fistula (1; Goldenberg et al., 2000).

In this Israeli study, 8 deaths were directly related to the tracheostomy. Immediate or intraoperative complications included intraoperative hemorrhage, air embolism, apnea, damage due to adjacent structures, and intraoperative fire. Early postoperative complications included postoperative hemorrhage, tube dislodgement or obstruction, subcutaneous emphysema, pneumothorax, pneumomediastinum, and infection. Late postoperative complications included hemorrhage due to granulation or tracheoinnominate artery fistula, tracheal stenosis, tracheocutaneous fistula, and tracheoesophageal fistula.

Let us consider each of these complications and the corresponding methods to prevent and/or treat them.

Intraoperative Complications

Intraoperative complications include hemorrhage (usually from the anterior jugular veins, the thyroid isthmus, or vascular variants such as the thyroid ima artery), the creation of a false passage, electrocautery-induced airway fire, and surgical injury to adjacent structures.

The inability to ventilate immediately after placement of the tracheostomy tube suggests the tube has entered a false passage, usually anterior to the tracheal wall or, rarely, posterior to the trachea into the esophagus. Passing a soft suction catheter into the newly placed tracheostomy tube helps recognize false passage cannulation. Also, all retractors and cricoid hooks should be kept in place until successful cannulation is confirmed to allow for an immediate reattempt at cannulation should difficulties arise.

Hemorrhage

Hemorrhage can occur as a result of laceration of major blood vessels in the neck during the procedure. Tracheotomies that are placed lower than usual—below the fourth tracheal ring—have a higher incidence of damage to the innominate artery. Minor bleeding is far more common and is estimated to occur in up to 40% of cases.

Intraoperative hemorrhage most commonly results from injury to the anterior jugular veins early in the dissection, especially during emergent procedures, or to the thyroid isthmus later in the dissection during attempts to mobilize it from the anterior tracheal wall or during attempts to divide and ligate it. High-riding innominate arteries present a significant risk of severe hemorrhage when the dissection is carried inferiorly.

Prevention. Finger palpation in the substernal region should, therefore, always precede instrumentation to rule out prominent pulses in this region. Bleeding can be minimized by carefully identifying and staying in the midline, cautiously dissecting layer by layer, and maintaining a well-lit operative field and retraction of the soft tissues. Patient position and neck extension should be optimized. If local anesthesia is used, the procedure should not be started until the vasoconstrictive agent in the local anesthetic has taken effect. Structures such as the anterior jugular vein and the thyroid isthmus should be carefully identified in order to avoid inadvertent trauma and bleeding. An aberrant innominate artery may traverse anterior to the trachea in the field of dissection, making it vulnerable to laceration and potentially life-threatening hemorrhage (Grant, Dempsey, Harrison, & Jones, 2006).

Management. After the insertion of the tracheostomy tube, the surgical wound should be carefully inspected for any bleeding sources. Increases in blood pressure—either as a result of coughing caused by tube insertion or recovery of normal blood pressure after relative hypotension during anesthesia—can disguise apparent bleeding sources during the procedure itself. If necessary, the tracheostomy tube should be removed to allow for better inspection of the surgical field for the source of bleeding. Superficial sources of bleeding can be addressed by mobilizing the flange on the tracheostomy tube while leaving the cannula in the trachea. Merely packing the wound to obtain hemostasis carries the risk of causing subcutaneous emphysema in the postoperative period.

Pneumothorax

Pneumothorax is usually the result of a traumatic puncture of the pleura. It is more common in pediatric tracheotomy, where the pulmonary apices are relatively elevated and therefore more vulnerable within the lower neck. In adults, this complication usually involves the rupture of a pulmonary bleb in a patient struggling to breathe during an awake, emergency tracheotomy. Pneumothorax can also result from damage to the posterior tracheal wall during the tracheal incision or during insertion of the tracheotomy tube. More commonly, the tracheostomy tube can be inadvertently inserted between the anterior tracheal wall and the anterior mediastinum. The insertion of the tube into this false passage results in worsening respiratory status after tube insertion and can be confirmed by the inability to pass a flexible suction catheter into the tracheal lumen. While some suggest obtaining postoperative radiographs on all tracheotomy patients, published data suggests this is unnecessary in routine, uncomplicated, elective cases (Smith, Grillone, & Fuleihan, 1999). These authors suggest restricting chest radiographs to emergency procedures, difficult procedures, or patients exhibiting signs or symptoms of pneumothorax.

Prevention. Pneumothorax is best prevented by establishing an airway before performing a tracheotomy and by restricting the dissection to the midline. The tracheostomy tube should be inserted under direct visualization and good illumination. The ability to suction tracheal contents via a flexible suction catheter should be immediately confirmed after placement of the tracheostomy tube. End-tidal CO_2 should be confirmed by the anesthesiologist as soon as possible. Insufflation through the tracheostomy tube should be delayed until these confirmatory measures can be performed to avoid insufflating the mediastinum. If there remains any doubt about the placement of the tube, retractors can be placed within the stoma to maintain its patency while the tracheostomy tube is removed and replaced under direct visualization.

Management. When pneumothorax is symptomatic, it should be treated by inserting a chest tube.

Intraoperative Fire

Although flammable anesthetic agents are no longer used, fire in the operating room continues to be a concern, particularly with tracheotomy. Although rare, airway fires are potentially devastating occurrences. There are approximately 100 intraoperative fires annually in the United States; 10 to 20 are deemed serious, and 2 directly result in death. Seventy percent of these fires are related to the use of electrocautery near a high concentration of oxygen (Daane & Toth,

2005; Rinder, 2008; Weber, Hargunani, & Wax, 2006). The "fire triangle" consists of the three elements necessary to initiate a fire: heat, fuel, and an oxidizer. Procedures involving the head and neck are at particular risk because all the elements of this triangle are in close proximity (Weber et al.). Once they start, surgical fires spread rapidly (Daane & Toth).

A number of different objects and fluids used in the operating room are flammable and can serve as a fuel source. Tincture of benzoin has ignited with the use of cautery during wound closure (Axelrod, Kusnetz, & Rosenberg, 1993). Sutures packed in isopropyl alcohol and the packaging material may be flammable. Likewise, skin preparations that include alcohol provide highly flammable residue (Plumlee, 1973). Gauze sponges have acted as fuel in many reported fires (Axelrod et al., 1993; Blanchard, 1987). Draping material (Stouffer, 1992) and tape (Nicholson, 1974) can also ignite if the oxygen tension is high enough. Although surgical drapes must be flame retardant, many other materials are flammable and serve as a fuel source if a sufficiently high oxygen tension exists. Endotracheal tubes are generally made of PVC because of its low implant toxicity and pliability. PVC endotracheal tubes are known to ignite in oxygen-rich environments but have been shown to be flammable in oxygen concentrations as low as 25% (deRichmond & Bruley, 1993; Wolf & Simpson, 1987).

It is essential that only cuffed endotracheal tubes be used during tracheotomy in order to prevent oxygen from leaking into the zone where the trachea is entered. When entering the trachea, every effort should be made to avoid puncturing the cuff. This can be accomplished by pushing the tube further down the trachea, close to the carina (Marsh & Riley, 1992; Michels & Stott, 1994; Wilson, Igbaseimokumo, & Martin, 1994). This may require fiber-optic bronchoscopic visualization to confirm the endotracheal tube is placed as close to the carina as possible. An additional precaution is to inflate the tracheal cuff with saline to prevent ignition should the cuff come into contact with an electrocautery source (Sosis & Dillon, 1991).

Prevention. Prevention of operative fires is the responsibility of each member of the surgical team. Communication between the surgeon and anesthesiologist is essential. Extreme care should be taken not to use cautery close to the trachea after entering it. Concentrations of oxygen in excess of 50% FiO_2 (fraction of inspired oxygen) have been shown to support airway fires (Thompson et al., 1998). The fractional concentration of oxygen should therefore be kept as low as possible during tracheotomy.

All personnel should be aware that an airway fire can occur during tracheotomy, whether at the bedside or in the operating room. Saline should be available at all times to help extinguish a fire. A fire extinguisher should also be available (Daane & Toth, 2005). Other recommended guidelines for the prevention of surgical fires during tracheotomy include the following:

- Keep the cautery unit in the holster when not in use.
- Use a nonconductive plastic clamp to attach cautery to the surgical field.
- Adjust cautery settings to prevent sparks.
- Disconnect power to high-intensity light sources when not in use.
- Never allow fiber-optic cables to come into contact with flammable materials.

- Advance the endotracheal tube close to the carina (24–25 cm from the teeth in the average male).
- Use saline to inflate the endotracheal tube cuff. Ensure there is no leak of anesthetic gas past the cuff.
- Never use cautery to enter the trachea.
- Avoid nitrous oxide or any flammable anesthetic agents.
- Avoid tenting surgical drapes to prevent the accumulation of oxygen.
- Avoid alcohol-based skin preparations and petroleum-based eye products.
- Stop supplemental oxygen at least 1 minute before using cautery.
- If bleeding occurs once the trachea has been incised, ensure the airway is secured and then use diathermy while suctioning to clear oxygen from the wound.
- Use an incise drape to isolate head and neck incisions from flammable vapors below the drape.
- Use fire-retardant surgical drapes.
- Wet all gauze sponges and cotton pledgets.
- Use suction to scavenge gases from the mouth.

Weber and others (2006) also suggest that prevention consists of the removal of one of the elements of the fire triangle. This includes shaving the entire neck and shoulders of a patient with excess body hair; enabling adequate drying of the prep solution; and decreasing oxygen delivery if tolerated, lessening the amount of oxygen in the operative field.

Management. In the event of an airway fire, the following steps should be taken:

- Stop the flow of oxygen to the endotracheal tube.
- Remove the endotracheal tube.
- Flood the field with fluids, if appropriate. Consider flushing saline down the endotracheal tube to extinguish any intraluminal fire (Wolf, Sidebotham, & Stern, 1994).
- Mask ventilate with 100% oxygen.
- Reintubate as soon as possible.
- Consider PEEP, continued ventilator support, and high-dose steroids.
- Call for immediate consultation by an otolaryngologist to evaluate the extent of the airway burn.

Air Embolism

Air embolism results from the aspiration of a volume of air through any rent in venous circulation. It is particularly liable to occur during neck surgery, as deep inspiratory movements of the chest—similar to awake tracheotomy—produce markedly negative venous pressure in the veins in the neck. This predisposes the patient to a sudden indrawing of air into any tears in the venous structures. This is more likely to occur in awake tracheotomy, where respiratory obstruction can result in significant distention of the cervical venous circulation. Air that enters the venous system is transported through the pulmonary circulation to the right atrium and ventricle. From there, it can continue on to the pulmonary arteries, where it may cause interference with gas exchange, cardiac arrhythmias, pulmonary hypertension, and even cardiac failure and arrest. A large bolus of air entering the venous system can cause an air lock in the right atrium and ventricle, leading to outflow obstruction, decreased pulmonary venous return, and subsequent decreased left ventricular preload and cardiac output. Intermediate amounts of air collect in the pulmonary circulation and produce a pulmonary vascular injury manifested by pre- and postcapillary pulmonary vasoconstriction, pulmonary hypertension, endothelial injury, and permeability pulmonary edema. Subsequent ventilation-perfusion mismatch can cause right to left shunting and increased arterial hypoxia and hypercapnia. Small amounts of air do not produce symptoms because the air is broken up and absorbed from circulation. Although classical teaching states that more than 5 ml/kg of air (intravenous) is required for a significant injury (including shock and cardiac arrest), complications secondary to as little as 10–20 ml of air (the length of an unprimed intravenous infusion set) have been reported. Further, as little as 0.5 ml of air in the left anterior descending coronary artery has been shown to lead to ventricular fibrillation (Agarwal, Kumar, Chavali, & Mestri, 2009; Hartveit, Lystad, & Minken, 1968).

Death from air embolism after tracheostomy is extremely rare. Asherson (1958) described an early postoperative death from air embolism in an 18-month-old child who passed away suddenly a few hours after tracheostomy. The procedure had been performed under general anesthesia. The veins in the neck were notably engorged, and there was profuse hemorrhage. The patient coughed immediately after extubation, and the venous hemorrhage from the lower aspect of the wound was controlled by gauze packing. The patient left the operating room in stable condition and was breathing spontaneously but coughing occasionally. Four hours later, the patient died suddenly and without warning. Upon autopsy, the right heart was shown to be filled with air and the cerebral arteries with air bubbles.

Prevention. To avoid this potentially lethal complication, all venous hemorrhage should be completely controlled. A nonslipping ligature should be used (e.g., silk). Care should be taken to avoid trauma to the inferior thyroid veins. Also, if feasible, tracheotomy above the thyroid isthmus could help avoid trauma in cases of significant venous engorgement.

Management. Once air embolism is suspected, the procedure in progress should be terminated immediately.

- Administer 100% oxygen and intubate for significant respiratory distress or refractory hypoxemia. Oxygen may reduce bubble size by increasing the gradient for nitrogen to move out.
- Promptly place patient in Trendelenburg (head down) position and rotate toward the left lateral decubitus position. This maneuver helps trap air in the apex of the ventricle, prevents its ejection into the pulmonary arterial system, and maintains right ventricular output.
- Maintain systemic arterial pressure with fluid resuscitation and vasopressors/beta-adrenergic agents if necessary.

- Consider transfer to a hyperbaric chamber. Potential benefits of this therapy include (a) the compression of existing air bubbles, (b) the establishment of a high diffusion gradient to speed the dissolution of existing bubbles, and (c) improved oxygenation of ischemic tissues and lowered intracranial pressure.
- Circulatory collapse should be addressed with cardiopulmonary resuscitation and potentially the aforementioned more invasive procedures.

Early Postoperative Complications

Tracheostomy Tube Displacement and Loss of Airway

The tracheostomy patient requires vigilant care to prevent complications, especially in the first several days post-op. Casserly, Lang, Fenton, and Walsh (2007) showed that health care professionals lack knowledge of what to do in the event of inadvertent decannulation. One of the most hazardous complications of a tracheostomy is inadvertent decannulation occurring before the tract between the skin and the trachea has matured, approximately 5 to 6 days after the procedure. If the stoma has not yet matured, the tissue planes collapse upon each other when the tracheostomy tube is removed. Inadvertent decannulation before a stable tract has formed can, therefore, result in a loss of airway. Several factors can predispose a patient to tube dislodgement, including: (a) loosening the straps and or sutures securing the tracheotomy tube in place, particularly with resolution of subcutaneous emphysema or edema of the neck; (b) the use of adjustable-length tracheostomy tubes; (c) excessive coughing; (d) excessive movements of an agitated, uncooperative, confused, or undersedated patient; and (e) an overweight patient with an elongated tract from skin to trachea resulting in an improperly fitting tube.

Tracheostomy tube displacement may not always be immediately evident, especially if the patient's airway obstruction was incomplete and the patient was not dependent on positive-pressure ventilation. In these situations, displacement may present with respiratory distress and the inability to pass a suction catheter instead of respiratory arrest and death.

Prevention. While the incidence of tube displacement is low, it has a high mortality rate. Care should be taken to secure the tracheostomy tube with sutures placed through the neck flange and with snug-fitting tracheostomy ties. Tube security should be regularly checked, and transporting the patient should be minimized as much as possible in the early postoperative period. Tube security should also be checked prior to moving the patient in any way, and care should be taken to relieve any added weight or traction from the ventilator tubing.

Management. When the airway is lost due to tube displacement in the early postoperative period, a mature stoma has not yet developed. Tissue planes collapse, and emergency efforts to replace the tube are not advised because of the likely development of a false passage. Rather, the immediate management of a lost airway in a patient with an immature stoma should include mask ventilation until an oral endotracheal airway can be established. The tracheotomy can then be revised under more controlled conditions, including adequate lighting, personnel, and equipment. If traction stay sutures were placed, the traction on these sutures will spread the skin edges and bring the stoma up to the level of the opening in the skin (Parnes & Myers, 1997; Walvekar & Myers, 2008).

Tube Obstruction

In a patient with a tracheostomy, the most frequent cause of respiratory or cardiac arrest is tube obstruction. Tube obstruction secondary to mucus plugs, blood clots, or tube displacement can occur in the early postoperative period. Mucus plugs are one of the most frequent complications of tracheostomies. Because the upper airway is bypassed, patients are at risk for the drying of secretions, which can lead to mucus plugs. Adequate measures to mobilize secretions are of the utmost concern in managing the patient with a tracheostomy.

Prevention. Obstruction may be minimized by attentive nursing care that includes frequent suctioning, adequate hydration, and the use of humidified oxygen. The prevention of obstruction is markedly facilitated by the use of tracheostomy tubes with inner cannulas, which allow regular inspection and cleaning. The two primary interventions to prevent the development of mucus plugs are adequate hydration and promoting mobility of secretions. Adequate hydration is necessary to keep secretions thin and mobile so they can be easily coughed or suctioned. This can be a challenge in a patient whose fluid status may be restricted for other reasons. HMEs can be effective in helping humidify secretions; however, these devices can become easily clogged with secretions.

While they provide some comfort to mucous membranes, high-humidity tracheostomy collars are not a source of hydration. Heated humidity, on the other hand, has been shown to be four times more effective than HMEs (Epstein, 2005).

Management. Mucus plugs are most often a respiratory emergency and usually present as acute dyspnea. Figure 10.1 is an algorithm for the management of airway obstruction. Immediate treatment measures include checking the inner cannula for the obstruction. If the inner cannula is clear, the obstruction may be further into the airway, in which case deep suctioning is necessary. This can be accompanied by vigorous use of the manual resuscitation bag in order to promote vigorous coughing and oxygenate a patient in distress. If there is difficulty passing a suction catheter or the manual resuscitation bag meets resistance, the clinician should be highly suspicious of secretions narrowing the diameter of the lumen of the tube. If the aforementioned measures have not relieved the obstruction, the entire tracheostomy tube should be changed. Frequently, a large mucus plug will be removed with the tracheostomy tube. If this does not relieve the obstruction, the clinician should remove the tracheostomy tube and suction directly into the mature stoma. Bronchoscopy can be used to identify and remove mucus plugs that are deep in the tracheobronchial tree. In patients for whom it is not contraindicated, the Heimlich maneuver can be considered to "bring a mucus plug into reach."

10.1

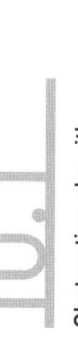

Obstruction algorithm.

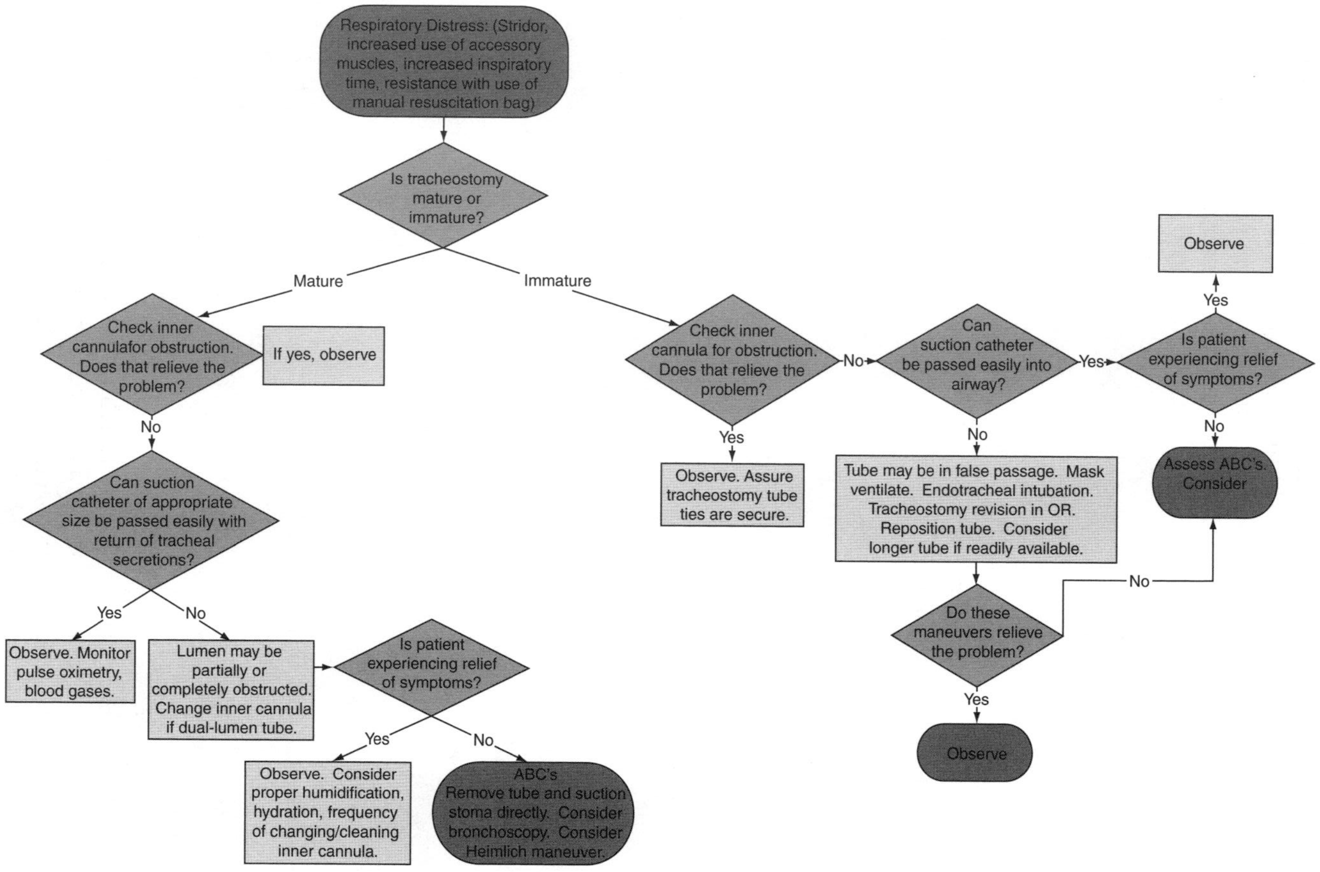

Internal Stomal Erosion

Internal stomal erosion occurs because of undue force creating outward pull or torque, most often as a result of the traction of the ventilator tubing against the trachea. These traction forces are magnified when more weight is added to the tubing system, including closed suction systems and in-line humidifiers.

Excessive traction can enlarge the stoma to the extent that the entire shaft of the tracheostomy tube as well as most of the cuff is visible within the stoma. Excessive outward traction can also produce enough force to cause inadvertent decannulation.

Prevention. Excessive force against the stoma must be minimized by adequately supporting the ventilator tubing and removing unneeded equipment. Unless the patient is hemodynamically unstable, a closed suction system should be removed. Unnecessary in-line features should also be removed, relocated, or minimized. When moving the patient in any way, the ventilator tubing should always be checked for excessive traction. To minimize traction when providing care, patients should always be first turned toward the ventilator and then turned away. When patients are positioned facing away from the ventilator, extra care must be taken to minimize traction forces.

Management. A longer tracheostomy tube may be required to avoid further trauma to the distal aspect of the stoma. The wound can then granulate and heal from within. If the integrity of the cartilaginous framework of the trachea has been compromised, the patient may require stenting or resection of the affected portion of the trachea in order to allow for decannulation.

External Stomal Erosion

External stomal erosion occurs as a result of inward pressure from the neck flange digging into the tissues of the neck. It can be exacerbated by flexion of the neck or added weight—such as in-line devices and closed suction systems—pushing on the neck flange.

Prevention. In the case of external stomal erosion, prevention and treatment are the same. The neck should be maintained in neutral position, and any added weight that creates inward pressure should be eliminated. In some cases, the erosion is so deep that packing may be required to eliminate drainage and allow the tissues to heal.

Management. The first step in treating external stomal erosion is relieving the pressure that caused it. Local wound care is important to avoid infection. Necrotic tissue should be carefully debrided with regular wet to dry dressings. Semipermeable dressings can be used to retain moisture and encourage cell growth. Dressings also provide a barrier between the tracheotomy tube flange and the peristomal skin.

Hemorrhage

Hemorrhage can result from bleeding from ligated thyroid isthmus, erosion into nearby blood vessels, or bleeding from granulation tissue or the tracheal wall from aggressive suctioning. Postoperative bleeding can occur after the vasoconstrictive effect of local anesthesia has worn off or from elevated blood pressure in a previously hypotensive patient. Delaney, Bagshaw, and Nalos (2006) reported the incidence of clinically relevant bleeding at 5.7%, with similar rates seen in both open and percutaneous tracheotomy.

Prevention. Bleeding after a tracheostomy may be prevented by careful dissection and attention to details.

Management. Brisk bleeding can arise from veins of thyroid tissue lacerated during surgery and should be managed by a return to the operative setting for wound exploration. Prolonged oozing should make the surgeon suspect a coagulopathy. If oozing is limited, and the patient has a cuffed tracheotomy tube, the wound can be lightly packed.

Infection

A tracheostomy is considered a clean contaminated wound. The reported incidence of infection is highly dependent upon the criteria for infection in the individual study considered. Indeed, while the rate of stomal infection was reported to be as high as 36% by Stauffer, Olson, and Petty (1981), the incidence of cellulitis and purulence has generally been reported at 3% to 8% (Delaney et al., 2006). Stomal infection usually manifests as an indolent infection, mild cellulitis, or granulation tissue. Serious infections such as mediastinitis, fasciitis, abscess, and clavicular osteomyelitis are rare. When they do occur, they can result in loss of tracheal tissue, large air leaks, and hemorrhage (Snow, Richardson, & Flint, 1981).

The peristomal region is quickly colonized with multiple species of organisms. Over 85% of tracheostomies have been shown to be colonized with *Pseudomonas,* for instance (Myers, Stool, & Johnson, 1985). It is believed that the tracheostomy results in a contaminated wound that secondarily infects a larynx injured from an endotracheal tube or other acute process resulting in chronic mucosal ulceration. This predisposes the patient to the formation of scar tissue, granuloma, and stricture.

The role of antibiotic prophylaxis is highly controversial. On one hand, Sasaki, Horiuchi, and Koss (1979) demonstrated in animal studies that perioperative prophylaxis with systemic antibiotics and povidone-iodine reduced bacterial growth and laryngeal damage. Other studies concluded that perioperative antibiotics merely selected for resistant pathogenic organisms and decreased the numbers of normal skin flora, such as beta-hemolytic streptococcus and *Staphylococcus epidermidis.* Some have also suggested that the use of gauze induces secondary wound injury and prevents wound healing (Tsunezuka, Suzuki, Nitta, & Oda, 2005). The use of fibrous wound dressings such as Aquacel (carboxymethylcellulose natrium sheet) and antimicrobial drain sponges (polyhexamethylene biguanide) can be used as adjuncts in controlling peristomal wound infections (Motta & Trigilia, 2005; Tsunezuka et al.).

The tracheostomy tube can also be viewed as a type of indwelling catheter that accumulates debris and serves as a source of infection similar to urological and intravascular catheters. The formation of a biofilm on polymer surfaces through colonization by *Staphylococcus epidermidis* has been recently recognized as a source of infection. The biofilm present on catheter surfaces plays an important role in the pathogenicity of the infecting organism by protecting the embedded staphylococci and reducing the efficacy of host defenses and antimicrobial killing (Mack, 1999; von Eiff, Heilmann, & Peters, 1999).

Prevention. Avoiding colonization is impossible. Meticulous hygiene involving careful suctioning; care of the stoma; cleaning the inner cannula; and regular changes of the stomal dressing, tracheostomy tube holder, and tracheostomy tube is necessary to decrease the burden of crust and debris, thereby reducing bacterial loads. Traction sutures should be removed with the first tracheostomy tube change when the tract has matured (3–5 days).

Management. True necrotizing wound infections with purulence and surrounding cellulitis should be treated with culture-specific antibiotic and local care with frequent debridement.

Subcutaneous Emphysema

The incidence of subcutaneous emphysema after tracheostomy ranges from 1% to 4% (Durbin, 2005). Air can be forced into a subcutaneous tissue plane during tube placement if the patient frequently coughs intra- or postoperatively. This complication is more likely if an uncuffed tracheostomy tube is used; if the tracheostomy wound is closed with sutures; or if it is packed, especially in the context of an uncuffed tracheostomy tube causing air to pass from the airway into the subcutaneous peristomal tissues.

Subcutaneous emphysema is usually mild and manifests as an area of crepitus in the region of the skin surrounding the tracheostomy site. Rarely, it may present more extensively with swelling of the entire body, which can occur with forceful use of the manual resuscitation bag with an immature stoma.

Prevention. There are several methods to avoid subcutaneous emphysema from tracheostomy placement. Securing the airway with endotracheal intubation prior to tube placement allows the administration of general anesthesia and prevents coughing in the awake patient. Another method is avoiding excessive dissection in the pretracheal plane or lateral to the trachea. Finally, the clinician should avoid closing the skin incision when a tracheotomy wound is packed to allow air to escape the trachea.

Management. Most cases of subcutaneous emphysema can be managed expectantly as the trapped air is usually resorbed spontaneously in the body over a few days. If the wound is sutured closed, the sutures should be removed; if the wound is packed, the packing should be removed. An uncuffed tracheostomy tube should be replaced with a cuffed tube.

Pneumomediastinum

Pneumomediastinum is the accumulation of air within the thoracic cavity, potentially resulting in decreased cardiac output and cardiovascular collapse and difficulty ventilating. It is a well-recognized complication following tracheotomy, especially in children; it is reported to occur in up to 43% of those older than 12 months and 28% of those younger than 12 months (Kremer, Botos-Kremer, Eckel, & Schlöndorff, 2002). The accepted mechanism occurs during forceful inspiratory movements of respiratory obstruction, when high negative intrathoracic pressures are developed. Through the incision of the skin and cervical fascia, an initial pathway is established for the aspiration of air through the wound edges into the mediastinum.

Prevention. The development of pneumomediastinum seems related to the extent of peritracheal dissection during the procedure (Rabuzzi & Reed, 1971). Dissection along the anterior wall of the trachea should therefore be minimized. As with pneumothorax, prevention depends on being able to establish an airway, either through endotracheal intubation or rigid bronchoscopy, prior to performing the tracheotomy.

Management. The treatment of pneumomediastinum depends on the amount of air present. A small amount of air noted on a postoperative chest x-ray in an asymptomatic patient will be reabsorbed spontaneously and warrants no specific treatment. For larger volumes of air or in the symptomatic patient, a chest tube may be required. Symptoms include coughing, shortness of breath, and chest pain that is often pleuritic and occasionally radiates to the neck, back, or shoulders.

Postobstructive Pulmonary Edema

Postobstructive pulmonary edema, also referred to as negative pressure pulmonary edema, occurs in a variety of circumstances. Although the cause is not clear, the common denominator for its development is hypoxia associated with airway obstruction. Negative intrapleural pressure is the primary pathologic event and develops against a closed glottis with catecholamine activation (Weymuller, 1998). This negative intrapleural pressure promotes the translocation of blood from systemic to pulmonary circulation, which further increases pulmonary microvascular pressures. When the obstruction is relieved, either via surgical airway or endotracheal tube placement, the pulmonary edema becomes evident either immediately or within hours.

Prevention. Although there are no effective means of prevention, knowledge of the risk factors and recognition of the symptoms are important. Factors that increase the risk for postobstructive pulmonary edema include obstructive sleep apnea and acute airway obstruction secondary to croup, epiglottitis, or tumor.

Management. Prompt recognition and treatment are essential and include oxygenation, PEEP, and diuretics.

Late Postoperative Complications

Epstein (2005) provided a good review of the late postoperative complications of tracheostomy, which typically occur after the first postoperative week.

They include tracheoinnominate fistula, tracheoesophageal or tracheocutaneous fistula, granulation tissue, tracheomalacia, and tracheal stenosis.

Tracheoinnominate Fistula/Hemorrhage

Tracheoinnominate fistula is a rare complication, with a reported incidence of 0.7% (Scalise, Prunk, Healy, & Votto, 2005). The peak incidence occurs between 1 and 3 weeks after the initial tracheotomy procedure. Risk factors include low placement of the tracheostomy tube (below the fourth tracheal ring), excessive tube movement, hypotension causing decreased capillary pressure, sepsis, corticosteroids, malnutrition, and diabetes (Heffner, 2005; Singh et al., 2007). The hallmark sign of a tracheoinnominate fistula is a sentinel hemorrhage, which is followed some time later by massive bleeding. The patient should be taken to the operating room for an endoscopic evaluation of the airway, and an immediate thoracotomy can be performed if massive hemorrhage occurs (Heffner, 2005).

Prevention. The best way to reduce incidence of tracheoinnominate fistula is to prevent the risk factors. Low placement of the stoma should be avoided. Hypotension should be minimized. The tracheostomy tube should be of optimal size so the cuff can be centralized within the trachea, which will also eliminate excessive angulation and anterior movement of the tube against the trachea. Cuff pressures should be monitored to avoid overinflation (Singh et al., 2007).

Management. Bleeding from a tracheoinnominate fistula is the most feared complication and carries a mortality rate above 80% (Goldenberg et al., 2000). The rupture of an innominate artery can present unexpectedly as sudden onset, fatal hemorrhage from the stoma. Occasionally, warning signs of this complication become evident, either as a sentinel bleed—a self-limited episode of bright red blood from the tracheostomy—or as a pulsatile tracheostomy tube caused by the proximity of the tube to the innominate artery.

If massive hemorrhage is the initial presenting symptom, the cuff should be immediately overinflated to tamponade the bleeding. This may, however, require reintubation with an endotracheal tube and positioning the cuff over the area of the fistula. The patient should then undergo an immediate thoracotomy and ligation of the artery.

Tracheoesophageal Fistula

Tracheoesophageal fistula (TEF) is another rare complication following tracheotomy, with an estimated incidence of 1% (Epstein, 2005). This complication usually occurs with prolonged excessive cuff pressure or when a malpositioned tracheostomy tube exerts pressure on the posterior wall, especially with an indwelling nasogastric tube. TEF can also develop after a penetrating injury to the posterior tracheal wall at the time of surgery. TEF is suspected when there are copious secretions, recurrent aspiration, a persistent cuff leak, severe gastric distention, or gastric contents presenting through the tracheostomy. Diagnosis is made with contrast esophagography or direct visualization with bronchoscopy (Sue & Susanto, 2003).

Prevention. Efforts to ensure the proper fit of the tracheostomy tube within the airway are necessary to prevent TEF. Patients with both nasogastric and tracheostomy tubes should be monitored closely to ensure that cuff pressures are within acceptable limits.

Management. If the mediastinum is involved in a secondary suppurative process, thoracotomy or CT-guided drainage may be necessary to drain the wound. If the process is isolated within the cervical region, it may be drained through a neck incision. With adequate drainage of the suppurative process, treatment with antibiotics, and attention to proper nutrition, a fistula may close spontaneously. If conservative measures are unsuccessful, stenting of the esophagus and trachea may alleviate symptoms.

Tracheocutaneous Fistula

Tracheocutaneous fistula (TCF) represents the failure of the tracheostomy stoma to close following decannulation. This results when the squamous epithelial surfaces of the peristomal skin and endotracheal mucosa heal to one another, creating an uninterrupted epithelial tract. The incidence of TCF ranges from 3.3% to 42% (Mohan, Kashyap, & Verma, 2003). The result is continued drainage of mucus onto the anterior chest wall, especially with cough, which can cause skin irritation and poor cosmesis. TCF also decreases the efficiency of the patient's cough, promoting recurrent aspiration. By tethering the laryngotracheal complex to the overlying skin, TCF also impairs swallowing, which is dependent on adequate laryngeal elevation. Fistula formation occurs more often after long-term tracheostomy and has a reported rate of 70% in those who have a tracheostomy tube for over 16 weeks (Bent & Smith, 1998).

Stomas generally close by secondary intention within 1 week of decannulation; however, it has been reported that up to 29% of all decannulated patients develop a persistent stoma. Epithelialization and/or infection of the tract can cause this failure to close. Atrophy and adhesion of the subcutaneous tissue can also occur, resulting in a depressed scar (Stanton, Kademani, Patel, & Foote, 2004).

Prevention. TCF occurs more often in patients with long-term tracheotomy tube placement. Avoiding this complication is, therefore, most often a function of preventing unnecessarily prolonged tube placement.

Management. The closure of the fistula may be possible via cautery and curettage of the tract. Cases in which the tract fails to close within 6 months, however, require operative closure (see Figure 10.2). Both the scar and fistula are addressed at the same time. The scar is excised via a horizontally oriented elliptical incision encompassing the fistula. The flaps are raised to release adherent scar tissue, and the squamous epithelium of the tract immediately adjacent to the trachea are left intact and inverted with a purse-string suture so the trachea is lined with squamous epithelium. The skin surrounding the tract is widely undermined. The strap muscles, which are frequently involved in the fistulous tract, are released and reapproximated in the midline. Joining the muscle in the midline fills the depressed area of the tract and, more importantly, separates

10.2

Surgical repair of tracheocutaneous fistula. (A) Scar from tracheostomy is excised down to fistula. (B) Skin flaps superior and inferior to the incision are undermined and strap muscles are dissected.

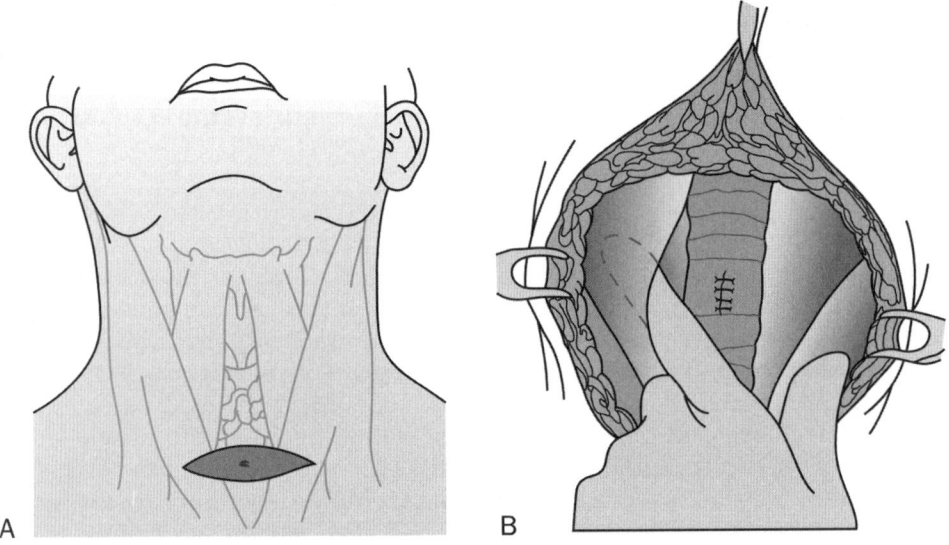

the laryngotracheal complex from the overlying skin, enabling the elevation of the complex during swallowing.

Complications of TCF closure include hematoma, infection, keloid formation, and subcutaneous emphysema (Bent & Smith, 1998). Rarely, subcutaneous emphysema develops into a well-defined air pocket located anterior to the trachea. These pockets are referred to as pneumatoceles, pretracheal air cysts, tracheoceles, or aeroceles. Treatment consists of simple drainage and the application of a pressure dressing and is performed in an outpatient setting. In cases where the aerocele presents months after the closure of the tracheocele, mucosalization has usually occurred and requires complete excision.

Complications of TCF closure are avoided by minimizing coughing after closure of the fistula as well as by placing a small drain to evacuate any air accumulation under the flaps during the immediate postoperative period.

Stomal Granulation Tissue

Granuloma formation after tracheotomy is very common due to the high rate of bacterial colonization of the stoma and the constant mechanical irritation associated with the motion of the tube. The incidence of granulation tissue has been estimated at 80% and is thought to be exacerbated by gastroesophageal reflux disease (GERD; Yaremchuk, 2003). Granulation tissue can cause bleeding, especially in patients who have experienced altered coagulation profiles, difficulty with a tracheostomy tube change, a decannulation delay, or obstruction of the tracheostomy tube or trachea itself. The tracheostomy tube can be considered a foreign body that elicits an inflammatory reaction because of its motion due to swallowing and the pulsatile effect from positive-pressure mechanical ventilation. At the stoma, a mucocutaneous junction allows contact with the skin and moisture from the mucosa of the trachea. The debris that accumulates around the tracheostomy tube can be a source of bacterial colonization and infection. The common problem of granulation tissue is a response to the irritation from indwelling tubes and catheters.

Prevention. Meticulous skin care and antimicrobial and corticosteroid preparations play important roles in decreasing the burden of bacterial contamination as well as the resultant inflammatory reaction that promotes granulation tissue formation. Yaremchuk (2003) concluded that instituting a program of regular tracheostomy tube changes causes a statistically significant decrease in the episodes of granulation tissue requiring operative intervention. According to her study, frequent tube changes also appear to decrease the likelihood of forming granulation tissue or inflammation at the stoma. The study did not determine whether tracheostomy tube changes more frequently than once every 2 weeks would eliminate the problem entirely or whether a certain subset of patients would require less frequent changes.

Management. Although some granulomas may resolve spontaneously, topical silver nitrate cauterization, inhaled beclomethasone, treatment of GERD, or surgical removal is usually required.

When granulation tissue becomes obstructive and prevents ventilatory support, surgical intervention is recommended. The use of bronchoscopic equipment in conjunction with sharp dissection has been described as a safe, reliable method for removing suprastomal granulation tissue (Fang, Lee, & Li, 2005). Simple eversion of the granulation tissue through the stoma with a skin hook and blind resection may lead to hemorrhage and incomplete excision. Using a CO_2 laser through the ventilating bronchoscope to ablate tracheal granulation tissue has also been described (Andrews & Horowitz, 1980). No studies have been performed to assess the efficacy of each treatment in a specific patient population.

Tracheomalacia

Tracheomalacia, or a weakening of the tracheal wall, results from ischemic injury to the trachea followed by chondritis and the subsequent destruction and necrosis of supporting tracheal cartilage (Feist, Johnson, & Wilson, 1975; Sue & Susanto, 2003). Such injury can result from either direct pressure from the tracheostomy tube itself or from its cuff. Recommended cuff pressures for tracheostomy tubes are normally less than 20 mm Hg to decrease the chance of ischemic injury to the tracheal mucosa (Andrews & Pearson, 1961). When overinflated, the cuff places increased pressure on the mucosa of the trachea, causing ischemic injury.

With the loss of airway support, the compliant tracheal airway collapses during expiration. This can result in expiratory airflow limitation, air trapping, and retained respiratory secretions. In addition, the loss of cartilaginous support may cause the trachea to be compressed by surrounding structures. In the acute setting, tracheomalacia may present as a failure to wean from mechanical ventilation. Alternatively, it may present as dyspnea in a patient with a history of previous tracheostomy. Diagnosis of tracheomalacia depends on a high index of suspicion. Bronchoscopy can reveal excessive expiratory collapse of the trachea in the patient on mechanical ventilation. In the spontaneously breathing patient, the flow-volume loop shows evidence of variable intrathoracic obstruction. Another approach is dynamic CT scan images of the trachea, which can depict expiratory tracheal collapse (Aquino et al., 2001).

Prevention. The single most important preventative strategy is to monitor cuff pressure and ensure it remains below 20 mm Hg. If obtaining an adequate seal with normal cuff pressure is not possible, a diagnosis of tracheomalacia should be considered rather than increasing the cuff pressure. A bronchoscopic examination should be performed to confirm the diagnosis.

Management. The treatment of tracheomalacia depends upon the severity of expiratory upper-airway obstruction (Feist et al., 1975). In mild cases, a conservative approach may be best. Any associated COPD should be optimally treated first. The placement of a longer tracheostomy tube (to bypass the region of expiratory collapse) facilitates ventilation and also moves the cuff away from the affected area to prevent further injury and allow for healing. In more severe cases, therapeutic options include stenting, tracheal resection, or tracheoplasty.

Tracheal Stenosis

Stenosis of the trachea can occur at the stoma, superior to the stoma, at the level of the cuff, or at the tip of the tube. The primary cause of stenosis is mucosal ischemia. One study (Pena et al., 2001) found that 89% of patients with subglottic stenosis had previously had a tracheostomy for at least 17 days. Substantial stenosis of the trachea at any location can be treated either surgically or by stenting (Rana, Pendem, Pogodzinski, Hubmayr, & Gajic, 2005).

Tracheal and subglottic stenosis are well recognized complications of tracheostomy. Their reported incidence varies and ranges from 0.6% to 21% (Sarper, Ayten, Eser, Ozbudak, & Demircan, 2005). Stenosis is categorized into suprastomal, stomal, or infrastomal and is considered clinically relevant when the diameter is reduced by more than 50% (Sue & Susanto, 2003). Suprastomal or subglottic stenosis is thought to be caused by damage to the cricoid cartilage followed by cricoiditis and bacterial infection resulting in cartilage destruction and scar formation. A report by Raghuraman, Rajan, Marzouk, Mullhi, and Smith (2005) reveals that stenosis secondary to PDT occurs earlier and is more commonly subglottic. This is thought to be due to the tracheal puncture site being more superiorly located compared to the open tracheotomy site.

Stenosis at the stomal level may be due to infection, peristomal chondritis, or an excessively large tracheotomy tube or overaggressive dilation of the stoma at the time of the procedure. Stomal stenosis is more common in patients who remain ventilator dependent because traction of the ventilator tubing against the tube causes ulceration of the stoma. Infrastomal stenosis most commonly occurs where the cuff comes in contact with the endoluminal tracheal mucosa. Alternatively, it can occur at the tip of the tube rubbing against the wall of the trachea if the tube lies within the trachea at an abnormal angle.

At the level of the cuff, high pressure leads to ischemia of the mucosa, which, in turn, leads to mucosal edema and ulceration. As ulceration deepens, normal ciliary flow is interrupted, and mucociliary stasis promotes secondary infection and perichondritis. With further infection, chondritis and cartilaginous necrosis develop. Healing occurs by secondary intention with granulation tissue proliferation in the area of ulceration and the deposition of fibrous tissue in the submucosa. Primary intention healing is hindered by poor blood supply to the cartilage and the constant motion of the laryngotracheal complex associated with swallowing and head movement. The use of high-volume, low-pressure cuffs has markedly decreased the incidence of this type of injury. The chosen tube size should allow an air leak at 20 cm H_2O pressure, if possible. Placement of a nasogastric tube with a tracheotomy tube can also increase pressure on the mucosa in the posterior trachea and should be avoided when possible.

Tracheal stenosis is caused by the pressure of the cuff, or the tube itself, against the trachea. This pressure injury causes commissural scarring and can result in necrosis. One study (Sarper et al., 2005) examined incidence of tracheal stenosis over a 19-year period. The study followed 45 patients who were identified with postintubation tracheal stenosis: 38 had tracheal stenosis, and 7 had infraglottic stenosis. Causes and risk factors varied by approach, which was either open surgical tracheotomy or percutaneous tracheotomy. Risk factors for stenosis after open tracheotomy included infection at the stoma site (10), cervical soft tissue trauma (6), urgent tracheotomy (4), pediatric age group (2), and hypotension (3). Risk factors for stenosis after the percutaneous approach included high tracheostomy (5), tracheal or cartilage damage (1), infection at the stoma site (2), and hypotension (1).

Goldenberg and colleagues (2000) reported that the leading complication in their 10-year sample of 1,130 patients was tracheal stenosis. They also reported that all the patients who developed tracheal stenosis had previously had an endotracheal tube in situ for at least 12 days prior to tracheotomy and that this was directly related to the subsequent stenosis.

Previous studies have reported that the most common site of tracheal stenosis is at the level of the cuff. However, Sarper and others (2005) found only a 31% rate of stenosis at the level of the cuff and a 64% rate of stenosis at the stoma. Two patients in their study had double stenosis at both the stoma and cuff. Stenosis can be a fixed scar, or it can manifest as functional stenosis due to tracheomalacia, which can narrow the tracheal wall during coughing or forced expiration (Heffner, 2005).

An undersized tracheostomy tube can contribute to overinflation of the cuff in order to provide an adequate seal. Symptoms of stenosis are often unrecognizable until the narrowing approaches 5 mm, when the patient may develop stridor. If patients fail to wean after a period of chronic ventilation, they should be evaluated for tracheal stenosis. It takes an 80% narrowing of the trachea before spirometry can detect evidence of tracheal stenosis (Heffner, 2005).

Prevention. Damaged cartilage is the most common cause for stenosis at the stoma site. The stoma should not be made too large, nor should there be too much force exerted when inserting the tube. Excessive movement of the tube within an overly large stoma can produce damage to the tissue around the stoma (Heffner, 2005). Wound sepsis and trauma to the tracheal area also affect wound healing. Sarper and others (2005) found that 42% of their cases of stomal stenosis following open tracheotomy were due to wound sepsis.

Keeping the cuff pressure less than 20 cm H$_2$O can help prevent stenosis at the level of the cuff (Rana et al., 2005). Subglottic stenosis can be prevented with early weaning and aggressive efforts toward decannulation.

High tracheotomy should be avoided, and careful placement of the stoma should be guided by bronchoscopy. Other prevention measures include the use

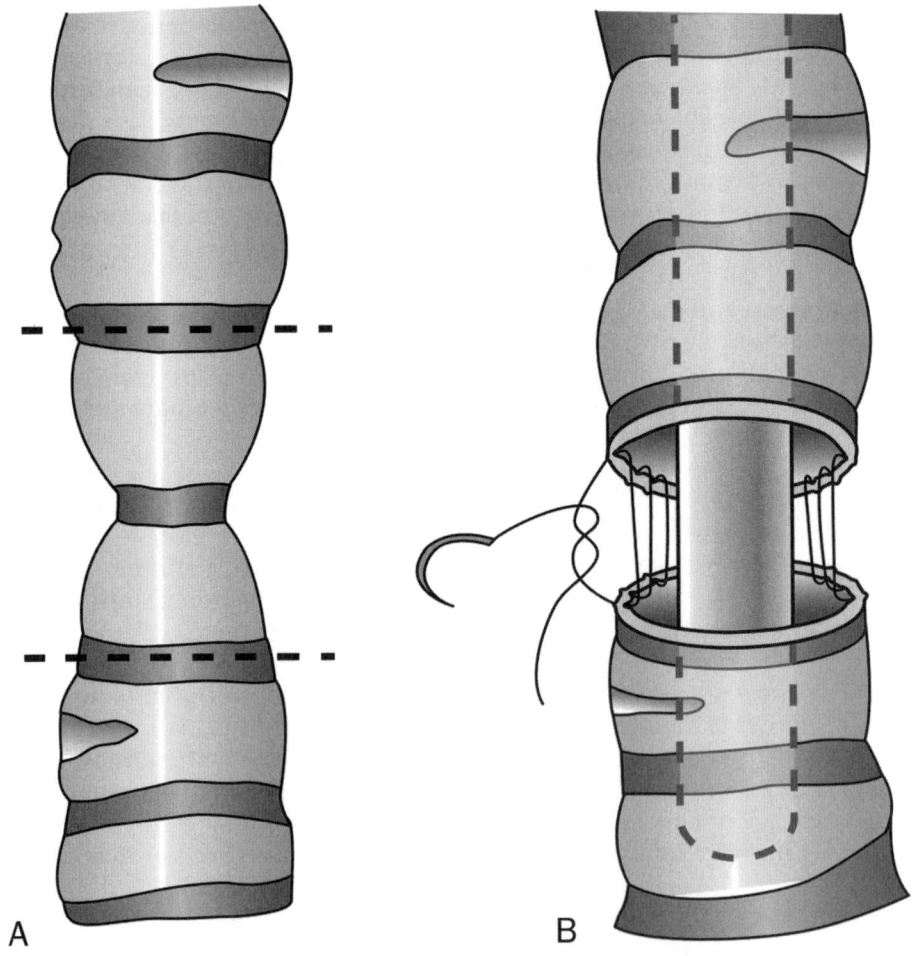

10.3

Surgical repair of tracheal stenosis. (A) Area of tracheal stenosis is identified. (B) Portion of trachea has been resected and closure is begun. Note insertion of anode endotracheal tube through the anastomosis.

of large-volume, low-pressure cuffs; the avoidance of large apertures; the elimination of heavy equipment connected to the tube; and meticulous nursing care (Sarper et al., 2005).

Management. Resection of the trachea may be necessary (see Figure 10.3), especially in those who have multiple stenoses. Complications are low for tracheal lesions but are significantly higher for laryngotracheal resections. In one study, the most common late complication of tracheal resection was granulation tissue at the suture line (Sarper et al., 2005).

Summary

Numerous complications can result from the placement of a tracheostomy. Although there is an overlap, complications are typically categorized as immediate or intraoperative; early (during the first postoperative week); or later. Many complications can be prevented by attention to detail and meticulous care. Good intraoperative communication between the surgeon and anesthesiologist is essential. During the first postoperative week, tube security is a priority to prevent inadvertent decannulation. Many of the later complications can be prevented by minimizing cuff pressure to avoid sequelae including stenosis, tracheomalacia, and granulation tissue. Knowledge of potential complications promotes quick action in the event of an emergency.

Key Points

- Complications of tracheotomy can be encountered in the intraoperative as well as the early and late postoperative periods. Adherence to preventive measures may avoid these complications.
- Tube displacement and loss of airway can occur before the stoma has matured (prior to the fifth postoperative day).
- Signs of tube displacement include resistance with the use of the manual resuscitation bag, the inability to pass a suction catheter, subcutaneous emphysema, and the inability to obtain an end-tidal CO_2 measurement.
- Mucus plugs are very common and can be prevented by adequate hydration and effective mobilization of secretions.
- There is a high incidence of tracheal stenosis that can be lessened by maintaining optimal cuff pressures.

References

Agarwal, S. S., Kumar, L., Chavali, K. H., & Mestri, S. C. (2009). Fatal venous air embolism following intravenous infusion. *Journal of Forensic Sciences, 54*(3), doi: 10.1111/j.1556-4029.2009.01004.628–684.

Andrews, A. H., Jr., & Horowitz, S. L. (1980). Bronchoscopic CO_2 laser surgery. *Lasers in Surgery and Medicine, 1*(1), 35–45.

Andrews, M., & Pearson, F. C. (1961). Incidence and pathogenesis of tracheal injury following cuffed tube tracheostomy with assisted ventilation: Analysis of a 2-year prospective study. *Annals of Surgery, 173,* 249–254.

Aquino, S. L., Shepard, J. A., Ginns, L. C., Moore, R. H., Halpern, E., Grillo, H. C., et al. (2001). Acquired tracheomalacia: Detection by expiratory CT scan. *Journal of Computer Assisted Tomography, 25*(3), 394–399.

Asherson, N. (1958). Tracheostomy: Sudden death from delayed air embolism. *Journal of Laryngology & Otology, 72,* 743–745.

Axelrod, E. H., Kusnetz, A. B., & Rosenberg, M. K. (1993). Operating room fires initiated by hot wire cautery. *Anesthesiology, 79,* 1123–1126.

Bent, J. P., III, & Smith, R. J. (1998). Aerocele after tracheocutaneous fistula closure. *International Journal of Pediatric Otorhinolaryngology, 42*(3), 257–261.

Blanchard, D. L. (1987). Fire in surgery. *Ophthalmic Plastic and Reconstructive Surgery, 3,* 59.

Casserly, P., Lang, E., Fenton, J. E., & Walsh, M. (2007). Assessment of healthcare professionals' knowledge of managing emergency complications in patients with a tracheostomy. *British Journal of Anaesthesia, 99,* 380–383.

Daane, S. P., & Toth, B. A. (2005). Fire in the operating room: Principles and prevention. *Plastic and Reconstructive Surgery, 115*(5), 73e–75e.

Dane, T. E., & King, E. G. (1975). A prospective study of complications after tracheostomy for assisted ventilation. *Chest, 67*(4), 398–404.

Delaney, A., Bagshaw, S. M., & Nalos, M. (2006). Percutaneous dilatational tracheostomy versus surgical tracheostomy in critically ill patients: A systematic review and meta-analysis. *Critical Care, 10*(2), R55.

DeLeyn, P., Bedert, L., Delcroix, M., Depuydt, P., Lauwers, G., Sokolov, Y., et al. (2007). Tracheotomy: Clinical review and guidelines. *European Journal of Cardio-thoracic Surgery, 32,* 412–421.

deRichmond, A. L., & Bruley, M. E. (1993). Head and neck surgical fires. In D. W. Eisele (Ed.), *Complications in head and neck surgery.* St. Louis, MO: Mosby-Year Book.

Durbin, C. G., Jr. (2005). Early complications of tracheostomy. *Respiratory Care, 50*(4), 511–515.

Epstein, S. K. (2005). Late complications of tracheostomy. *Respiratory Care, 50*(4), 542–549.

Fang, T. J., Lee, L. I., & Li, H. Y. (2005). Powered instrumentation in the treatment of tracheal granulation tissue for decannulation. *Otolaryngology Head and Neck Surgery, 133*(4), 520–524.

Feist, J. H., Johnson, T. H., & Wilson, R. J. (1975). Acquired tracheomalacia: Etiology and differential diagnosis. *Chest, 68*(3), 340–345.

Francois, B., Clavel, M., Desachy, A., Puyraud, S., Roustan, J., & Vignon, P. (2003). Complications of tracheostomy performed in the ICU: Subthyroid tracheostomy vs. surgical cricothyroidotomy. *Chest, 123*(1), 151–158.

Goldenberg, D., Ari, E. G., Golz, A., Danino, J., Netzer, A., & Joachims, H. Z. (2000). Tracheotomy complications: A retrospective study of 1130 cases. *Otololaryngology Head and Neck Surgery, 123*(4), 495–500.

Grant, C. A., Dempsey, G., Harrison, J., & Jones, T. (2006). Tracheo-innominate artery fistula after percutaneous tracheostomy: Three case reports and a clinical review. *British Journal of Anaesthesia, 96,* 127–131.

Hartveit, F., Lystad, H., & Minken, A. (1968). The pathology of venous air embolism. *British Journal of Experimental Pathology, 49*(1), 81–86.

Heffner, J. E. (2005). Management of the chronically ventilated patient with a tracheostomy. *Chronic Respiratory Disease, 2,* 151–161.

Henderson, C. G., Harrington, R. L., Izenberg, S., Dyess, D. L., & Silver, F. M. (1995). Tracheocele after routine tracheostomy. *Otolaryngology Head and Neck Surgery, 113,* 489–490.

Kremer, B., Botos-Kremer, A. I., Eckel, H. E., & Schlöndorff, G. (2002). Indications, complications, and surgical techniques for pediatric tracheostomies—An update. *Journal of Pediatric Surgery Nov, 37*(11), 1556–1562.

Mack, C. (1999). Molecular mechanisms of *Staphylococcus epidermidis* biofilm formation. *Journal of Hospital Infection, 43,* S113–S125.

Marsh, B., & Riley, R. H. (1992). Double-lumen tube fire during tracheostomy. *Anesthesiology, 76*(3), 480–481.

Michels, A. M., & Stott, S. (1994). Explosion of tracheal tube during tracheostomy. *Anaesthesia, 49*(12), 1104.

Mohan, V. K., Kashyap, L., & Verma, S. (2003). Life threatening subcutaneous emphysema following surgical repair of tracheocutaneous fistula. *Paediatric Anaesthesia, 13*(4), 339–341.

Motta, G. J., & Trigilia, D. (2005). The effect of an antimicrobial drain sponge dressing on specific bacterial isolates at tracheostomy sites. *Ostomy Wound Management, 51*(1), 60–62, 64–66.

Myers, E. N., Stool, S. E., & Johnson, J. T. (1985). Technique of tracheotomy. In E. N. Myers, S. E. Stool, & J. T. Johnson (Eds.), *Tracheotomy* (pp. 113–124). New York: Churchill Livingston.

Neema, P. K., & Manikandan, S. (2005). Tracheostomy and its variants. *Indian Journal of Anaesthesia, 49*(4), 323–327.

Nicholson, M. J. (1974). Case history number 82: "Nonflammable" fires in the operating room. *Anesthesia and Analgesia, 54,* 152–153.

Parnes, S. M., & Myers, E. N. (1997). Traction sutures in a tracheostomy using a ligature passer. *Transactions. Section on Otolaryngology. American Academy of Ophthalmology and Otolaryngology, 82,* 479.

Pena, J., Cicero, R., Marin, J., Ramirez, M., Cruz, S., & Navarro, F. (2001). Laryngotracheal reconstruction in subglottic stenosis: An ancient problem still present. *Otolaryngology. Head and Neck Surgery, 125*(4), 397–400.

Plumlee, J. E. (1973). Operating-room flash fire from use of cautery after aerosol spray: A case report. *Anesthesia and Analgesia, 52,* 202–203.

Rabuzzi, D. D., & Reed, G. F. (1971). Intrathoracic complications following tracheotomy in children. *Laryngoscope, 81*(6), 939–946.

Raghuraman, G., Rajan, S., Marzouk, J. K., Mullhi, D., & Smith, F. G. (2005). Is tracheal stenosis caused by percutaneous tracheostomy different from by surgical tracheostomy? *Chest, 127*(3), 879–885.

Rana, S., Pendem, S., Pogodzinski, M. S., Hubmayr, R. D., & Gajic, O. (2005). Tracheostomy in critically ill patients. *Mayo Clinic Proceedings, 80*(12), 1632–1638.

Rinder, C. S. (2008). Fire safety in the operating room. *Current Opinion in Anaesthesiology, 21*(6), 790–795.

Sarper, A., Ayten, A., Eser, I., Ozbudak, O., & Demircan, A. (2005). Tracheal stenosis after tracheostomy or intubation: Review with special regard to cause and management. *Texas Heart Institute Journal, 32*(2), 154–158.

Sasaki, C. T., Horiuchi, M., & Koss, N. (1979). Tracheostomy-related subglottic stenosis: Bacteriologic pathogenesis. *Laryngoscope, 89*(6, Pt. 1), 857–865.

Scalise, P., Prunk, S. R., Healy, D., & Votto, J. (2005). The incidence of tracheoarterial fistula in patients with chronic tracheostomy tubes: A retrospective study of 544 patients in a long-term care facility. *Chest, 128*(6), 3906–3909.

Singh, A., Kazi, R., DeCordova, J., Nutting, C. M., Clarke, P., Harrington, K. J., et al. (2008). Multidimensional assessment of voice after vertical partial laryngectomy: A comparison with normal and total laryngectomy voice. *Journal of Voice, 22*(6), 740–745.

Singh, N., Fung, A., & Cole, I. E. (2007). Innominate artery hemorrhage following tracheostomy. *Otolaryngology—Head and Neck Surgery, 136*(4S), S68–S72.

Smith, D. K., Grillone, G. A., & Fuleihan, N. (1999). Use of postoperative chest x-ray after elective adult tracheotomy. *Otolaryngology—Head and Neck Surgery, 120*(6), 848–851.

Snow, N., Richardson, J. D., & Flint, L. M. (1981). Management of necrotizing tracheotomy infections. *Journal of Thoracic Cardiovascular Surgery, 82*(3), 341–344.

Sosis, M. B., & Dillon, F. X. (1991). Saline-filled cuffs help prevent laser-induced polyvinylchloride endotracheal tube fires. *Anesthesia and Analgesia, 72*(2), 187–189.

St. John, R. E., & Malen, J. F. (2004). Contemporary issues in adult tracheostomy management. *Critical Care Nursing Clinics of North America, 16*(3), 413–430.

Stanton, D. C., Kademani, D., Patel, C., & Foote, J. W. (2004). Management of post-tracheotomy scars and persistent tracheocutaneous fistulas with dermal interpositional fat graft. *Journal of Oral and Maxillofacial Surgery, 62,* 514–517.

Stauffer, J. L., Olson, D. E., & Petty, T. L. (1981). Complications and consequences of endotracheal intubation and tracheotomy: A prospective study of 150 critically ill adult patients. *American Journal of Medicine, 70,* 65–76.

Stouffer, D. L. (1992). Fires during surgery: Two fatal incidents in Los Angeles. *Journal of Burn Care Rehabilitation, 13,* 114–117.

Sue, R. D., & Susanto, I. (2003). Long-term complications of artificial airways. *Clinics in Chest Medicine, 24*(3), 457–471.

Thompson, J. W., Colin, W., Snowden, T., Hengesteg, A., Stocks, R. M., & Watson, S. P. (1998). Fire in the operating room during tracheostomy. *Southern Medical Journal, 91*(3), 243–247.

Tsunezuka, Y., Suzuki, M., Nitta, K., & Oda, M. (2005). The use of fibrous wound dressing sheets made of carboxymethylcellulose natrium in the postoperative management of tracheostomy. *Kyobu Geka, 58*(12), 1063–1067.

von Eiff, C., Heilmann, C., & Peters, G. (1999). New aspects in the molecular basis of polymer-associated infections due to staphylococci. *European Journal of Clinical Microbiology and Infectious Diseases, 18,* 843–846.

Waldron, J., Padgham, N. D., & Hurley, S. E. (1990). Complications of emergency and elective tracheostomy: A retrospective study of 150 consecutive cases. *Annals of the Royal College of Surgeons of England, 72*(4), 218–220.

Walvekar, R. R., & Myers, E. N. (2008). Technique and complications of tracheostomy in adults. In E. N. Myers & J. T. Johnson (Eds.), *Tracheotomy: Airway management, communication, and swallowing* (2nd ed., pp. 35–67). San Diego, CA: Plural Publishing.

Watanakunakorn, C. (1989). Successful novel drainage treatment of mediastinal abscess complicating tracheostomy. *Chest, 96*(4), 946–948.

Weber, S. M., Hargunani, C. A., & Wax, M. K. (2006). Duraprep and the risk of fire during tracheostomy. *Head and Neck, 28,* 649–652.

Weymuller, E. A., Jr. (1998). Acute airway management. In C. W. Cummings (Ed.), *Otolaryngology. Head and neck surgery* (3rd ed.). St. Louis, MO: Mosby-Year Book.

Wilson, P. T., Igbaseimokumo, U., & Martin, J. (1994). Ignition of the tracheal tube during tracheostomy. *Anaesthesia, 49*(8), 734–735.

Wolf, G. L., Sidebotham, G. W., & Stern, J. B. (1994). Intraluminal flame spread in tracheal tubes. *Laryngoscope, 104,* 874–879.

Wolf, G. L., & Simpson, J. I. (1987). Flammability of endotracheal tubes in oxygen and nitrous oxide enriched atmosphere. *Anesthesiology, 67,* 236–239.

Wright, S. E., & Van Dahm, K. (2003). Long-term care of the tracheostomy patient. *Clinics in Chest Medicine, 24,* 473–487.

Yaremchuk, K. (2003). Regular tracheostomy tube changes to prevent formation of granulation tissue. *Laryngoscope, 113,* 1–10.

Downsizing and Decannulation

Linda L. Morris

Unless a tracheostomy is placed for irreversible conditions, the clinician must always consider the goal of decannulation. The decannulation process does have some risk, but there are several benefits. Not only is the tube itself a foreign object irritating the airway, but it also interferes with swallowing, coughing, and phonation. There are psychosocial issues associated with the presence of a tracheostomy tube, including loss of control, anxiety, and an inability to communicate (Christopher, 2005), all of which can create frustration at best and severe depression at worst.

Planning for downsizing and decannulation should begin as soon as the patient has recovered from the immediate postoperative period and is looking toward the first tracheostomy change. Downsizing is the gradual process of decreasing the size of the tracheostomy tube, usually with the eventual goal of decannulation. Downsizing has several advantages, including decreasing long-term complications such as tracheal stenosis and tracheomalacia as well as improving swallow and decreasing the risk of aspiration. Another theoretical advantage to the downsizing process is minimizing scarring; however, no studies to date have discussed the appearance of scarring related to downsizing.

Assessment for downsizing should begin with a thorough review of the medical record and discussion with the primary care practitioner and the surgeon who placed the tracheostomy. When the medical condition has stabilized and there are no factors that necessitate continued cannulation, planning for decannulation should take place. Decannulation should be considered when the reason for tracheostomy placement is resolved, when airway secretions have abated, and when mechanical ventilation is no longer required (Christopher, 2005).

Factors to Consider Prior to Decannulation

It is important to consider the reason for the placement of the tracheostomy in the plan for downsizing and decannulation. Decannulation of patients who have had a prolonged period of mechanical ventilation is markedly different from decannulation in those who have had a resolution of an upper airway obstruction (Christopher, 2005). This is because those who have had a prolonged period of mechanical ventilation also have other comorbidities to consider as well as poor respiratory reserve. These patients are also likely to be deconditioned and may have limited ability to protect their airway.

A retrospective study by the National Association of Long-Term Hospitals (NALTH) found that 54% of patients were able to discontinue mechanical ventilation support after a prolonged period, but only 59% of those weaned were ultimately decannulated (Scheinhorn et al., 2007). O'Connor, Kirby, Terrin, Hill, and White (2009) studied the process of decannulation in patients who had received prolonged mechanical ventilation in 23 long-term-care hospitals. They found that within a median of 45 days after tracheostomy placement, decannulation was successful in 35% of patients. The patients who were decannulated successfully had tracheostomy tubes placed earlier and had shorter stays in the acute care hospital. Three years later, 35% of all patients were alive, including 62% of those who were decannulated.

Resistance and Work of Breathing

The prolonged placement of an endotracheal tube and subsequent tracheostomy interferes with the normal airway-protective mechanisms of cough and swallow. The disadvantages of tracheostomy include loss of the upper airway for ventilation, loss of laryngeal function, and imposed resistance of the artificial airway (Moscovici da Cruz, et al., 2002). The presence of a tracheostomy tube interferes with the normal swallowing mechanism. The vocal cords in the larynx are bypassed by the tracheostomy tube, which interferes with effective coughing and partial regulation of breathing. When the vocal cords are partially closed, subglottic pressure is maintained, and physiologic PEEP maintains airway patency. Subglottic pressure also contributes to effective swallowing and reduction of the risk of aspiration. Intrinsic PEEP is lost with a tracheostomy tube (Christopher, 2005). Furthermore, the laryngeal blast that produces an effective cough is lost.

Compared to endotracheal tubes, tracheostomy tubes have been associated with significant reductions in airflow resistance, work of breathing, and intrinsic

PEEP (Diehl, El Atrous, Touchard, Lemaire, & Brochard, 1999; Rumbak et al., 1997). Diehl and colleagues demonstrated a decrease in these measures comparing tracheostomy to mechanical ventilation through an endotracheal tube. Moscovici da Cruz and colleagues (2002) showed this difference by comparing spontaneously breathing nonintubated patients to patients with tracheostomies. Presumably, this difference is due to decreases in airflow resistance (Rumbak et al.).

The primary factors involved in resistance and work of breathing are the following (Pierson, 2005):

1. The larger the diameter, the lower the resistance.
2. The shorter the tube, the lower the resistance.
3. Secretions within the walls of the tube increase resistance.
4. The sharper the curve of the tube, the greater the resistance.
5. Higher gas flows require increased pressure.

The small radius and curvature of a tracheostomy tube increase turbulence and airway resistance. However, when compared to endotracheal tubes, these effects are offset by the tracheostomy tube's short length, which results in an overall lowering of airway resistance and muscle loading. In addition, secretions within the lumen of the tracheostomy tube also increase resistance, but the ease of suctioning and removable inner cannulas mitigate this effect (MacIntyre et al., 2001).

Downsizing allows more air to pass around the outside of the tracheostomy tube rather than through the tube. A progressively smaller size promotes this gradual increase in airflow around the tube (see Figure 11.1). The patient gradually becomes reacquainted with air passing through the upper airway. The general principle during downsizing is that, as the tube gets smaller, it is more difficult to breathe through it but easier to breathe around it. With each change in tube size comes a change in airway dynamics. If the patient is breathing *through* a smaller tube, airway resistance increases. If the patient is breathing *around* a smaller tube, airway resistance decreases. The caveat here is that the tube itself creates an increasingly hindering obstruction as the ratio of tube size to airway diameter increases. This explains why some patients who do not tolerate capping can be successfully decannulated (Gao et al., 2008).

It is estimated that up to 10% (Frutos-Vivar et al., 2005; Kollef, Ahrens, & William, 1999; Stelfox et al., 2008) to 16.9% (Cox, Carson, Holmes, Howard, & Carey, 2004) of all mechanically ventilated patients receive a tracheostomy, and this trend appears to be increasing. Cox and co-investigators reviewed a 10-year database comprising 144,875 patients requiring mechanical ventilation. Approximately one-third of these mechanically ventilated patients (49,872) required longer ventilator support (greater than or equal to 4 days). Approximately one-fifth of these patients who required prolonged mechanical ventilation (9,794) underwent a tracheostomy. Of interest is that the incidence of tracheostomy placement increased 200% over the 10-year duration of their study.

Aerodynamics not only change during the downsizing process but also after decannulation. Chadda and others (2002) found that tidal volume increased without any change in respiratory rate, inspiratory time, or arterial pCO_2. A return to mouth breathing resulted in a 17.5% increase in tidal volume.

11.1

Airflow through a smaller tube compared to a larger one. Note less resistance with breathing through a larger tube. As the tube gets smaller, resistance (and, hence, work of breathing) increases.

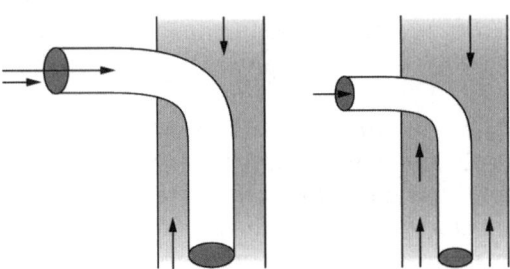

These changes were due to a significant increase in physiologic dead space and were associated with a significant increase in work of breathing. However, Dellweg, Barchfeld, Haidl, Appelhans, and Kohler (2007) found that decannulation resulted in increased or decreased respiratory burden depending on upper airway morphology and pathology. Upper airway morphology was shaped by anatomy, position, muscle tone, secretions, infection, edema, or the presence of an artificial airway. Moscovici da Cruz and investigators (2002) studied seven patients with head and neck cancer and also found that upper airway resistance changed with individual differences in airway morphology.

Cannulation Times

The course and outcome following tracheostomy varies with the reason for intubation. One Australian group (Leung, Campbell, MacGregor, & Berkowitz, 2003) retrospectively studied all patients in their ICU over 1 year. Of 100 patients who had tracheostomies during that time, 35 were admitted for respiratory causes, 35 for neurologic conditions, 17 due to trauma, and the remaining 13 for cardiovascular, gastrointestinal, sepsis, and metabolic complications. The authors found that 47 patients required tracheostomies because of prolonged mechanical ventilation, 45 for bronchial hygiene or the risk of aspiration, and 8 for an unstable or obstructed airway. During the study period, 37 patients died, 30 of whom had the tracheostomy tube in place. Seventy patients were successfully decannulated; 63 survived and 7 died after being decannulated for at least 1 week. Total cannulation times varied with the reasons for tracheostomy tube placement. As expected, the authors noted that cannulation times were longer for neurologic than for respiratory diagnoses and even shorter for trauma. Median cannulation time was 25 days, but 3 patients had cannulation times longer than 6 months.

Leung and coauthors (2003) noted that patients with unstable airways were cannulated for a mean of 13 days. Those with prolonged mechanical ventilation were cannulated for a mean of 25 days, and those with aspiration were cannulated for a mean of 33 days. Comparatively, Dellweg and colleagues (2007) reported an average cannulation time of 37 days, and Rumbak and coauthors (1997) reported an average intubation/cannulation time of 2.4 weeks.

O'Connor and co-investigators (2009) studied patients on prolonged mechanical ventilation. In their study of 135 patients, 58 (43%) were successfully liberated from mechanical ventilation and 81% (47/58) of those weaned were ultimately decannulated. Mean time to decannulation was 45 days. Of those who were weaned, 23% were not decannulated because of an ongoing need for airway protection. In their study, the most common diagnoses were pneumonia, COPD, and septic shock. The median time to the placement of a tracheostomy was 18 days after translaryngeal intubation. A survival analysis found that 35% of patients were alive 3.5 years later. Those who were decannulated had improved survival compared with those who remained on mechanical ventilation ($p = 0.11$).

Cannulation times in children tend to be even longer. Kontzoglou and colleagues (2006) reported an average cannulation time of 26.4 months. Other studies reported a mean cannulation time of 21.6 months (Gray, Todd, & Jacobs, 1998; Zenk, et al., 2008). Furthermore, the duration of the decannulation process is also longer in children. Waddell, Appleford, Dunning, Papsin, and Bailey (1997) described a detailed protocol for decannulation in children that took up to 11 days. This prolonged decannulation schedule could be due to the much longer cannulation times. This study involved children with tracheostomy tubes in place for a mean of 3.5 years who had more complex airway issues. Nonetheless, it is important to consider several factors when planning for decannulation in children. More discussion on decannulation in children can be found in chapter 8.

Reason for Initial Placement of Tracheostomy

The most important factor when considering decannulation is the initial reason for tracheostomy placement. If the primary issues are not resolved, attempts to downsize and decannulate will not be successful. Factors affecting the decision to place a tracheostomy are the same factors affecting the decision to decannulate. An easy way to remember the indications for the placement of an artificial airway is the acronym VOPS: ventilation, obstruction, protection, and secretions (Shapiro, Harrison, Kacmarek, & Cane, 1985).

Ventilation. Patients who continue to require any form of positive-pressure ventilation will benefit from continued use of the tracheostomy. Noninvasive means of positive-pressure ventilation are often met with other complications—such as gastric insufflation, discomfort, and air leak—that can contribute to less than optimal delivery of volume. If the tracheostomy was placed because of the need for prolonged mechanical ventilation, it is usually safe to consider downsizing and decannulation as soon as the patient has been liberated from *continuous* positive-pressure ventilation for at least 24 hours.

Obstruction. Depending on the nature of the obstruction, the tracheostomy tube can usually be decannulated after the obstruction is relieved. A direct view of the trachea is often indicated if obstruction is suspected or documented.

Causes of obstruction include vocal cord paralysis, head or neck masses, edema after prolonged surgery (especially in the prone position), granulation tissue, stenosis, and obstructive sleep apnea.

Protection. The two primary mechanisms that contribute to airway protection are an adequate cough and an adequate swallow. Patients who cannot protect their airway require a cuffed tracheostomy tube, but even an inflated cuff provides imperfect protection.

Cough effectiveness should be evaluated during the downsizing and decannulation process. Failure to produce an adequate cough can result in atelectasis, inspissation of secretions, or tube obstruction because of the incomplete clearance of secretions. The clinical measure of cough effectiveness is vital capacity, and a normal measurement is considered to be 70 ml/kg ideal body weight (Adams & Lim, 2003). The accepted minimum vital capacity is considered to be 15 ml/kg ideal body weight; below this point, patients are unable to effectively clear secretions. A regression equation has been described for calculating accepted minimum vital capacity based on gender, age, and height (Douce, 2003); however, a simpler formula to calculate ideal body weight is used most often:

$$\text{female: 5 feet} = 100 \text{ pounds; male: 5 feet} = 105 \text{ pounds}$$

Add 5 pounds for each inch over 5 feet. Convert pounds to kilograms by dividing by 2.2 and multiply by 15 ml/kg to find the minimum acceptable vital capacity in milliliters.

It is common for patients to be quite deconditioned after a long stay in the ICU, so a vigorous program of physical mobility is required to provide them with the strength to mobilize secretions themselves. When patients can effectively mobilize secretions on their own, they may no longer require suctioning.

Swallowing Function. Swallowing physiology provides intermittent alimentation and continuous airway protection. The action of swallowing consists of several phases. The oral phase consists of preparing the food for transport. This includes mastication and the addition of saliva to create a bolus. During the pharyngeal stage, the food bolus is pushed downward past the nasopharynx. As it enters the vallecular space, the epiglottis tilts downward. The muscles of the larynx contract, causing it to close tightly, and respiration momentarily ceases. The pharyngeal muscles constrict, and the tongue pushes the bolus posteriorly and downward, propelling it toward the esophagus. The cricopharyngeus muscle relaxes, and the anterior pharyngeal wall is pulled forward. This action allows the bolus to pass into the esophagus. During the esophageal stage, the bolus moves through the esophagus and into the stomach by peristalsis (Tippett, 2000).

Prolonged intubation interferes with the glottic mechanism, and it may take some time for normal function to return. This could explain the high incidence of aspiration in patients with tracheostomies, which has been reported by some authors as 69% (Cameron, Reynolds, & Zuidema, 1973) and 64.8%, with a reported range from 50%–87% (Ding & Logemann, 2005). An inflated cuff elevates during the swallow and desensitizes the larynx. In addition, it can bulge posteriorly and compress the esophagus. The tube can also partially interfere with the elevation of the larynx and its anterior movement during swallowing. This tethering effect is magnified with cuff inflation (Tippett, 2000). Silent (clinically nonobservable) aspiration is a common problem in patients with tracheostomies and has been reported to be 46.2%. Silent aspiration was significantly higher with an inflated cuff compared to a deflated cuff (Ding & Logemann).

Swallow physiology is different with various medical conditions. Patients with neuromuscular disorders show significantly greater frequencies of reduced tongue manipulation, slow oral transit, delayed pharyngeal triggering, and aspiration after the swallow. In contrast, patients with head and neck cancer show significantly higher frequencies of reduced laryngeal closure, aspiration during the swallow, and aspiration after the swallow (Ding & Logemann, 2005). Pooled salivary secretions are a predictor of dysphagia (McGowan, Gleason, Smith, Hirsch, & Shuldham, 2007; Murray, Langmore, Ginsberg, & Dostie, 1996). Gross, Tedla, and Ross (2007) found a significantly higher number of inhalations during the swallow in patients with a tracheostomy tube compared to normal controls without a tracheostomy tube. They concluded that this increased tendency to inhale during a swallow places patients with a tracheostomy at higher risk for aspiration. Finally, while the inflated cuff provides some measure of airway protection, it also interferes with the coughing mechanism. It has been implicated in contributing to aspiration because the larynx is desensitized due to the diversion of airflow through the tracheostomy tube.

Secretions. The failure of patients to manage secretions is a common reason for the continued placement of a tracheostomy tube. The underlying condition may contribute to the production of secretions, but it is often the tracheostomy itself that produces significant secretions (Wright & Van Dahm, 2003). Fortunately, secretions commonly decrease during the capping process. Chapter 7 outlines the management of secretions.

Tube Size

Tube size is an important consideration—both the size of the tube in situ and the size of the tube under consideration. When patients breathe *through* a cuffed tube, the general rule of thumb is to choose a tube with the largest inner diameter in order to minimize resistance and decrease airway pressures. As downsizing is considered, however, it is necessary to choose a tube with a smaller outer diameter in order to allow the patient to breathe more easily *around* the tube.

Future Need for Artificial Airway

Before decannulation is performed, there should be an inquiry into any impending need for an artificial airway. If a patient is scheduled for a surgical procedure within the next few days or weeks, it may be beneficial to wait until the recovery is complete.

Determining Readiness for Decannulation

There is no standard method to determine a patient's readiness for decannulation. Some rely on clinical judgment, some on endoscopy or radiography. Stelfox and others (2008) conducted a survey of physicians and respiratory therapists to determine usual practices regarding decannulation. They found that the most important factors influencing readiness for decannulation were the patient's level of consciousness, cough effectiveness, amount of secretions, and ability to tolerate tracheostomy tube capping. Of moderate importance were patient comorbidities, etiology of respiratory failure, swallowing function, respiratory rate, and oxygenation. Compared to respiratory therapists, physicians rated level of consciousness significantly more important and ability to tolerate tracheostomy tube capping significantly less important.

Capping is also called plugging, corking, or blocking; the principle is the same, but the means may be slightly different. They all involve obstructing the tube. With capping, the *uncuffed* tracheostomy tube is obstructed so the patient breathes around the tube rather than through it. The potential problem is that the blocked tube occupies a significant portion of the airway, depending on its size.

Gao and others (2008) developed a simple device for measuring airflow and subglottal pressure in order to determine a patient's readiness for decannulation. Two groups were compared: a decannulation group (deemed ready based on the usual clinical criteria of capping the tracheostomy tube for 24–48 hours) and a second group determined unsuitable for decannulation. The researchers took airflow measurements during shallow and deep breathing. A routine examination using a flexible fiberoptic bronchoscope determined the resolution of the initial anatomic reasons for tracheostomy placement as well as assessed any changes in the airway. The decision to decannulate was determined by a surgeon, who made the decision on clinical criteria but was uninformed of the airway resistance measurements. All patients were observed in the hospital for at least 24 hours after decannulation, and all were followed for 3 months by telephone.

All patients in the decannulation group were successfully decannulated without any breathing difficulties during the 3-month follow-up period. However, resistance was significantly higher in the group that was not decannulated on all measures of upper airway resistance: inspiratory resistance during shallow breathing, expiratory resistance during shallow breathing, inspiratory resistance during deep breathing, and expiratory resistance during deep breathing. The causes of this increased airway resistance were postoperative scarring, vocal cord paralysis, or neoplasms (Gao et al., 2008).

Turbulent airflow requires a greater pressure gradient than laminar flow. The irregular airways noted in the patients who were not decannulated generated more turbulent flow. The investigators found that glottis width was narrower in those patients who failed the protocol. Furthermore, they reported that some patients who could not tolerate plugging or capping were still ready for decannulation. The tube itself created a significant obstruction, and removal of the tube improved breathing. The authors suggested that an objective assessment of airway resistance could lead to quicker decannulation without the need for 24–48 hour capping and potentially decrease costs and length of stay.

There is no accepted definition for decannulation failure; however, Stelfox and colleagues (2008) found that most clinicians considered decannulation failure to be the reinsertion of an artificial airway between 48 to 96 hours after decannulation. In their study, respiratory therapists considered shorter time frames than physicians for defining decannulation failure: 48 hours versus 96 hours ($p = 0.002$). They also found significant differences in practice between those working in acute care facilities and those working in chronic care facilities (Stelfox et al.).

The decision to decannulate is based on clinical judgment and falls within a spectrum of approaches. The more methodical approach requires a host of clinical measures to determine the patient's readiness for decannulation and a very slow downsizing progression from one step to the next before the patient is actually decannulated. A trial-and-error approach is much more rapid and inherently riskier. There are no studies to determine the optimal duration for the process of decannulation. Choate, Barbetti, and Currey (2008) studied patients at a tertiary care hospital over a 4.5-year period and recorded a 4.8% decannulation failure rate (40 out of 823 decisions to decannulate). Stomal recannulation was required in 25 cases, whereas 15 cases resulted in reintubation. There was no associated mortality or other adverse events. The most common reason for decannulation failure was sputum retention. The authors advised that nursing staff should closely monitor newly decannulated patients for the initial 4 hours and for up to 24 hours after decannulation (Choate et al.).

Barnes, Barbetti, and Currey (1999) studied patients in a rehabilitation facility over 18 months to determine the duration of decannulation. The patients' disorders included spinal cord injury, traumatic brain injury, neuromuscular dysfunction, and ventilator-dependent respiratory failure. A protocol was developed, and an interdisciplinary team was established to implement the decannulation protocol. The team consisted of a respiratory therapist, a nurse practitioner, a primary nurse, and a physician. The study evaluated 93 patients, and 93.5% of them qualified for decannulation; however, 6.5% did not meet criteria because of a prolonged inability to protect their airway and continued ventilator support. All patients who qualified were eventually decannulated within 50 days. The average time for the entire decannulation process in an uncomplicated patient was 10 days, which represented 74% of their population.

Godwin and Heffner (1991) recommended several principles to guide the evaluation for decannulation, including adequate ventilatory reserve (spontaneous breathing for 24–48 hours), adequate nutritional state, patent upper airway, absence of bronchopulmonary infection and impending need for mechanical ventilation, adequate cough without suctioning, minimal aspiration, and medical stability.

Decannulation Protocol

There is no set protocol currently recommended for downsizing and decannulation. Some protocols simply recommend cuff deflation and assessment for movement of air around the cuff. Others recommend a fenestrated tracheostomy tube for an added boost of air. Still others recommend capping trials. Downsizing usually begins with cuff deflation, which serves two purposes: to assess airway protection and to assess the movement of air through the upper airway. Cuff deflation involves the admixture of room air, which lowers overall FiO_2 and creates the potential for hypoxemia. If significant hypoxemia results from cuff deflation, the clinician should reinflate the cuff and later reattempt downsizing when the patient can tolerate cuff deflation.

Christopher (2005) defined a period of physiologic decannulation as an interim step to evaluate patients with long-term tracheostomy. His study conducted evaluations for cough, secretions, and breathing through the upper airway around an occluded tracheostomy tube, as well as a capping trial period. Kubba, Cooke, and Hartley (2004) suggested that tolerating a blocked tube during the decannulation process is a test of the patient's reserve and may predict success after decannulation. There are no studies that have tested this notion; however, experience has shown it to be generally true.

The most conservative decannulation protocol was reported by Waddell and colleagues (1997) for children. Their protocol began with endoscopic evaluation of the airway. If no anatomical, physiologic, or medical concerns were identified, the child was observed for exercise tolerance for 2 days. If that evaluation was satisfactory, the tracheostomy tube would be replaced by a tube of a smaller size on each consecutive day. When the smallest tracheostomy tube was reached (for children, 3 mm internal diameter), it was left in place for 2 days and capped for 12 hours on the second morning. If that capping trial was tolerated, a 24-hour capping trial was attempted beginning the following morning. If successful, the tracheostomy would be decannulated and the stoma covered with a dry dressing. Following decannulation, the child was observed on the ward for at least 3 more days and discharged the fourth day after decannulation. Depending on the number of steps involved in downsizing, the process took up to 11 days.

Some authors have suggested that bronchoscopy should be a routine part of a decannulation protocol; however, Rumbak and colleagues (1997) supported their hypothesis that routine bronchoscopy was unnecessary. They studied 75 patients clinically ready to be decannulated. All those patients underwent a tracheostomy occlusion protocol followed by bronchoscopy. They deflated the cuff on a fenestrated tracheostomy tube and occluded it. Patients who developed respiratory distress while the tube was occluded were considered to have failed the protocol. In the study, 84% of patients tolerated the protocol, and 16% failed. Bronchoscopy revealed that all patients had some degree of tracheal injury; however, those who failed the protocol had clinically more significant tracheal obstruction to airflow. The authors concluded that patients who successfully pass the occlusion protocol could be safely decannulated without undergoing bronchoscopy. Conversely, they also suggested that those who fail an occlusion protocol should undergo bronchoscopic evaluation.

Gao and others (2008) used a protocol of capping the tracheostomy tube for 24–48 hours. St. John and Malen (2004) reported their decannulation protocol began with a formal swallow evaluation in order to assess for anatomic narrowing or obstruction of the upper airway as well as swallowing function. They recommended endoscopy to assess the function of the vocal cords. When patients could breathe spontaneously and swallow safely, they recommended a low-profile cuffed, metal, or cuffless tube during the transition period. When the patient could tolerate a speaking valve for several days with activity, the patient was downsized to a cuffless tracheostomy tube that was capped. The patient was decannulated when able to tolerate capping for 48 hours with no further need for suctioning or positive-pressure ventilation.

Lewarski (2005) and Heffner (2005) discussed a rapid "one-step" decannulation protocol that began with assessment for decannulation 48 hours after the patient was liberated from mechanical ventilation. The first step was cuff deflation while assessing for signs of aspiration, at which point the tube was occluded to assess for ease of breathing around the tube. The immediate onset of stridor or the inability to breathe comfortably indicated obstruction or that the tube was too large for the airway, which warranted further bronchoscopic evaluation. If the patient tolerated tube occlusion, it was capped for 30 minutes. If the patient tolerated this brief capping trial, decannulation would be performed, and the patient would be observed for 24–48 hours. However, Heffner acknowledged that most patients benefit from a more systematic approach for downsizing.

Godwin and Heffner (1991) began their decannulation protocol with cuff deflation after 24–48 hours of spontaneous ventilation. If there was no immediate evidence of aspiration with cuff deflation, the patient was observed for the next 24 hours with the cuff deflated. At that point, the authors offered several options for decannulation. The tube could be occluded and the patient observed for 12–24 hours. If the patient did not tolerate tube occlusion, a fenestrated tracheostomy tube could be placed. Another option applied progressively smaller cuffless tubes. The smallest tube could be placed and capped for a period of time before decannulation. A third option is a tracheostomy button, which offers the advantage of the use of the upper airway but without the resistance of breathing around a plugged tube.

Rather than abruptly downsizing the tracheostomy, some practitioners prefer to use progressive corking. Corks of different sizes reduce the tube's effective diameter by first blocking one-quarter, then one-half, and then three-quarters of the tube and finally providing total occlusion of the opening as tolerated. However, Gray and others (1998) recommended against this practice because one patient aspirated portions of cork.

In a lung model, Hussy and Bishop (1996) recommended the use of a fenestrated tracheostomy tube to avoid the significant work of breathing involved with a nonfenestrated tube. Christopher (2005) described the use of a small-diameter fenestrated or nonfenestrated capped tube with the cuff deflated but also cautioned about the development of granulation tissue. He suggested the interim use of a speaking valve to redirect air to the upper airway but acknowledged that "functional decannulation" would likely not be achieved with this method.

Other practitioners advocate the use of a fenestrated tracheostomy to aid in decannulation; however, this practice may produce granulation tissue within the fenestration if the patient is not properly fitted. Not only would this defeat the purpose of the fenestrated tube, but it might result in a potential complication requiring surgical intervention. For a discussion on proper fitting of a fenestrated tracheostomy tube, see chapter 4.

Still other practitioners use peak cough flow as a predictor of success with decannulation. Bach and Saporito (1996) studied patients with neuromuscular ventilatory insufficiency and found the only independent predictor of success was peak cough flow. When peak cough flow was at least 160 liters per minute, patients were more likely to have success with decannulation. Normally, a pre-cough inspiration is approximately 85%–90% of total lung capacity. Then the glottis closes and intrathoracic pressure increases to generate a normal peak cough flow of 360–1,000 liters per minute. Total expiratory volume during normal coughing is approximately 2.3 liters (Bach and Saporito). Patients with neuromuscular disease, however, are often unable to generate sufficient cough effectiveness due to their decreased ability to inflate the lungs, abdominal muscle weakness (weakened expiration), and their inability to adduct the vocal cords and close the glottis in order to generate a deep breath.

Tobin and Santamaria (2008) reported that the creation of a tracheostomy review team led to shorter decannulation time and length of stay. Patients were decannulated when they could tolerate 24 hours of cuff deflation with the use of either a speaking valve or tube occlusion and could clear secretions without suctioning. Norwood, Spiers, Bailiss, and Sayers (2004) also reported patient outcomes after the implementation of a tracheostomy team. They found that ICU decannulation rate increased (14%–34%), ICU death with tubes in place decreased (43%–16%), and fewer patients were transferred to the wards with their tubes still in situ (39%–18%). Interestingly, time to decannulation did not change between the two groups. They did not describe their decannulation protocol; however, they did report that 25% of the patients were discharged to the wards with a mini-tracheostomy tube in place, which resulted in a significant reduction in complications.

Cameron and researchers (2009) showed the impact of a multidisciplinary team on patients with spinal cord injury. The team consisted of clinical nurse consultants, physiotherapists, speech pathologists, and physicians who visited patients twice weekly and provided consultation, support, and education on other days as needed. After implementation of the team, they reported a reduced length of stay (from 60 to 41.5 days), a decrease in duration of cannulation (from 22.5 to 16.5 days), and an eight-fold reduction in cost of care. In addition, time to phonation was decreased from 130 to 10 days.

Dellweg and others (2007) studied patients who had failed at least one attempt at decannulation. Their protocol used a tracheostomy retrainer, a device not available in the United States that appears similar to a tracheostomy button in that it does not compromise the lumen of the trachea or contribute to airway resistance. These devices provide a functional decannulation because there is no occluded tube within the airway around which the patient must breathe. Out of 25 patients, only two did not tolerate this trial; others had only a slight increase in inspiratory time, but work of breathing, compliance, and resistance were unchanged.

For most adult patients in an inpatient hospital setting, the following methodical approach to decannulation has proven effective and successful to this author. See Figure 11.2 for a downsizing algorithm.

1. Ensure resolution of the initial reason for tracheostomy tube placement (VOPS).
2. Exclude immediate future need of artificial airway. Patients scheduled for a surgical procedure in the near future may benefit from continued cannulation.
3. Determine need for positive-pressure ventilation.
   - Delivery of positive-pressure breaths during breathing treatments.
   - Need for intermittent nocturnal positive-pressure ventilation.

11.2

Downsizing algorithm.

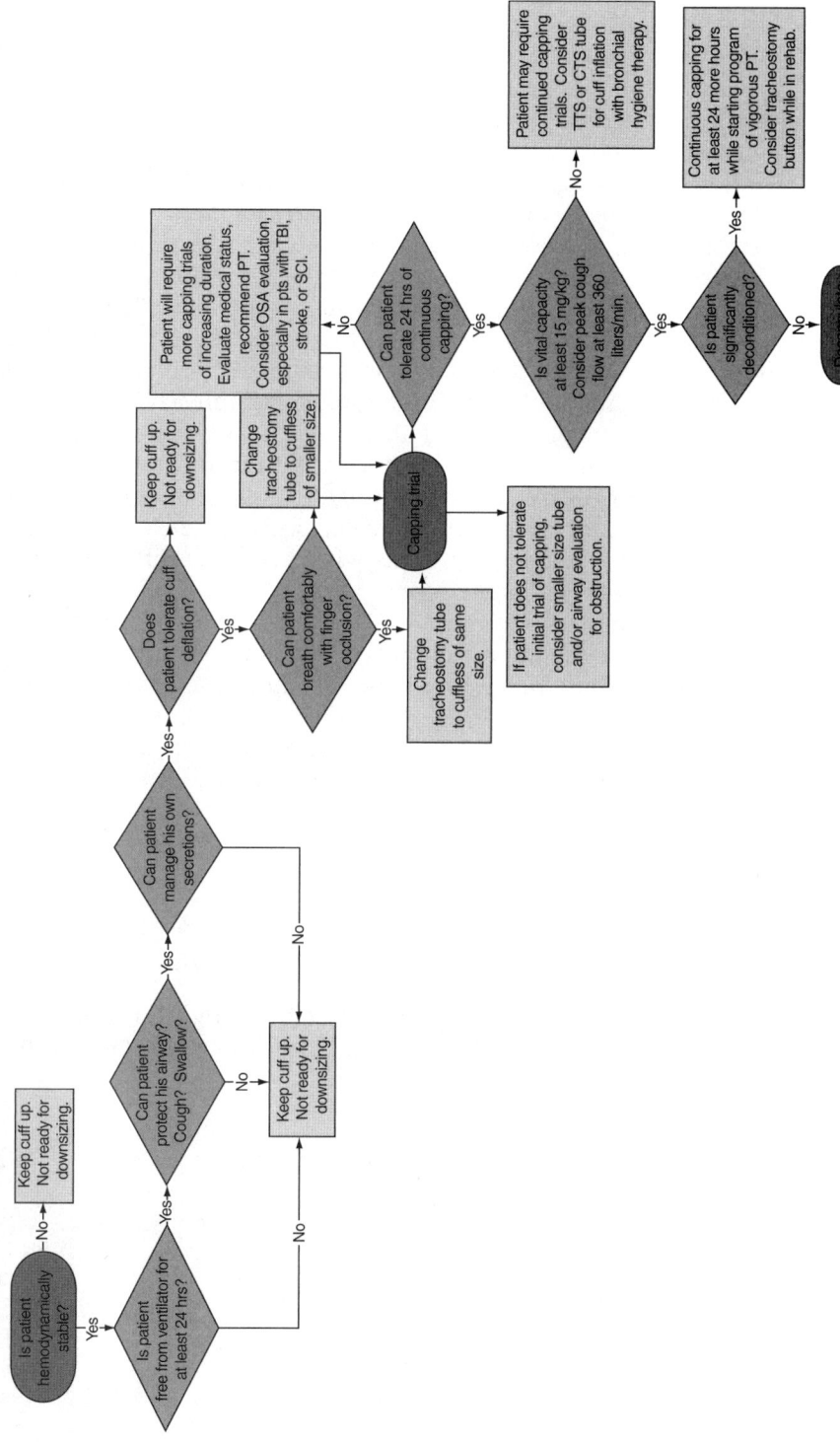

4. Examine size and type of tracheostomy tube in situ.
5. Evaluate bedside swallow.
   - Patients not alert enough to follow commands may be difficult to downsize.
   - Patients unable to swallow their own saliva are unlikely to be downsized successfully.
   - Patients with significant central neurological deficits may be challenging to downsize, which is discussed further in chapter 12.
6. Perform deep subglottic suctioning to remove secretions above the cuff.
7. Deflate the cuff. Instruct patients that the sensation will be unusual because of the unfamiliar feeling of air moving through their upper airway.
8. Occlude the airway with a gloved finger and assess ease of air movement (with cuff deflated). Within two or three breaths, it is usually evident when patients are unable to tolerate digital occlusion. The clinician will observe signs of air hunger and feel pulling against his or her finger as the patient takes a strong inspiratory effort. For this reason, it is important to inform patients prior to this maneuver to gain their cooperation and trust. If patients are able to tolerate finger occlusion, they will be able to breathe easily around the deflated cuff. Patients will have more difficulty when breathing around the cuff of a larger tube.
   - If the patient is not able to tolerate finger occlusion, the tracheostomy tube may be too large, the folds of the deflated cuff may create too much resistance, or other upper airway factors might be obstructing airflow. See Figure 11.3.
9. Observe for significant deconditioning. For patients who have been confined to bed rest for long periods of time and are quite weak, Step 7 is generally

11.3

Deflated cuff compared to cuffless tube of the same size. On left, note increased resistance to airflow around folds of deflated cuff. On right, note laminar airflow around cuffless tube.

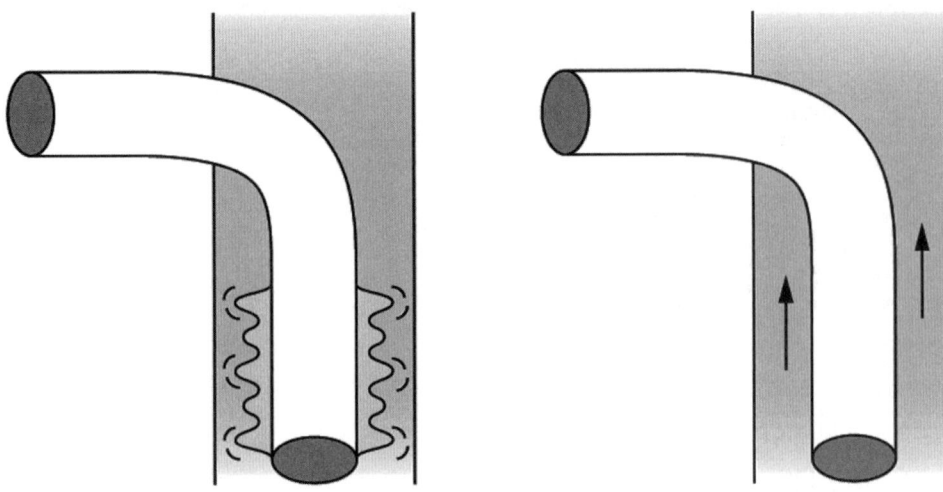

followed with at least a 24-hour period of cuff deflation. In this way, the patient can be observed for a longer time, and the cuff can be easily reinflated in case of respiratory distress or desaturation. However, if the patient is relatively strong, cooperative, and anxious to proceed, a prolonged cuff deflation is usually unnecessary.
10. Consider formal swallow evaluation by a speech language pathologist.
11. Evaluate amount and thickness of secretions.
    - Large amounts of thick secretions will require a dual-cannula tube.
    - Minimal secretions will likely indicate a single-cannula tube.
12. Test ventilation and phonation without tube.
    - With the tracheostomy tube removed from the stoma, determine if the tube is a source of obstruction and airway resistance.
    - Occlude the stoma with a gauze pad and assess for ease of ventilation. If the patient is unable to breathe easily with the stoma occluded, capping will not be tolerated.
    - Allow the patient to inspire through the stoma, and then occlude upon expiration. This action simulates a speaking valve.
    - If the patient experiences dyspnea with these maneuvers, endoscopic examination can reveal a source of obstruction.
13. Replace (downsize) the tracheostomy tube with one with a smaller outer diameter.
    - Steps 1–11 will help determine the type of tube to place.
    - Generally, a cuffless tube of the same or smaller external diameter is sufficient.
    - If intermittent positive-pressure ventilation is required, Bivona TTS or Arcadia CTS tubes would be good choices, especially for the patient who desires to speak.
14. Test readiness to cap.
    - Digitally occlude downsized cuffless tube.
    - If the patient tolerates digital occlusion, cap the tracheostomy tube. *A cuffed tracheostomy tube should never be capped, even when the cuff is completely deflated.* The only exceptions to this rule are the Bivona TTS and Arcadia CTS tubes, whose low-profile cuffs are designed to be capped when deflated.
    - If the patient is unable to tolerate digital occlusion, use timed occlusion to simulate a speaking valve. Allow the patient to inspire through the tube, and then occlude it on expiration. The patient's comfort with this intermittent occlusion signals his or her readiness for a speaking valve. Upper airway endoscopic inspection should then exclude any obstructions to airflow.
    - If the patient tolerates capping, supply oxygen by nasal cannula to guarantee saturation greater than 92%.
    - If the patient uses a speaking valve, deliver oxygen by high-humidity tracheostomy collar.
15. Cap tracheostomy tube continuously for 24–48 hours.
    - If patient is unable to tolerate continuous capping, then cap for progressively increasing lengths of time, especially in patients who received prolonged mechanical ventilation support.
    - The goal is to keep the tube capped continuously for 24–48 hours.
    - Remove cap in case of respiratory distress or desaturation and then suction vigorously and return to high-humidity tracheostomy collar.

- Attempt another capping trial later that day or the following day.
- Monitor with continuous pulse oximetry.
16. Measure vital capacity.
    - Vital capacity is an objective measure of cough strength. Vital capacity should be high enough to ensure the patient is able to protect his or her airway. Normal vital capacity is 60–70 ml/kg of body weight (Morgan, Mikhail, & Murray, 2003).
    - Monitor vital capacity measurements during downsizing and always prior to decannulation.
    - Consider decannulation if vital capacity is greater than 15 ml/kg of (ideal) body weight—approximately 1 liter for most adults.
    - Patients who do not meet minimum vital capacity criteria will benefit from a vigorous exercise program in a rehabilitation center. The patient should remain cannulated during the rehabilitation period and later assessed for decannulation. A tracheostomy button may be beneficial to avoid obstruction within the airway during functional decannulation. See chapter 4 for further discussion on fitting a tracheostomy button.
17. Decannulate.
    - Cover the stoma with a gauze dressing.
    - If the patient tolerates the first 24 hours of continuous capping (without respiratory distress or desaturation) and has a vital capacity greater than 15 ml/kg, decannulate.
    - If patient can tolerate 24 hours of continuous capping but has a vital capacity less than 15 ml/kg, extend continuous capping for another 24 hours.
    - At the same time, begin a vigorous program of physical therapy to improve cough strength and mobility of secretions.

After Decannulation

It is important to discuss with patients the expected course after decannulation. Patients need to know that they will likely be unable to phonate without digital pressure over the stoma until the stoma heals completely. Phonation without the need for digital pressure can be facilitated by placing a bulky dressing snugly over the stoma. Patients should be instructed to change the dressing twice daily and inspect the stoma for healing and any signs of redness or drainage. Drainage could be a sign of a stomal infection and will often delay complete closure of the stoma. After decannulation, a mature stoma closes slowly. Johnson, Wagner, and Sigler (1988) reported that closure of the stoma took an average of 3 to 4 days, with a range of 1 to 26 days. Experience has shown that stomal diameter can shrink by nearly 50% within 12 hours of decannulation.

Occasionally, patients will panic when they realize the tracheostomy tube has been removed and they are unable to speak after decannulation. This is a well-described phenomenon referred to as "decannulation panic" and is most commonly seen in children (Black, Baldwin, & Johns, 1984; Eber & Oberwaldner, 2006). One author reported that this panic could be attributable to the sudden increase in airway resistance and dead space that occurs after decannulation. Gray and others (1998) suggested that more gradual downsizing prior to decannulation does not provoke decannulation panic; however, this author has seen decannulation panic in an adult despite a rather conservative (lengthy) downsizing process. Sherlock, Wilson, and Exley (2009) reported that two of eight patients reported panic attacks after decannulation: "Having got rid of [the tracheostomy tube] which was my heart's desire at the time, it just turned out to be my worst nightmare, for a couple of days anyway. But the panic attacks lasted 2 or 3 days....I was frightened to go to sleep."

Decannulation in Children

Decannulation appears to have more significance upon speech production in children. A child's age at decannulation may determine whether or not there are delays with speech and language (Kraemer, Plante, & Green, 2005). Simon, Fowler, and Handler (1983) found that children decannulated between birth and 3 months of age demonstrated normal speech patterns. However, children decannulated between 12 to 47 months developed difficulties with speech and language (Simon et al.). It is thought that children decannulated before 1 year of age may have a better chance at normal speech than those decannulated in their second year (Kraemer et al.).

Decannulation Failure

Occasionally, patients who have been decannulated must be recannulated or reintubated within a relatively short period of time. This situation is called decannulation failure. It is difficult to determine a priori whether or not a patient will require recannulation, but the downsizing process usually identifies patients who may have difficulty.

Summary

Downsizing and decannulation should be a planned and systematic process with the clinician paying attention to the initial reason for the placement of the tracheostomy tube (VOPS). For many patients, a simple capping trial is a reasonable test to ensure a safe return to physiologic breathing through the upper airway. However, the tube itself creates an obstruction within the airway, and some patients require a more thoughtful and systematic approach to downsizing and decannulation. Given the shorter length of stay in acute care hospitals, this process is often delayed until the patient has transferred to a less acute level of care. Chapter 12 discusses some specific issues involved in a more long-term approach to downsizing and decannulation in the chronic care and rehabilitation setting.

Key Points

- The issues that led to the placement of the tracheostomy must be resolved before decannulation is considered.

- As a tracheostomy tube gets smaller, it is more difficult to breathe through it and easier to breathe around it.
- A planned and systematic approach to downsizing and decannulation usually prevents decannulation failure.
- Deconditioned patients often require a vigorous program of physical exercise prior to decannulation to improve cough strength and ensure airway protection.

References

Adams, A. B., & Lim, S. (2003). Monitoring and management of the patient in the intensive care unit. In R. L. Wilkins, J. K. Stoller, & C. L. Scanlan (Eds.), *Egan's fundamentals of respiratory care* (8th ed., pp. 1081–1119). St. Louis, MO: Mosby.

Bach, J. R., & Saporito, L. R. (1996). Criteria for extubation and tracheostomy tube removal for patients with ventilatory failure: A different approach to weaning. *Chest, 110,* 1566–1571.

Barnes, W. M., Warner, R. C., & Krassen, J. (1999). Utilization of a tracheostomy weaning protocol in the acute rehabilitation hospital. *Respiratory Care, 44*(10), 1262.

Black, R. J., Baldwin, D. L., & Johns, A. N. (1984). Tracheostomy "decannulation panic" in children: Fact or fiction? *Journal of Laryngology and Otology, 98*(3), 297–304.

Cameron, J. L., Reynolds, J., & Zuidema, G. D. (1973). Aspiration in patients with tracheostomies. *Surgery, Gynecology and Obstetrics, 136*(1), 68–70.

Cameron, T. S., McKinstry, A., Burt, S. K., Howard, M. E., Bellomo, R., Brown, D. J., et al. (2009). Outcomes of patients with spinal cord injury before and after introduction of an interdisciplinary tracheostomy team. *Critical Care Resuscitation, 11*(1), 14–19.

Chadda, K., Louis, B., Benalissa, L., Annane, D., Gajdos, P., Raphael, J. C., et al. (2002). Physiological effects of decannulation in tracheostomized patients. *Intensive Care Medicine, 28*(12), 1761–1767.

Choate, K., Barbetti, J., & Currey, J. (2008). Tracheostomy decannulation failure rate following critical illness: A prospective descriptive study. *Australian Critical Care, 22*(1), 8–15.

Christopher, K. L. (2005). Tracheostomy decannulation. *Respiratory Care, 50*(4), 538–541.

Cox, C. E., Carson, S. S., Holmes, G. M., Howard, A., & Carey, T. S. (2004). Increase in tracheostomy for prolonged mechanical ventilation in North Carolina, 1993–2002. *Critical Care Medicine, 32*(11), 2219–2226.

Dellweg, D., Barchfeld, T., Haidl, P., Appelhans, P., & Kohler, D. (2007). Tracheostomy decannulation: Implication on respiratory mechanics. *Head and Neck, 29,* 1121–1127.

Diehl, J. L., El Atrous, S., Touchard, D., Lemaire, F., & Brochard, L. (1999). Changes in the work of breathing induced by tracheotomy in ventilator-dependent patients. *American Journal of Respiratory Critical Care Medicine, 159,* 383–388.

Ding, R., & Logemann, J. A. (2005). Swallow physiology in patients with trach cuff inflated or deflated: A retrospective study. *Head and Neck, 27,* 809–813.

Douce, F. H. (2003). Pulmonary function testing. In R. L. Wilkins, J. K. Stoller, & C. L. Scanlan (Eds.), *Egan's fundamentals of respiratory care* (8th ed., pp. 391–425). St. Louis, MO: Mosby.

Eber, E., & Oberwaldner, B. (2006). Tracheostomy care in the hospital. *Paediatric Respiratory Reviews, 7,* 175–184.

Frutos-Vivar, F., Esteban, A., Apeztequia, C., Anzueto, A., Nightengale, P., Gonzalez, M., et al. International Mechanical Ventilation Study Group. (2005). Outcome of mechanically ventilated patients who require tracheostomy. *Critical Care Medicine, 33*(2), 290–298.

Gao, C., Zhou, L., Wei, C., Hoffman, M. R., Li, C., & Jiang, J. J. (2008). The evaluation of physiologic decannulation readiness according to upper airway resistance measurement. *Otolaryngology—Head and Neck Surgery, 139*(4), 535–540.

Godwin, J. E., & Heffner, J. E. (1991). Special critical care considerations in tracheostomy management. *Clinics in Chest Medicine, 12*(3), 573–583.

Gray, R. F., Todd, N. W., & Jacobs, I. N. (1998). Tracheostomy decannulation in children: Approaches and techniques. *Laryngoscope, 108,* 8–12.

Gross, R. D., Tedla, M., & Ross, S. B. (2007). Breathing-swallowing pattern in tracheostomy vs. controls. *Otolaryngology—Head and Neck Surgery, 137*(2S), P170.

Heffner, J. E. (2005). Management of the chronically ventilated patient with a tracheostomy. *Chronic Respiriratory Disease, 2,* 151–161.

Hussey, J. D., & Bishop, M. J. (1996). Pressures required to move gas through the native airway in the presence of a fenestrated vs. a nonfenestrated tracheostomy tube. *Chest, 110*(2), 494–497.

Johnson, J. T., Wagner, R. L., & Sigler, B. A. (1988). Disposable inner cannula tracheostomy tube: A prospective clinical trial. *Otolaryngology—Head and Neck Surgery, 99*(1), 83–84.

Kollef, M. H., Ahrens, T. S., & William, S. (1999). Clinical predictors and outcomes for patients requiring tracheostomy in the intensive care unit. *Critical Care Medicine, 27*(9), 1714–1720.

Kontzoglou, G., Petropoulos, I., Noussios, G., Skouras, A., Benis, N., & Karagiannidis, K. (2006). Decannulation in children after long-term tracheostomy. *B-ENT, 2*(1), 13–15.

Kraemer, R., Plante, E., & Green, G. E. (2005). Changes in speech and language development of a young child after decannulation. *Journal of Communication Disorders, 38,* 349–358.

Kubba, H., Cooke, J., & Hartley, B. (2004). Can we develop a protocol for the safe decannulation of tracheostomies in children less than 18 months old? *International Journal of Pediatric Otorhinolaryngology, 68*(7), 935–937.

Leung, R., Campbell, D., MacGregor, L., & Berkowitz, R. G. (2003). Decannulation and survival following tracheostomy in an intensive care unit. *Annals of Otology, Rhinology and Laryngology, 112,* 853–858.

Lewarski, J. S. (2005). Long-term care of the patient with a tracheostomy. *Respiratory Care, 50*(4), 534–537.

MacIntyre, N. R., Cook, D. J., Ely, E. W., Jr, Epstein, S. K., Fink, J. B., Heffner, J. E., et al. (2001). Evidence-based guidelines for weaning and discontinuing ventilatory support: A collective task force facilitated by the American College of Chest Physicians; the American Association for Respiratory Care; and the American College of Critical Care Medicine. *Chest, 120*(6, Suppl.), 375S–395S.

McGowan, S. L., Gleason, M., Smith, M., Hirsch, N., & Shuldham, C. M. (2007). A pilot study of fiberoptic endoscopic evaluation of swallowing in patients with cuffed tracheostomies in neurological intensive care. *Neurocritical Care, 6*(2), 90–93.

Morgan, G. E., Jr., Mikhail, M. S., & Murray, M. J. (2003). Respiratory physiology: The effects of anesthesia. In G. E. Morgan, Jr., M. S. Mikhail, & M. J. Murray (Eds.), *Clinical anesthesiology* (4th ed.). Retrieved from http://www.accessmedicine.com

Moscovi da Cruz, V., Demarzo, S. E., Sobrinho, J. B., Amato, M. B., Kowalski, L. P., & Deheinzelin, D. (2002). Effects of tracheotomy on respiratory mechanics in spontaneously breathing patients. *European Respiratory Journal, 20,* 112–117.

Murray, L., Langmore, S., Ginsberg, S., & Dostie, A. (1996). The significance of accumulated oropharyngeal secretions and swallowing frequency in predicting aspiration. *Dysphagia, 11,* 99–103.

Norwood, M. G., Spiers, P., Bailiss, J., & Sayers, R. D. (2004). Evaluation of the role of a specialist tracheostomy service: From critical care to outreach and beyond. *Postgraduate Medicine Journal, 80*(946), 478–480.

O'Connor, H. H., Kirby, K. J., Terrin, N., Hill, N. S., & White, A. C. (2009). Decannulation following tracheostomy for prolonged mechanical ventilation. *Journal of Intensive Care Medicine, 24*(3), 187–194.

Pierson, D. J. (2005). Tracheostomy and weaning. *Respiratory Care, 50*(4), 526–533.

Rumbak, M. J., Graves, A. E., Scott, M. P., Sporn, G. K., Walsh, F. W., Anderson, W. M., et al. (1997). Tracheostomy occlusion protocol predicts significant obstruction to air flow in patients requiring prolonged mechanical ventilation. *Critical Care Medicine, 25*(3), 413–417.

Scheinhorn, D. J., Hassenpflug, M. S., Votto, J. J., Chao, D. C., Epstein, S. K., Doig, G. S., et al. (2007). Ventilator Outcomes Study Group. Ventilator-dependent survivors of catastrophic illness transferred to 23 long-term care hospitals for weaning from prolonged mechanical ventilation. *Chest, 131*(1), 76–84.

Shapiro, B. A., Harrison, R. A., Kacmarek, R. M., & Cane, R. D. (1985). *Clinical application of respiratory care* (3rd ed.). Chicago: Yearbook Medical Publishers.

Sherlock, Z. V., Wilson, J. A., & Exley, C. (2009). Tracheostomy in the acute setting: Patient experiences and information needs. *Journal of Critical Care* (e-pub ahead of print: doi:10.1016/j.jcrc.2008.10.007).

Simon, B. M., Fowler, S. M., & Handler, S. D. (1983). Communication development of young children with long-term tracheostomies. Preliminary report. *International Journal of Pediatric Otolaryngology, 6,* 37–50.

St. John, R. E., & Malen, J. F. (2004). Contemporary issues in adult tracheostomy management. *Critical Care Nursing Clinics of North America, 16*(3), 413–430.

Stelfox, H. T., Crimi, S., Berra, L., Noto, A., Schmidt, U., Bigatello, L. M., et al. (2008). Determinants of tracheostomy decannulation: An international survey. *Critical Care, 12*(1), R26.

Tippett, D. C. (2000). Swallowing, tracheostomy, and ventilator dependency. In D. C. Tippett (Ed.), *Tracheostomy and ventilator dependency: Management of breathing, speaking, and swallowing.* New York: Thieme.

Tobin, A. E., & Santamaria, J. D. (2008). An intensivist-led tracheostomy review team is associated with shorter decannulation time and length of stay: A prospective cohort study. *Critical Care, 12*(2), R48.

Waddell, A., Appleford, R., Dunning, C., Papsin, B. C., & Bailey, C. M. (1997). The Great Ormond Street protocol for ward decannulation of children with tracheostomy: Increasing safety and decreasing cost. *International Journal of Pediatric Otorhinolaryngology, 39*(2), 111–118.

Wright, S. E., & Van Dahm, K. (2003). Long-term care of the tracheostomy patient. *Clinics in Chest Medicine, 24,* 473–487.

Zenk, J., Fyrmpas, G., Zimmerman, T., Koch, M., Constantinidis, J., & Iro, H. (2008). Tracheostomy in young patients: Indications and long-term outcome. *European Archives of Otorhinolaryngology, 266*(5), 705–711.

12

Rehabilitation and Recovery

John Parson and
Linda L. Morris

Patients who are discharged from the hospital with a tracheostomy have many needs. They need information in order to provide proper care for themselves. They need appropriate supplies. They need support and encouragement. They need confidence in their ability to manage themselves and knowledge of what to do in an emergency. And they often need someone to care for them when they are unable to do it for themselves.

Discharge Disposition of Patients With Tracheostomies

There is little research that identifies the discharge disposition of tracheostomy patients when they leave the hospital. Tobin and Santamaria (2008) conducted a single-institution study in Australia and found that over 4 years there were 4,561 total admissions to the ICU; 446 of them required a tracheostomy. Median time to tracheostomy placement was 5 days. In the course of the study, 280 patients were discharged from the ICU to the wards with a tracheostomy in situ, while 8 patients discharged to the wards required a tracheostomy for nocturnal positive-pressure ventilation. Of these 280 patients, 93% were discharged alive, and 7% died in the hospital. Survivors were discharged from the hospital to home (21%), to a rehabilitation unit or long-term care facility (70%), or to an aged-care facility (2%). Overall, 86% were decannulated prior to discharge; of the 14% of patients who were not decannulated prior to discharge, 67% died and 33% were transferred to a rehabilitation unit or long-term facility.

Frutos-Vivar and others (2005) conducted a multicenter trial of ICU patients in 20 countries over the course of 1 month. During that time, 546 patients received a tracheostomy, and the median time to tracheotomy was 12 days. This group reflected 10.7% of their total population of 5,183.

There are limited options for patient disposition with a tracheostomy and a multitude of factors to consider when planning for discharge. The usual options are to discharge the patient to home (or to the home of a family member), an extended care facility, a rehabilitation facility, or a skilled nursing facility. Each of these destinations has its own set of requirements and limitations.

Qualifying for Admission to Acute Rehabilitation

In order to qualify for an acute rehabilitation stay, the patient must be able to participate in therapy for up to 3 hours per day. Patients who are unable to tolerate such a rigorous program can qualify for sub-acute rehabilitation. The purpose of a rehabilitation program is for the patient to participate in therapy and, thus, improve his or her function and activities of daily living. Rehabilitation includes physical therapy, speech therapy, and occupational therapy. Patients who are unable to benefit from therapy are likely to be cared for in a skilled nursing facility or at home. The scope of this chapter is to highlight the considerations involved when a patient with a tracheostomy is discharged to a rehabilitation facility or to home.

Tracheostomy in Acute Rehabilitation

Tracheostomy patients admitted to the acute rehabilitation setting should have their artificial airway issues approached with the same systematic and ongoing evaluation as those in the acute care setting. With length of stay increasingly compromised in the acute care setting, addressing the continued need for a tracheostomy tube is often deferred to the next level of care.

A multitude of injuries and illnesses can result in the placement of an artificial airway. A large percentage of patients admitted for acute rehabilitation can have their tracheostomy tubes safely progressed and ultimately removed. Regardless of the admitting illness or injury, the tracheostomy tube originally would have been placed for one or more of four indications. Those indications, which cannot be overemphasized, are the following (Shapiro, Harrison, Kacmarek, & Cane, 1985):

- The need for positive-pressure mechanical ventilation
- The need for tracheal suctioning
- The need to relieve upper airway obstruction
- The need for airway protection

The clinician should revisit these indications regularly and carefully consider the pros and cons of progressing the tracheostomy tube. Clinicians often focus on one indication and fail to consider the others. Common mistakes are focusing only on *airway protection* and overlooking potential *airway obstruction* or evaluating *upper airway obstruction* but failing to consider *bronchial hygiene*. A multidisciplinary approach helps prioritize these indications.

Progressing the Airway: Taking the First Step

Progressing the tracheostomy tube need not always be a prolonged process provided the clinician has adequately addressed the ongoing indications. Weaning the patient from the tracheostomy tube using a multistep process and utilizing many devices is often unnecessary. If no clear indication remains at any given point in the acute rehabilitation process, decannulation may be carried out quickly and with few, or no, intermediate steps. The prolonged delay of decannulation with no clear indication remaining can lead to the well-documented sequelae associated with tracheostomy tubes (Grillo, Cooper, Geffin, & Pontoppidan, 1971; Kastanos, Estopa Miro, Marin Perez, Xaubet Mir, & Aqusti-Vidal, 1983; Law, Barnhart, Rowlett, de la Rocha, & Lowenberg, 1993). In contrast, there are patients who *will* require a careful, multistep process to safely advance their airway. It is important for the clinician to know the difference between the one-step and the multistep process.

Choosing the Optimal Tracheostomy Tube

Equally important in the acute rehabilitation setting is carefully considering the optimal tracheostomy device for the patient at various stages of the rehabilitation process. Commonly, patients admitted to the acute rehabilitation setting with a tracheostomy tube in place have whatever appliance is most commonly used at the referring acute care hospital. A standard, dual-cannula, cuffed tracheostomy tube, in one of a few sizes, is typical. The type of product used commonly depends on purchasing contracts established by an individual institution.

A one-size-fits-all approach may suffice for short-term airway management but is rarely optimal for those needing a long-term tracheostomy. A poorly fitting tracheostomy tube can also lead to a variety of potentially serious problems (Schmidt et al., 2008). Many products by various manufacturers have become available in the past several years and can address most patient needs. Customized tracheostomy tubes are becoming increasingly unnecessary because a wide selection of standard tubes is currently available. Most manufacturers, however, will customize a tube if needed. Customized tracheostomy tubes can be created with virtually any combination of diameter, length, flange, and cuff variation. Custom products, of course, are considerably more costly than standard products and require additional time to obtain.

Evaluating the Need for Airway Protection

Historically, the tracheostomy tube cuff has been implicated in many of the problems associated with tracheostomy tubes (Grillo et al., 1971; Guyton,

Banner, & Kirby, 1991; Kastanos et al., 1983). A logical first step in tube evaluation is evaluating the need for an inflated cuff to protect the airway. The concept of sealing off the trachea with an inflated cuff to protect the airway is self-evident, but controversy exists over when, and for how long, this process should be applied. Additionally, it is clear that airway protection with a cuff remains an imperfect solution to the problem of aspiration; as yet, there is no ideal solution (Dullenkopf, Gerber, & Weiss, 2003).

In the critical care setting, the serious risks and consequences of aspiration appropriately take priority, and cuff inflation for airway protection remains standard. In the acute rehabilitation setting and beyond, other priorities may prevail. Patient disorders that *might* warrant protection with a cuff include dysphagia as a result of stroke, traumatic brain injury, or other pathologies.

When deciding to keep a tracheostomy tube in place for airway protection, the clinician must carefully consider the pros and cons. Disadvantages include the inability to speak, the potential sequelae of a long-term inflated cuff, and the difficulty of maintaining a properly inflated cuff at home or in the extended care setting. The presence of a tracheostomy tube may also limit the discharge destination, as some extended care facilities may not be able to accommodate patients with tracheostomies.

The potential benefit of a cuffed tracheostomy tube in the chronic care setting for the prevention of aspiration pneumonia continues to be studied. The problem of VAP in the acute care setting is well recognized, but there is also an increased risk of VAP well after the tracheotomy procedure, especially 7–9 days into the postoperative period. This is especially true if fever is present and if continued sedation is necessary (Park, 2005). Cuff pressures must be maintained within the limits of capillary perfusion pressure to ensure the leakage of secretions around the cuff is minimized and pressures are low enough to prevent tracheal ischemia. Another important function of the cuff is as a seal for precise delivery of positive-pressure breaths. The latter point will be addressed later in the chapter.

Evaluating Need for Suctioning

Evaluating the need for tracheal suctioning is primarily a matter of evaluating the effectiveness of the patient's cough. Objective means of assessing the potential for a good cough include simple bedside measurements such as forced vital capacity and/or peak cough expiratory flow rate. Shapiro and others (1985), for example, established that patients with spinal cord injuries who had vital capacities equal to or greater than 15 ml/kg should be able to maintain adequate bronchial hygiene without a tracheostomy tube. Bach (1993) has noted that peak cough expiratory flows of at least 6 liters/second appear to be necessary for the reasonably effective elimination of airway secretions without intubation. The clinician must carefully consider, however, that these reduced measurements may only be adequate in conjunction with devices such as the mechanical in-exsufflator (Figure 12.1) or with manual secretion mobilization techniques, such as the diaphragmatic cough assist (Figure 12.2A–B).

Additionally, if the patient is ultimately to be discharged to home or to an extended care facility, the resources and skill of the caregivers at that destination must be carefully assessed. A patient whose bronchial hygiene might easily

12.1

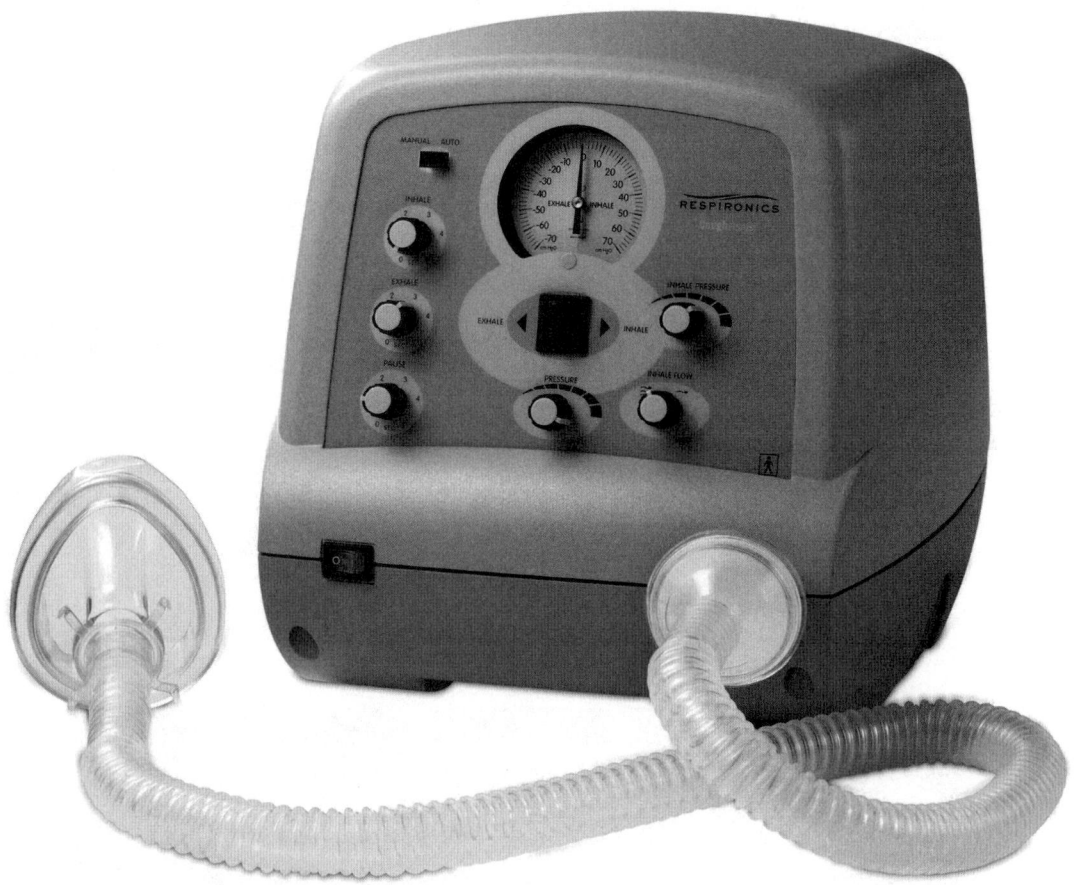

Photo of Emerson CoughAssist insufflator/exsufflator. Image courtesy of Philips Respironics (Murrysville, PA).

be managed without a tracheostomy tube in a health care setting might not fare well in the home care setting with less skilled help. All decisions made in the acute rehabilitation setting must be made with the discharge destination and available resources in mind.

Considerable thought should also be given to the expected course of a patient's condition. For example, a stable patient with a spinal cord injury whose ventilatory reserves might be expected to remain relatively stable or improve somewhat over time would be viewed differently from a patient with a progressive neuromuscular disease, where a steady decline might be expected. If there is any doubt about a patient's long-term need for a tracheostomy to manage secretions, the stoma can be maintained with a tracheostomy button. This would allow for the future replacement of a tracheostomy tube should one be needed

12.2

Manual ventilation with inflation hold requires a cuffed tracheostomy tube for best results. A tracheostomy tube with a low-volume, high-pressure cuff is ideal for patients with chronic but intermittent need for this maneuver. The tube is generally well tolerated for capping purposes, and it has a cuff that may be used for this maneuver or with a mechanical in-exsufflator. (A) Secretion mobilization using manual ventilation with inflation hold and chest physical therapy techniques. The clinician gives a large manual breath, followed by a short pause (inflation hold) while positioning his or her hand over the patient's chest. (B) The clinician simultaneously releases his or her grip on the manual ventilator to allow for exhalation while vibrating the chest wall to mobilize secretions.

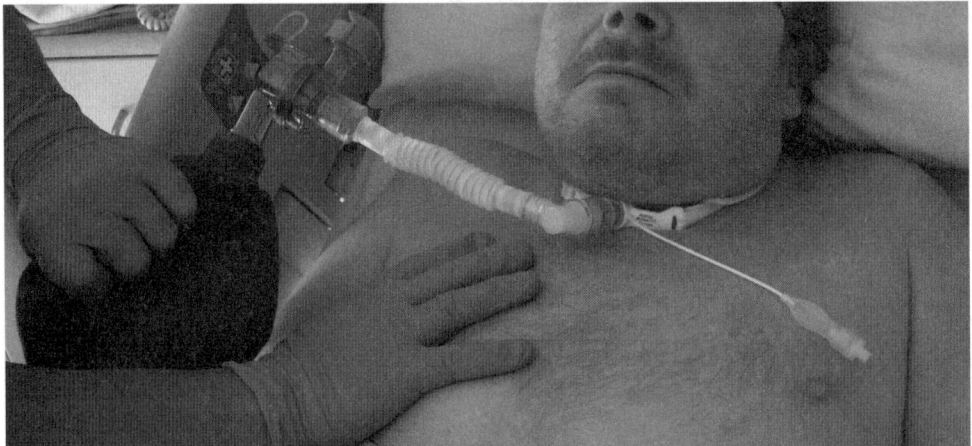

A

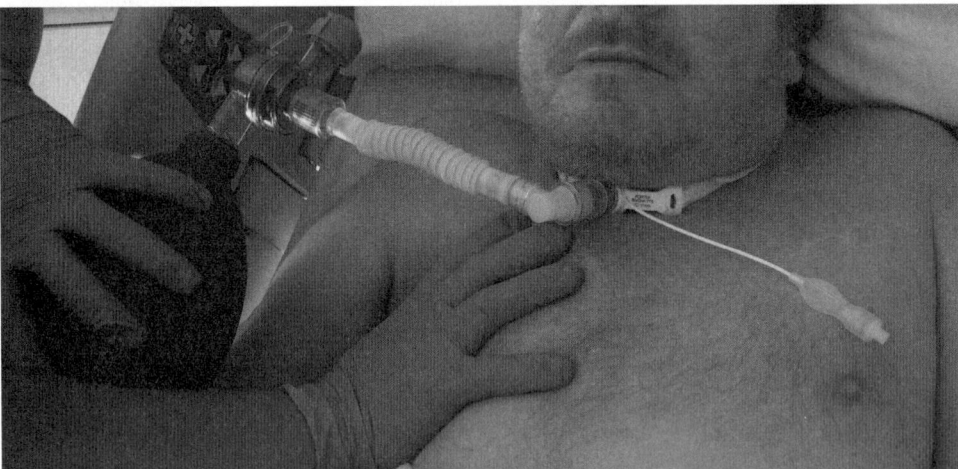

B

without requiring surgery. Tracheostomy buttons typically require cautious fitting by experienced clinicians. A well-formed stoma, free of irregularities and granulation tissue, is necessary to achieve a proper fit. Careful measurement of stoma length and diameter are essential (see chapter 4 for proper fitting

12.3

A properly fit tracheostomy button compared to a capped tracheostomy tube. Left: Tracheostomy button in place. Right: Capped cuffless tracheostomy tube in place. Note the much greater space the capped tracheostomy tube occupies within the airway compared to the tracheostomy button.

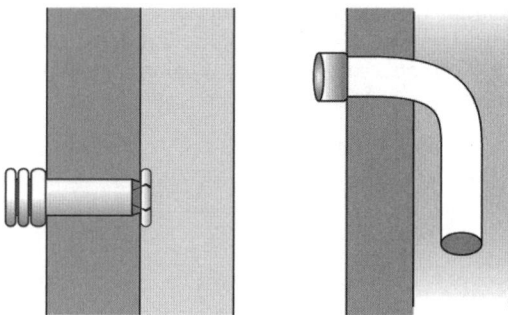

of a tracheostomy button). A tracheostomy button fitted too short allows the posterior portion of the stoma to close, resulting in the inability to place a tracheostomy tube should one be needed. A tracheostomy button fitted too long protrudes into the tracheal lumen, potentially causing an airway obstruction (see Figure 4.11).

Several benefits result from the placement of a tracheostomy button. A cross-sectional diagram comparing a tracheostomy button to a tracheostomy tube demonstrates the difference in space allocation within the tracheal lumen by each of the two devices (Figure 12.3). If a patient is being assessed for the ability to cough and clear secretions, this difference might be critical. Attempting to assess the effectiveness of a patient's cough while a corked tracheostomy tube occupies a large part of the tracheal lumen might be an unfair trial. Secretions often get caught on the tracheostomy tube and cannot be mobilized into the oropharynx. A properly fitted tracheal button, however, will eliminate this problem.

If a tracheostomy button cannot be fitted properly, it may be best to maintain the stoma with a cuffless tracheostomy tube of the smallest reasonable size (typically a size 4 in an adult), thus facilitating the mobilization of secretions.

Adapting Choice of Tracheostomy Tube and Care Plans to Clinical Settings

Tracheostomy Tubes and Effective Bronchial Hygiene Therapy

The function of the tracheostomy tube exceeds the facilitation of suctioning in bronchial hygiene therapy. While all tracheostomy tubes can be used for suctioning, not all are optimal for bronchial hygiene therapy. A decision should be made between a cuffed and a cuffless tube. Often, patients with marginal

12.4

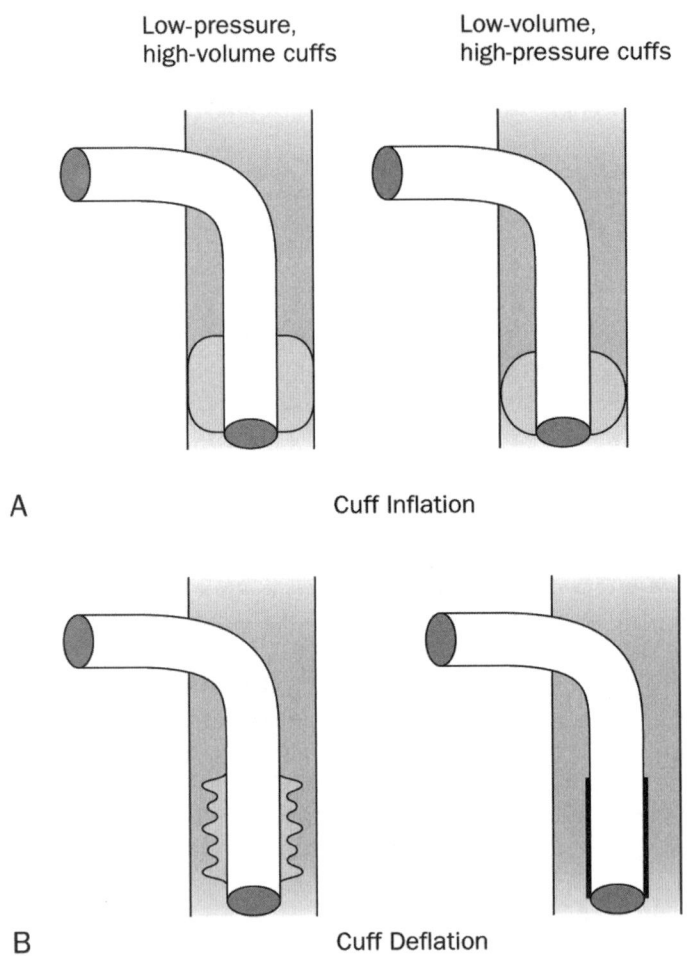

Inflation and deflation characteristics of high-volume, low-pressure cuffs compared to low-volume, high-pressure cuffs. (A) During cuff inflation, high-volume, low-pressure cuffs distribute pressure over larger surface area. With low-volume, high-pressure cuffs, pressure is concentrated into a very small surface area. (B) During cuff deflation, the folds of the deflated high-volume, low-pressure cuff occupy a large surface area and create resistance to airflow around the outside of the tracheostomy tube. In contrast, the deflated low-volume, high-pressure cuff lies snugly along the shaft of the tube, creating no resistance to airflow around the outside of the tube.

pulmonary reserves need suctioning as well as a cuffed tracheostomy tube to augment various secretion mobilization devices and techniques. Devices such as the mechanical in-exsufflator and techniques such as manual ventilation with inflation hold are best with a cuffed tube. The patient who can be capped or corked most of the time, but who requires periodic use of these devices or techniques, is often best served with a Bivona TTS or Arcadia CTS tracheostomy tube. Although they have low-profile cuffs, they do not create the resistance of traditional low-pressure cuffs (see Figure 12.4). Thus, the TTS and CTS are very well tolerated for capping provided the proper size outer diameter is used.

Strong Cough but Poor Cough Reflex

While it is essential to evaluate the mechanical *strength* of a cough, it is also important to assess the adequacy of the cough *reflex*. The neurologically impaired patient (as a result of stroke or traumatic brain injury [TBI]) may have a strong cough when initiated, but his or her cough reflex may be delayed or diminished. This may or may not be of clinical significance, but it must always be evaluated carefully. In spite of seeming chronically congested, the patient may well remain largely free of pulmonary complications such as atelectasis and pneumonia and may also oxygenate adequately. The clinical picture of rhonchi and congestion must be carefully evaluated when considering removal of the tracheostomy tube. Careful assessment over the course of inpatient rehabilitation can better predict the prolonged need for an airway.

Tracheostomy Tubes and Bronchorrhea

While the need to suction secretions is an indication for having a tracheostomy tube, its presence paradoxically may also *contribute* to secretion problems. The presence of a foreign body (tracheostomy tube), along with the repeated introduction of suction catheters into the airway, may be the cause of irritation and secretion production. Additionally, devices such as heated aerosol tracheostomy collars can add particulate water to the airway, further stimulating secretion production.

Therefore, the tracheostomy tube may be *a contribution to,* rather than *a treatment for,* the secretion problem. It is our experience that apparent secretion problems often subside or cease once the tracheostomy tube is progressed and patients are allowed to breathe in a more natural fashion, without suctioning. This can be especially notable in patients with an asthmatic history.

Providing Phonation for Patients Who Require Positive-Pressure Ventilation

The most common form of mechanical ventilatory support remains invasive, positive-pressure mechanical ventilation. While noninvasive, positive-pressure ventilation has grown and improved substantially in recent years, mechanical ventilation via tracheostomy tube often remains the best option for the patient needing long-term support. Ongoing patterns for ventilatory support (e.g., continuous versus nocturnal only) influence the choice of tracheostomy tube. Extensive literature exists on assessing patient readiness for weaning and will not be the focus of this discussion.

For the patient in need of continuous mechanical ventilatory support, phonation often determines the choice of tracheostomy tube. Acute medical disorders (e.g., pneumonia or hemodynamic instability) should be resolved before providing verbal communication for the tracheostomized patient. Speech while on mechanical ventilation requires adequate cardiopulmonary reserve, so the patient should be hemodynamically stable before attempting phonation.

Traditional mechanical ventilation with an inflated cuff delivers precise volume ventilation but does not allow for speech since exhaled airflow is diverted away from the vocal cords and through the expiratory limb of the ventilator. The ensuing detailed discussion offers a balance of various options that allow proper tracheostomy tube selection, adjustment of ventilator settings, and speech.

Leak Speech With a Deflated Tracheostomy Tube Cuff

For the patient requiring long-term invasive positive-pressure ventilation, leak speech with a deflated, or partially deflated, tracheostomy tube is often the quickest and safest way to achieve phonation. Tube size becomes an important choice when attempting phonation. The tube's outer diameter must allow enough airflow between the tube and the tracheal wall for air to reach the vocal cords and achieve phonation. A tube that is too small, however, may allow *too much* airflow past the tracheostomy tube and make adequate ventilation difficult when the cuff is deflated. Furthermore, a small tube may also create undesirably high peak airway pressures on the ventilator and impede adequate suctioning.

Achieving phonation in the chronically ventilated patient through leak speech usually requires a fine balance between adequate phonation and adequate ventilation. The tracheostomy tube cuff volume can usually be adjusted to achieve this balance if full deflation cannot be tolerated.

Equally important is coaching patients on how their speaking and breathing will be altered when the cuff is deflated. A patient's understanding of the central role of glottic control in balancing breathing and speech is essential. This can present a challenge to patients, who are likely unfamiliar with upper airway anatomy and may be overwhelmed by their new dependence on a mechanical ventilator. Often, patients in the early stages of this process allow too much air to escape through their upper airway. This may lead to shortness of breath, feelings of upper airway dryness, and hypercapnia. The patient's realization that vocal cord adduction can direct more air into his or her lungs often gives a much-needed feeling of control to the fearful patient experiencing air hunger. Coordination between the speech language pathologist and respiratory care practitioner is essential in this endeavor.

The careful adjustment of ventilator settings must accompany the leak speech approach. Phonation is limited by the airflow during the inspiratory cycle of the ventilator. Speaking during inspiration is, of course, opposite of what one normally does and, thus, requires relearning a new speech mechanism. The key components that ensure adequate and minimally interrupted phonation are a trialed ventilator rate, longer inspiratory times, and larger delivered tidal volumes. PEEP at varying settings has also been reported to improve speech during mechanical ventilation with cuff deflation (Hoit, Shea, & Banzett, 1994). It is important that the clinician not rely too much on a patient's glottic control for delivery of adequate volume. The size of the tracheostomy tube and the degree of cuff inflation, along with the ventilator settings, should be such that acceptable ventilation is achieved regardless of a patient's glottic manipulation.

Unlike using an inflated cuff, where volume delivery and arterial pCO_2 levels can be precisely tailored, the clinician will usually have to accept a range of clinically acceptable values once phonation with a deflated cuff is pursued.

Mechanical Ventilator Adjustment to Balance Speaking and Breathing

A mechanical ventilator set to deliver 8 breaths per minute, with an inspiratory time of 1 second, will only allow for approximately 8 seconds of speaking time per minute, which is usually unsatisfactory. A mechanical ventilator set at 12 breaths per minute, with an inspiratory time of 2 seconds, will allow for 24 seconds per minute of phonation, tripling the potential speaking time. It is very important, however, not to let the desire for adequate speech conflict with the other goals of mechanical ventilation. For example, higher ventilator rates, which might be preferable for speech, require *smaller* tidal volumes to maintain a desired pCO_2 level. However, smaller tidal volumes interfere with the prevention of atelectasis. Some authors have advocated the use of the pressure-control ventilation mode to automatically guarantee delivered volumes with leak speech (Gilgoff, Peng, & Keens, 1992). This approach may have merit, but our experience with modern, portable ventilators is that alarm settings can be difficult to adjust to safely accommodate this mode.

Leak Speech With Deflated Tracheostomy Tube Cuff and One-Way Valve

This method of allowing for speech in the chronically mechanically ventilated patient may allow for a more satisfactory speech pattern. This technique essentially *prevents* the patient's exhaled gas from following the normal pathway through the expiratory limb of the ventilator circuit. Thus, all exhaled gas flow must exit through the patient's upper airway. Optimally, the patient is taught to close his or her glottis during the inspiratory phase of the ventilator, receive the full ventilator breath, and then exhale and speak during the *expiratory cycle*. Hence, a normal pattern of speech is approximated. Keeping inspiratory pressures and flow rates modest will help the patient achieve this holding of the breath during inspiration. In contrast to leak speech without a one-way valve, this method should employ shorter inspiratory times and longer expiratory times, since speech occurs primarily during exhalation and all exhaled gas must be expelled before the next breath is delivered. Ventilator settings (e.g., mode, rate, inspiratory pressure, and flow rate) should be optimized by a methodical trial-and-error approach.

Precautions. Patients unfamiliar with this method initially require instruction, encouragement, and careful monitoring.

- *It is vital that the tracheostomy tube cuff never be reinflated while using the one-way valve, as the patient will not be able to exhale.*
- Choosing the proper tube size and type becomes very important as well as excluding any upper airway lesions that may obstruct airflow. This method requires the clinician to carefully assess if exhaled gas can flow

through the upper airway before the next breath is delivered. A failure to allow complete exhalation may lead to air trapping with consequences for increased intrathoracic pressures, decreased venous return, and hypotension.
- Humidification can become problematic with prolonged use of this technique, since an HME attached distal to the one-way valve renders it ineffective.

It is a good idea to assess the risks and benefits of the two options early on with each patient, and then choose one method. Switching from cuff deflation alone to cuff deflation with a one-way valve can be confusing to the patient and caretakers alike.

Other Options for Speaking While on a Mechanical Ventilator

Three types of tracheostomy tubes address the potential problems encountered with speech using a deflating cuff. One design has long been on the market, one has recently been introduced to the market, and one is described in literature but is presently unavailable. Each will be briefly discussed in the following section.

Categories of Tracheostomy Tubes

Speaking Tracheostomy Tubes. Speaking tracheostomy tubes have long been available but do not appear to have gained widespread acceptance. The design of these tubes is essentially the same as tubes with a subglottic suction port. A feature of these tubes is that a port is attached to an external flow of gas rather than to suction. This flow of gas is delivered above the cuff and moves through the upper airway to facilitate phonation. One limitation of this design is the possibility for the misdirection of airflow if this opening is improperly aligned within the tracheal lumen. Without proper alignment, air often exits primarily through the tracheal stoma. Additionally, this small line is prone to clogging with secretions, often rendering it useless. The need for an external gas source also creates limitations for the mobile, ventilator-dependent patient. This external supply of gas for phonation typically comes from portable air or oxygen cylinders or from a small air compressor. Patients who cannot use their hands to occlude this port are dependent on a caregiver for speech. Should a clinical scenario dictate the continuous inflation of a tracheostomy tube cuff, however, this tube design may be considered if phonation is to be attempted.

Blom Tracheostomy Tube System. The Blom tracheostomy tube system was recently introduced and promises another option for speech in the ventilator-dependent patient who needs an inflated cuff. In addition to a fenestrated outer cannula, this tube has a special inner cannula that allows delivery of the exhaled portion of the ventilator breath through the vocal cords. This design obviates the need for an external gas source as well as manual occlusion of the air delivery port. The potential benefit of this system is guaranteed volume delivery, which could not otherwise be achieved with a deflated cuff. The mechanics of this device must be fully appreciated by those using it. Training and experience are necessary to safely use this tube.

Voice Tracheostomy Tube. A newly designed device, though presently unavailable, promises to allow speech while preserving predictable volume ventilation (Nomori, 2004). Its clever design involves fenestrations placed at the cuff site in a single-cannula tube, which results in cuff inflation during mechanically delivered inspiration. During exhalation, the elastic cuff deflates, directing approximately 40% of the exhaled volume through the vocal fold and allowing speech.

Characteristics of Tracheostomy Tubes

Size. The size of the tracheostomy tube will have an impact on airflow resistance and cuff-related complications. A small inner diameter may cause excessively high ventilating pressures and increase resistance to spontaneous breathing. A high-volume, low-pressure cuff, if mismatched to the tracheal diameter, may act as a *high-pressure* cuff (Guyton et al., 1991).

Ease of Changing. In the patient who is completely dependent on ventilator support—such as the patient with a high-level spinal cord injury—it is critical that the tube be easily reinserted should it become dislodged. A high-volume, low-pressure cuff can occasionally be difficult to reinsert because, even when deflated, it takes up considerable space and may not easily pass through a stoma that has closed tightly around the outer cannula. By contrast, a low-volume, high-pressure cuff (e.g., the Bivona TTS or Arcadia CTS) can typically be reinserted with much less difficulty and trauma. This can be advantageous for the patient who is a difficult tracheostomy tube change and is critically dependent on mechanical ventilation. Complications from long-term or improper use of these cuffs have been described previously.

Dual- Versus Single-Cannula. The ideal tracheostomy tube should have an inner cannula. However, the desirable features of some single-cannula tubes may outweigh the advantage of an inner cannula. One advantage is the increased inner diameter of a single-lumen tube relative to the outer diameter. Another advantage is the increased flexibility of many single-cannula tubes that accommodate variations in anatomy.

With a single-cannula tube, attention should be given to proper humidification and a prescribed tube-changing schedule to avoid obstruction and a narrowing of the tube's inner diameter. By comparison, an obstruction of a dual-cannula tube can be easily remedied by changing the inner cannula. However, a clogged single-lumen tube may only be remedied by changing the entire appliance.

Evaluating the Need for Relief of Upper Airway Obstruction

When the clinician decides to progress the tracheostomy tube and allow the patient to breathe through his or her native upper airway, it is essential to exclude upper airway lesions, particularly in patients with long-term tubes. At minimum, a simple bedside evaluation should be performed to assess patency of the upper airway; however, a fiber-optic exam may be of value before decannulation (Law et al., 1993). Informing patients about these evaluation options is essential to minimize anxiety and fear. Coughing and minor discomfort as well as a sensation of difficulty breathing may all be encountered.

The initial step should be clearing secretions above and below the cuff. In a patient with a strong cough, the cuff may be slowly deflated to allow the patient to expel the respiratory secretions. In a patient with a weaker cough, it is helpful to deliver a large breath with a manual ventilator while simultaneously deflating the tube cuff. The large exhaled volume will facilitate blowing the accumulated secretions above the cuff into the oropharynx. It may take a few moments for the patient to adjust to the deflated cuff. The clinician should then occlude the tube digitally to assess airflow through the upper airway and look for the following signs of increased airway resistance:

- Stridor
- Prolonged inspiratory phase
- Use of accessory muscles of inspiration
- Intercostal retractions
- Subjective complaints

It is important to remember that any of these signs and symptoms could be attributed to an oversized device, which does not permit sufficient airflow around it. An oversized tube would typically have a larger than 10 mm outer diameter in an adult. In some adults, a smaller tube may contribute to significant airway resistance, especially a completely deflated high-volume, low-pressure cuff.

Eliminate the Tracheostomy Tube as a Source of the Problem

In order to exclude the tube as the cause of obstruction, the clinician must remove the tracheostomy tube and reassess airflow. Only clinicians experienced in *replacing* airways should *remove* airways. Initial preparation for the procedure includes having immediately available a tube of similar size, a tube one size smaller, and a cuffless tube. The latter two can usually be placed if the original tube proves difficult to reinsert.

When the tube is removed, the clinician should cover the open stoma securely with sterile gauze, apply finger pressure, and assess for upper airway resistance. If no airway resistance is noted, the clinician can reasonably assume that tracheostomy type or size is the problem.

Eliminate Soft Tissue Upper Airway Obstruction as a Source of the Problem

Should the obstruction remain, one additional maneuver can be performed in select patients. While one clinician covers the tracheal stoma, another can perform a chin lift. If this maneuver eliminates the obstruction, soft tissue might be the cause. At this point, the tracheostomy tube of choice should be replaced and left uncapped, and a subsequent plan should be discussed. Upper airway endoscopy is warranted to verify causes of obstruction. In the patient with mild soft tissue upper airway obstruction, it may be appropriate to cork the tube while providing supervision for speech therapy sessions. Another option is the use of a one-way valve, which bypasses the soft tissue obstruction. Patients with a history of stroke and TBI have a high frequency of soft tissue upper airway obstruction.

Conclude the Bedside Clinical Evaluation

If bedside evaluations reveal no upper airway problem, the clinician may proceed to capping trials, once an appropriate tube has been chosen, in accordance with safety measures as dictated by the patient and institution. If signs of upper airway obstruction persist, the clinician should replace the tracheostomy tube and leave it uncapped. The patient should then be evaluated by an otolaryngologist before the tube is progressed. The incidence of obstructive airway lesions in patients with long-term tracheostomies has been reported as high as 67% (Law et al., 1993). Commonly acquired lesions include tracheal granuloma, tracheomalacia, tracheal stenosis, and vocal cord and laryngeal dysfunction.

Traumatic Brain Injury, Stroke, and Upper Airway Obstruction. Patients impaired by stroke, TBI, or anoxic brain injury often manifest soft tissue upper airway obstruction in the acute rehabilitation setting. In fact, increasing evidence links obstructive sleep apnea (OSA) syndrome as an independent risk factor for stroke (Martinez-Garcia et al., 2005; Yaggi et al., 2005). Soft tissue upper airway obstruction due to loss of pharyngeal muscle tone may occur during sleep or waking hours. Since an open tracheostomy tube is curative for the obstruction, the clinician must cautiously progress the tracheostomy tube in this patient population.

The primary supportive mode for patients with soft tissue upper airway obstruction is nasal CPAP. With this therapy, positive pressure throughout the ventilatory cycle acts to start the upper airway and relieve soft tissue obstruction. The main limitation to CPAP is the patient's level of alertness and tolerance. It is advisable to attempt nasal CPAP support before decannulation. If the patient does not tolerate the CPAP device, the tracheostomy tube can be left open. If the patient tolerates nasal CPAP, a tube suitable for corking must be fitted for proper titration of CPAP level. Following the decannulation of a patient using nasal CPAP, a period of suboptimal CPAP support is expected and should be compensated for while the stoma is closing. Positive airway pressure applied nasally can escape through an open tracheal stoma; therefore, the stoma should be sealed with an occlusive dressing until it closes. Discharge planning arrangements should accommodate the use of nasal CPAP.

Newer devices such as auto-titrating CPAP are increasingly available in the acute rehabilitation setting and beyond. It is always advisable to consult with a sleep disorder team for diagnosis, optimal choice of CPAP titration device, and monitoring of CPAP support.

Considerations for Transitioning Tracheostomy Tubes

The progression of tracheostomy tubes warrants consideration of several important factors, including presence or absence of cuffs, structure of the tubes, and technique of downsizing. A description of the impact of those factors is provided in the following sections.

Cuffless Tracheostomy Tubes

Cuffless tracheostomy tubes offer an advantage during corking or capping maneuvers because they offer less airway resistance. Regardless, they may be less than ideal with nocturnal ventilation needs and significant bronchial hygiene problems.

TTS Tracheostomy Tubes

The Bivona TTS tracheostomy tube has a low-volume, high-pressure cuff. Consequently, the clinician must pay attention to cuff pressure to avoid tracheal wall damage from long-term exposure to high cuff pressures.

Fenestrated Tracheostomy Tubes

Fenestrated tracheostomy tubes can be used to transition toward decannulation. Their potential advantages during this transitional phase have been introduced elsewhere (see chapters 6 and 11); however, the frequent challenges of properly positioning these tubes warrant careful observation of the following:

- Fenestrated tubes should be properly fit so the fenestration is located centrally within the tracheal lumen to allow airflow between the upper and lower airways.
- Proper positioning of the fenestration should be periodically checked by removing the inner cannula or cap and illuminating the opening with a light source. No tissue should compromise the window.
- Changes in patient position, coughing, and too much or too little gauze under the tube are factors that alter the placement of the fenestration within the airway.
- A window in the outer cannula often allows tissue growth into the opening.

One-Way Valves

One-way valves (see chapter 6, Table 6.3) can play a role in the progression of an artificial airway. They allow inspiration through the tube and direct exhalation through the upper airway. Therefore, an upper airway obstruction should be evaluated prior to the use of a one-way valve. In an attempt to allow patients to phonate, clinicians often use one-way valves with improper tubes, which do not allow easy exhalation. Therefore, a completely deflated cuff and a tube of appropriate size must be used to allow easy airflow between tube and the trachea. Any signs of air trapping should signal an end to the use of a one-way valve until further assessments of tube size and upper airway patency are carried out. Patients can usually be safely capped without a one-way valve as long as the cuffless tube is of proper type and size. The advantage of routine capping over the use of one-way valves is the restoration of normal upper airway humidification of inspired air. Prolonged use of one-way valves without supplemental humidification leads to the formation of thick, inspissated secretions and atelectasis. However, some conditions—such as mild, soft tissue obstruction in the neurologically compromised patient—might benefit from using a one-way valve.

Downsizing Tracheostomy Tubes

Downsizing tracheostomy tubes can play an important role in the progression toward capping and decannulation; thus, the following implications should be considered:

- Increased work of breathing: An increase in airway resistance will occur when the patient breathes through a smaller tube, particularly if the cuff is inflated.
- Adequate removal of secretions: With tube downsizing, the size of the suction catheter will also need to be downsized so it is not a source of obstruction. However, a smaller suction catheter may not be adequate to evacuate thick secretions.
- Appropriate monitoring of cuff pressure: When used to achieve a proper seal, an overinflated low-pressure, high-volume cuff has the effect of a high-pressure cuff. Thus, close attention to all cuff pressure is important, particularly when repeated inflation is necessary.

Discharge to Home

The majority of tracheostomized patients can be decannulated during their acute care stay; however, there are always those who cannot. Cox, Carson, Holmes, Howard, and Carey (2004) reviewed a 10-year database of 144,875 patients who required mechanical ventilation in the state of North Carolina. Of 49,872 patients who required intubation for more than 4 days, nearly 10,000 underwent a tracheostomy. Not only did the rate of tracheostomy increase 200% over the 10-year duration, but also significantly fewer tracheostomized patients were discharged home.

Patients who use oxygen in the hospital must undergo a desaturation trial within 2 days prior to discharge. Patients are monitored with a pulse oximeter at rest and when the oxygen supplement is removed. If there is no desaturation at rest, the patient is tested during exertion. If the patient desaturates to 88% or less on exertion, he or she qualifies for home oxygen use. Detailed qualifications for the use of long-term oxygen are provided by the Centers for Medicare and Medicaid Services (http://www.cms.hhs.gov/MedicareApprovedFacilitie/02_o2 trial.asp).

Patients who transition to home with tracheostomy tubes warrant careful planning for transition of care. The American Thoracic Society published guidelines that help chart the long-term care of these patients (ATS, 2000; DeLeyn et al., 2007).

Discharge Planning

The Extended Care Information Network (ECIN) is a national database that connects patients with vendors. Hospitals and vendors subscribe to this service. When patients require medical equipment and services at home, the discharge planner matches the patient's insurance coverage with that of appropriate subscribing vendors. Patients must be given a choice of vendors. Discharge planners should be given a list of the required supplies in order to procure them from appropriate vendors long before the date of discharge. The discharge planner or case manager is usually responsible for investigating what is covered by the patient's insurance company, including home care services and supply companies.

All equipment should be delivered in the home prior to discharge. It is advisable to have emergency equipment delivered to the patient's bedside for availability during transport. These essential supplies include a manual resuscitation bag for ventilation, a suction machine, suction catheters, and two extra tracheostomy tubes (same size as the patient's and one size smaller).

The entire family should be educated to provide routine as well as emergency care. Routine care includes suctioning, cleaning the inner cannula, cleaning the stoma, and changing the tracheostomy tube ties or holder. While doing routine care, patients and family members should be taught to observe color and odor changes to secretions, the presence of fever, an increase in respiratory rate, or bleeding and report these signs to their care provider. Emergency care includes the management of respiratory distress—most likely a mucus plug. In addition to calling the emergency response system, family members should be taught emergency procedures such as basic life support and the Heimlich maneuver.

When a patient with a tracheostomy is discharged home, a back-up plan should be in place to mobilize prompt and appropriate assistance. Local emergency response personnel should be notified in advance about patients with tracheostomies and their addresses. They should be provided with pertinent medical history and shown how to access the house. This will give paramedics advance notice of what to expect upon arrival, and they will be able to save precious minutes in an emergency, especially since the patient will likely be unable to speak.

It is also important to make the power company aware that vital emergency equipment—such as suction machines, oxygen extractors, and ventilators—is in the home. In this way, patients and caregivers can be notified in advance of any planned power interruptions.

Home Discharge Checklist

- Teach patient and family about tracheostomy care and managing emergencies
- Organize planned discussion among family members regarding shared responsibilities or schedule for care
- Order supplies
- Arrange for home nursing supervision of care
- Complete electrical assessment
- Complete oxygen desaturation test to determine requirement for home oxygen

Care for Patients at Home

There are several factors to consider when a patient is discharged home. Is the patient physically able to manage the care of the tracheostomy? Does the patient live alone, or is there someone at home who can assist? When a discharged patient with a tracheostomy is otherwise healthy and strong, he can easily resume a relatively normal life. If the patient is weakened because of disease or disability, destinations other than home should be considered. A ventilator-dependent patient will likely require professional assistance, and consideration should be given for the patient's placement in a specialized facility. This care is a daunting task but should not overcome a sense of duty, responsibility, or love for a family member. Normal home life is disrupted, and the focus of all activity becomes the care of the patient. There is no reprieve unless arrangements are made for respite care. Clearly, one person cannot provide round-the-clock care (Warren et al., 2004). Continuous professional care at home is a prohibitive out-of-pocket expense not covered by payors, whereas approximately 80% of durable medical equipment cost is covered by Medicare and most insurance companies.

Tracheostomy Care and Supplies at Home

Care and Cleaning. In contrast to the hospital setting, care of the tracheostomy at home is done with clean rather than sterile technique. Table 12.1 outlines teaching points for tracheostomy care at home. Patients and caregivers should be taught to clean or change the inner cannula at least twice per day, and more often if necessary. Specific cleaning instructions depend on the type of tube. Inner cannulas made of polyvinyl chloride can typically be cleaned using hydrogen peroxide, which is not recommended for metal or silicone tubes. The

---

12.1 Teaching Points for Routine and Emergency Tracheostomy Care at Home

- Patients with a tracheostomy have a tendency to develop mucus plugs.
- Use clean technique at home.
- Check and clean the inner cannula at least twice per day (refer to the manufacturer's recommendations).
- Clean the stoma with cotton swabs.
- Change tracheostomy tube holder as needed.
- Change entire tracheostomy tube every 2 months (refer to the manufacturer's recommendations).
- Increase fluids as tolerated to keep secretions thin and mobile.
- Suction as needed to remove secretions.
- Minimize cuff pressure.
- Add humidity as needed.

manufacturer's recommendations should be consulted regarding specific cleaning procedures. The purpose of cleaning or changing the inner cannula is to keep it free from obstructing secretions. The stoma should also be assessed and cleaned twice per day with cotton-tipped swabs soaked in saline or water. To prevent infection and ensure the integrity of the tube, the entire tracheostomy tube should be changed every 2 months.

The most common cause of cardiac arrest from airway obstruction in the patient with a tracheostomy is mucus plugs. In order to prevent mucus plugs, secretions must remain thin and mobile. The patient must be optimally hydrated and participate in a program of physical mobility. Bedridden patients can perform active or passive range-of-motion exercises. It is essential that secretions are mobilized regularly, and regular suctioning is indicated for patients whose cough is ineffective. Routine saline lavage is not recommended as fully discussed in chapter 7.

Patients and their caregivers must ensure the tracheostomy tube is regularly changed. Tube changes can be accomplished during an office visit; however, many patients and caregivers are comfortable changing tubes on their own. A standard (noncustomized) plastic tracheostomy tube should be changed at least every 2 months. Backman and others (2009) demonstrated that polymeric tubes that remained in the trachea for 3–6 months acquired major surface degradation. The tubes in the study were made of polyvinyl chloride, polyurethane, and silicone. The investigators recommended these tubes be changed after no more than 3 months of use. Stainless steel and silver tracheostomy tubes can last a lifetime with regular care. Bivona Fome-Cuf and Arcadia Foam Cuff tubes are made of silicone but should be changed monthly because of the accumulation of moisture and debris, which can cause hardening of the cuff and make removal difficult.

Emergency Care at Home. The most common respiratory emergency for the tracheostomy patient at home is mucus plugs causing obstruction within the airway, which is manifested as respiratory distress. The patient and caretakers should be taught to do the following:

1. Check the inner cannula for obstruction.
2. Suction deeply.
3. Use the manual resuscitation bag for rescue breathing.
4. Change the entire tracheostomy tube.
5. Perform the Heimlich maneuver.

If no immediate relief is noted, emergency personnel should be summoned for assistance.

Reimbursement and Medicare Support for Equipment and Supplies. The availability of medical supplies should be periodically checked. A standard Medicare allowance for tracheostomy supplies [includes a limited supply of suction catheters, inner cannulas, tracheostomy care kits, and so forth (Table 12.2)]. Extra supplies can be provided if the patient has a letter of medical necessity. Table 12.3 identifies the Medicare coverage for tracheostomy supplies. Table 12.4 lists the 2009 approximate costs for tracheostomy supplies.

12.2 Tracheostomy Care Supplies

Gloves
2 each solution basins
Tracheostomy tube brush
Drape
4×4 gauze sponges
Pipe cleaners
4×4 nonwoven tracheostomy dressings (precut)
Cotton-tipped applicators
Hydrogen peroxide
Sterile water
Tracheostomy holder or cotton twill tape

12.3 Medicare Allowance for Tracheostomy Supplies

Item	Maximum Allowed	Frequency
Suction machine	1	N/A
Yankauer suction catheter	12	Monthly
Suction catheter	90	Monthly
Tracheostomy tube	1	Monthly
Inner cannula	30	Monthly
Speaking valve	1	Per 6 months
Tracheostomy tube tie holder	30	Monthly
Tracheostomy care kits	30	Monthly
Tracheostomy mask/collar	1	Monthly

Payment for equipment varies between payors. Durable medical equipment is covered at 80% by Medicare. Aerosol and HMEs are covered by all payors. Medicare and private insurance companies cover manual resuscitation bags, but Medicaid does not. Gloves, peroxide, and normal saline are covered by Medicare and private insurance only, while Medicaid patients can obtain these items through their pharmacy.

Unfortunately, insurance regulations do not allow reimbursement for tracheostomy tube changes beyond a certain point in the postoperative period—namely, more than 2 weeks after the procedure. After that time, a tracheostomy tube change is usually billed through an office visit. For this reason, patients are

> ### 12.4 Average Cost of Tracheostomy Supplies (2009)
>
> Tracheostomy tubes:
> - Plastic tubes: $40–$120
> - Disposable inner cannulas (plastic): $3–$5
> - Stainless steel tubes: $80–$160
> - Silver tubes: $300–$1200
> - Custom tubes: $500+
>
> Tracheostomy ties: $3–$5
> Speaking valves: $60–$120
> Suction catheters: $0.50
> Drain sponges/dressings: $0.25 each
> Tracheostomy care kits: $2–$4

often given a prescription for the tracheostomy tube and are asked to bring it with them for the office visit.

Psychosocial Issues

The patient with a tracheostomy is likely to have numerous psychosocial concerns, including depression, quality of life, body image, and the presence of social support.

Depression. It is common for patients with tracheostomies to become depressed, but it is unknown whether this depression is due to the tracheostomy itself or the underlying conditions. It is well-known that patients with head and neck cancer, especially laryngectomy patients, become depressed (Murphy, Ridner, Wells, & Dietrich, 2007). This may manifest itself as poor self-care or avoidance of social activities (Bowers & Scase, 2007; Mason, Murty, Foster, & Bradley, 1992).

Prior to discharge, tracheostomy and laryngectomy patients should be counseled about the likelihood of depression. This is especially true with laryngectomy patients. Not only do these patients have an external reminder of cancer, but they are also grieving the loss of their voice, their natural method of communication, and a personal distinctive feature. Patients need to understand that depression is a natural reaction to what is often a devastating condition. When patients are not given any information about depression, they are often surprised by its onset and need guidance for its management, including medication and psychotherapy.

Brook (2009) provides an insightful discussion of his experience as a physician who underwent treatment for cancer of the neck. He described how depression and hopelessness were "strangely helpful and calming" as he faced his uncertain future and potentially poor outcome. He described his frustration at his inability to communicate effectively with the health care team and his fear at his inability to summon help when his laryngectomy tube was blocked.

Depression can manifest in the patient as poor self-care. For example, some patients prefer to remove their inner cannula rather than clean it. It is important to reinforce with these patients the purpose of the inner cannula and the fact that secretions will accumulate within the tube and create an obstruction. Guiding these patients to available resources for managing depression will improve long-term tracheostomy care.

Quality of Life. Quality of life data that are focused on patients with tracheostomies is not prevalent because of the confounding nature of their coexisting disorders (Hopkins, Whetstone, Foster, Blaney, & Morrison, 2009). Furthermore, it is difficult to accurately interpret these data, since it is generally known that health care professionals tend to underestimate patients' satisfaction with their lives and overestimate their dissatisfaction (Tippett & Vogelman, 2000).

In the nursing literature, reports of patients with head and neck cancer magnified concerns when they underwent tracheostomy. Restrictions based on the patient's underlying disabilities, and not necessarily the tracheostomy itself, define the patient's psychosocial reactions. Studies of chronic ventilator-dependent patients suggest that the ability to speak plays a large part in quality of life perceptions of patients with tracheostomies. One young, ventilator-dependent tetraplegic patient described his quality of life as follows:

> I feel more normal, less trapped in my body because I can take part—project my personality out of my body with my voice. So communication is important. It's certainly primary in my life and with my family. (Tippett & Vogelman, 2000)

Babin, Beyneir, LeGall, and Hitier (2009) studied quality of life in 150 patients before and after total laryngectomy. They found that there was a significant decrease in smoking, drinking, and dinner outings with friends at home and in restaurants but a significant increase in owning a pet and watching television. The authors concluded that the latter two findings were indicative of feelings of solitude among total laryngectomees and that voice deprivation and the stoma itself are limiting factors in social relationships that push patients into withdrawal.

Caregiver Burden. Ferrario, Zotti, Zaccaria, and Donner (2001) studied the burden on those caring for patients with tracheostomies. Their study used interviews with 63 caregivers who were given a family strain questionnaire; 40 of them repeated the questionnaire 1 year later. The greatest strain was felt by female caregivers. Among the caregivers, 84% reported that their patients experienced emotional distress such as embarrassment, shame, reduction of social contacts, and a feeling of being a burden on their families. A significant number (12 of 63) of these caregivers reported similar feelings themselves. Most caregivers reported restricted social and leisure activities. Very few ever went out to visit friends, to restaurants, or to the cinema. Nearly all caregivers (94.7%) reported they felt better when they were caring for their patients.

Despite the report that caregivers felt better in their role, many reported a sense of intolerance toward their patients. Some patients' wife-caregivers reported disgust with the physical proximity of their partners. Physical intimacy and exchanges of affection were sources of great distress, which also created feelings of guilt (Ferrario et al., 2001).

One study on quality of life in children and their parents found that the quality of life of the caregiver was significantly associated with that of the child. Parents were interviewed with the Pediatric Tracheotomy Health Status Questionnaire. The questionnaire focuses on four domains: physical symptoms of the child, frequency and financial impact of medical visits, quality of life of the child, and quality of life of the caregivers, most of whom were the parents. Most caregivers reported frequent disturbances in their own sleep. Most children woke at night and had at least one nocturnal choking episode per week, and 31% needed help breathing during the night, with 19% needing help every night (Hopkins et al., 2009).

Caring for a child with a tracheostomy has far-reaching effects on the emotional and physical well-being of family members as well as a significant impact on family relationships and the integrity of the family structure. There is a high incidence of divorce among parents of children with a tracheostomy, which places an added burden on the remaining parent. One British study showed that most families received no home nursing care; 73% of the responders did not work outside the home and cared for their child full time, which lowered annual household income. Interestingly, most parents rated the quality of life of their child as better than their own (Hopkins et al., 2009). A plan for respite care is a wise idea for caregivers caring for patients with a tracheostomy. Planned time off can help prevent burnout and nurture relationships between patient and caregiver.

Body Image. The face is considered of high importance in establishing body image perception. Mutilating injuries to the head and neck trigger profound changes that influence self-image, relationships with partners, sexuality, and social isolation. Gilony and others (2005) evaluated the effect of tracheostomy and decannulation on body image in noncancer patients. Patients in the study had a tracheostomy for at least 3 months and were grouped into three categories: those who were waiting for laryngotracheal reconstruction, those who had undergone successful decannulation, and a control group of noncannulated patients who were hospitalized for elective surgery with no obvious body defects. They compared long-term and short-term psychological effects. Those patients with tracheostomies in place had been cannulated for a mean of 38.7 months. The investigators found a significant reduction in life satisfaction in patients with tracheostomies in place. After decannulation, there was only mild improvement in life satisfaction and no improvement in body image. Personality tests also revealed that patients became more introverted after prolonged cannulation (Gilony et al., 2005).

Patients also report embarrassment with the tracheostomy tube. One patient reported that "people's eyes are drawn to the tracheostomy tube" (Morris, unpublished data). Bowers and Scase (2007) reported that one patient avoided social situations because it was "too embarrassing both for other people and me if I had to [give myself] suction." Another patient commented on the ugliness of the tube and its negative impact on her appearance (Sherlock, Wilson, & Exley, 2009).

Clinical Follow-Up

Patients with a tracheostomy who live at home should be followed up at regular intervals to ensure they remain otherwise healthy. Frequently, patients are followed up during an office visit; however, patients who are ventilator dependent and confined to bed may not be able to attend an office visit. In the latter patient, an efficient use of available resources might include ambulance transport for in-hospital care, particularly if there is a suspicion of a comorbid medical condition such as urinary tract infection or fever. Tracheostomy tube changes can take place during hospital care. Fortunately, there are now specialized home care nursing services that provide tracheostomy tube changes at home. Some coordination is required by the discharge planner to find an agency, but families are grateful for the convenience and peace of mind.

Summary

The purpose of rehabilitation is to optimize the patient's functional level after a long and complicated medical course. It takes patience, methodical planning, continuous assessment, and encouraging support to guide these patients toward optimal function. The debilitation that occurs over the course of a critical illness often takes weeks or months to resolve. As patients become stronger, they become increasingly able to protect their airway and manage secretions. Concurrently, their tracheostomy tube can be progressed. In the hospital, time to tracheostomy progression and decannulation is often short. By contrast, the process of recovery and tracheostomy tube progression after discharge can take weeks or months. Regardless of discharge destination, patients and their caregivers need information on safe management of the tracheostomy and proper responses to an emergency. Patients and caregivers need to learn good tracheostomy care and the importance of follow-up to prevent major complications.

Finally, caregivers and health professionals must not forget the impact of depression and body image on the recovery process. It is only through teamwork with a group of dedicated professionals that patients can reach their goals.

Key Points

- When progressing tracheostomy tubes, the clinician must always consider the need for mechanical ventilation, suctioning, airway obstruction, and airway protection.
- Patients with a history of stroke or TBI have a high frequency of soft tissue upper airway obstruction.
- Patients and their caregivers must be given predischarge instructions to become comfortable managing their care at home.
- Patients should be provided with clinical follow-up to manage tracheostomy-related issues.

References

American Thoracic Society. (2000). Care of the child with chronic tracheostomy. *American Journal of Respiritory Critical Care Medicine, 161,* 297–308.

Babin, E., Beyneir, D., LeGall, D., & Hitier, M. (2009). Psychosocial quality of life in patients after total laryngectomy. *Revue de Laryngologie Otologie Rhinologie (Bord), 130*(1), 29–34.

Bach, J. R. (1993). Mechanical insufflation-exsufflation comparison of peak expiratory flows with manually assisted and unassisted coughing. *Chest, 14,* 1553–1562.

Backman, S., Bjorling, G., Johansson, U. B., Lysdahl, M., Markstrom, A., Schedin, U., et al. (2009). Material wear of polymeric tracheostomy tubes: A six-month study. *Laryngoscope, 119*(4), 657–664.

Bowers, B., & Scase, C. (2007). Tracheostomy: Facilitating successful discharge from hospital to home. *British Journal of Nursing, 16*(8), 476–479.

Brook, I. (2009). A physician's experience as a cancer of the neck patient. *Surgical Oncology* (e-pub ahead of print: doi:10.1016/j.suronc.2009.05.005).

Cox, C. E., Carson, S. S., Holmes, G. M., Howard, A., & Carey, T. S. (2004). Increase in tracheostomy for prolonged mechanical ventilation in North Carolina, 1993–2002. *Critical Care Medicine, 32*(11), 2219–2226.

DeLeyn, P., Bedert, L., Delcroix, M., Depuydt, P., Lauwers, G., Sokolov, Y., et al. Belgian Association of Pneumology and Belgian Association of Cardiothoracic Surgery. (2007). Tracheotomy: Clinical review and guidelines. *European Journal of Cardio-Thoracic Surgery, 32,* 412–421.

Dullenkopf, A., Gerber, A., & Weiss, M. (2003). Fluid leakage past tracheal tube cuffs: Evaluation of the new Microcuff endotracheal tube. *Intensive Care Medicine, 29,* 1849–1853.

Ferrario, S. R., Zotti, A. M., Zaccaria, S., & Donner, C. F. (2001). Caregiver strain associated with tracheostomy in chronic respiratory failure. *Chest, 119*(5), 1498–1502.

Frutos-Vivar, F., Esteban, A., Apeztegula, C., Anzueto, A., Nightengale, P., Gonzalez, M., et al. International Mechanical Ventilation Study Group. (2005). Outcome of mechanically ventilated patients who require a tracheostomy. *Critical Care Medicine, 33*(2), 290–298.

Gilgoff, I. S., Peng, R. C., & Keens, T. G. (1992). Hypoventilation and apnea in children during mechanically assisted ventilation. *Chest, 101*(6), 1500–1506.

Gilony, D., Gilboa, D., Blumstein, T., Murad, H., Talmi, Y. P., Kronenberg, J., et al. (2005). Effects of tracheostomy on well-being and body image perceptions. *Otolaryngology Head and Neck Surgery, 133*(3), 366–371.

Grillo, H. C., Cooper, J. D., Geffin, B., & Pontoppidan, H. (1971). A low-pressure cuff for tracheostomy tubes to minimize tracheal injury. A comparative clinical trial. *Journal of Thoracic Cardiovascular Surgery, 62*(6), 898–907.

Guyton, D., Banner, M., & Kirby, R. (1991). High-volume, low-pressure cuffs: Are they always low pressure? *Chest, 100,* 1076–1081.

Hoit, J., Shea, S., & Banzett, R. (1994). Speech production during mechanical ventilation in tracheostomized individuals. *Journal of Speech and Hearing Research, 37,* 53–63.

Hopkins, C., Whetstone, S., Foster, T., Blaney, S., & Morrison, G. (2009). The impact of paediatric tracheostomy on both patient and parent. *International Journal of Pediatric Otorhinolaryngology, 73,* 15–20.

Kastanos, N., Estopa Miro, R., Marin Perez, A., Xaubet Mir, A., & Aqusti-Vidal, A. (1983). Laryngotracheal injury due to endotracheal intubation: Incidence, evolution, and predisposing factors. A prospective long-term study. *Critical Care Medicine, 11*(5), 362–367.

Law, J., Barnhart, K., Rowlett, W., de la Rocha, O., & Lowenberg, S. (1993). Increased frequency of obstructive airway abnormalities with long-term tracheostomy. *Chest, 104,* 136–138.

Martinez-Garcia, M., Galiano-Blancart, R., Roman-Sanchez, P., Soler-Cataluna, J. J., Cabero-Salt, L., & Salcedo-Maiques, E. (2005). Continuous positive airway pressure treatment in sleep apnea prevents new vascular events after ischemic stroke. *Chest, 128,* 2123–2129.

Mason, J., Murty, G. E., Foster, H., & Bradley, P. J. (1992). Tracheostomy self care: The Nottingham system. *Journal of Laryngology and Otology, 106*(8), 723–724.

Morris, L. L. (2009). [Outcome evaluation of patients with tracheostomies (short-term), #1429-007]. Unpublished data.

Murphy, B. A., Ridner, S., Wells, N., & Dietrich, M. (2007). Quality of life research in head and neck cancer: A review of the current state of the science. *Critical Reviews in Oncology/Hematology, 62,* 251–267.

Nomori, H. (2004). Tracheostomy tube enabling speech during mechanical ventilation. *Chest, 125*(3), 1046–1051.

Park, D. R. (2005). The microbiology of ventilator-associated pneumonia. *Respiratory Care, 50*(6), 742–765.

Schmidt, U., Hess, D., Kwo, J., Lagambina, S., Gettings, E., Khandwala, F., et al. (2008). Tracheostomy tube malposition in patients admitted to a respiratory acute care unit following prolonged ventilation. *Chest, 134*(2), 288–294.

Shapiro, B. A., Harrison, R. A., Kacmarek, R. M., & Cane, R. D. (1985). *Clinical application of respiratory care* (3rd ed.). Chicago: Yearbook Medical Publishers.

Sherlock, Z. V., Wilson, J. A., & Exley, C. (2009). Tracheostomy in the acute setting: Patient experience and information needs. *Journal of Critical Care* (e-pub ahead of print: doi:10.1016/j.jcrc.2008.10.007).

Tippett, D. C., & Vogelman, L. (2000). Communication, tracheostomy, and ventilator dependency. In D. C. Tippett (Ed.), *Tracheostomy and ventilator dependency*. New York: Thieme.

Tobin, A. E., & Santamaria, J. D. (2008). An intensivist-led tracheostomy review team is associated with shorter decannulation time and length of stay: A prospective cohort study. *Critical Care, 12*(2), R48.

Warren, M. L., Jarrett, C., Senegal, R., Parker, A., Kraus, J., & Hartgraves, D. (2004). An interdisciplinary approach to transitioning ventilator-dependent patients to home. *Journal of Nursing Care Quality, 19*(1), 67–73.

Yaggi, H. K., Concato, J., Kernan, W., Lichtman, J. H., Brass, L. M., & Mohsenin, V. (2005). Obstructive sleep apnea as a risk factor for stroke and death. *New England Journal of Medicine, 353,* 2034–2041.

Index

Activities of daily living, 235–236
Air embolism
  management of, 284–285
  prevention of, 284
  tracheostomy complicated by, 283–285
Airflow
  fenestrated tracheostomy tube, 188
  matching tube shape with, 144–145
  smaller tracheostomy tube size with, 143
  speaking valve, 189–190
Air-Lon laryngectomy tubes, 134
Air-Lon Tracheostomy Tube and Inhalation Set, 70–71
  diameters of, 122
Airway
  adult v. infant, 13–15
  anatomy of, 1–15
    epiglottis, 9–10
    larynx, 5–9
    mouth, 2–3
    nose, 2
    pharynx, 3–5
    thyroid cartilage, 10–11
    tongue, 3
    trachea, 11–13
  assessing resistance for artificial, 116–117
  decannulation dependent on need for artificial, 309
  humidification, 227–228
  indications for rehabilitation with placement of, 325
  leaks around cuff with, 166
  lower, 11–13
  matching tracheostomy tube shape with, 144–145
  obstruction of upper, evaluation for, 335–337
    soft tissue in, 336
    tracheostomy tube in, 336
  pressure differences with, 12
  pressures, 161–162
  protection, 119–120
    rehabilitation need based on evaluation of, 325–326
    strength of cough with, 119–120
    swallowing with, 120
  tube displacement/loss of, 285–286
  upper, 2–11, 335–337
American Academy of Otolaryngology, indication for tracheotomy defined by, 18
American Society of Anesthesiologists (ASA), 22
Anatomy
  airway, 1–15
  child airway, 13–15
  epiglottis, 9–10
  larynx, 5–9
    anterior view, 5
    arytenoid in, 5
    cricoid cartilage in, 5, 11
    cricothyroid ligament in, 5
    functional relevance, 6–9
    hyoid bone in, 4, 5
    pyramidal arytenoids cartilages in, 6
    recurrent laryngeal nerve in, 6–8
    sagittal view, 5
    thyrohyoid ligament in, 5
    thyroid cartilage in, 5, 10
    vocal cords in, 6–7
  mouth, 2–3
  nose, 2
  pharynx, 3–5
    functional relevance of, 3–5
    oropharyngeal muscle in, 3
  surgical, 25–26
    cricothyroid muscles in, 25
    sternal notch in, 25
    thyroid gland in, 26
  thyroid cartilage, 10–11

Anatomy *(continued)*
  tongue, 3
  trachea, 11–13
Anesthesia, 21–25
  complications with, 25
    hemorrhage, 25
    pneumothorax, 25
  cuff changes with, 172–173
  emergence from, 25
  equipment for, 22–23
  induction of, 23
  maintenance of, 23–25
  monitoring for, 23
  premedication for, 22
  preoperative evaluation for, 21–22
  technique, 22
Angioneurotic edema, 18, 19
Antidisconnect device, 110
Arcadia Adjustable-Neck Flange tracheostomy tubes, 79
  diameters of, 122
Arcadia Foam Cuff tracheostomy tubes, 67
  diameters of, 122
Arcadia Silicone Air Cuff tracheostomy tubes, 65
  diameters of, 122
Arcadia Silicone CTS Cuff tracheostomy tubes, 69
  capping of, 186
  diameters of, 123
  positive-pressure ventilation patients with, 197
Arcadia Silicone Cuffless tracheostomy tubes, 74
  diameters of, 122
Aryepiglottic fold, 4
Arytenoid, 5
ASA. *See* American Society of Anesthesiologists

Balloon valve, 42
Benzodiazepine, tracheostomy tube change with, 146
Bivona cap, 107
Bivona Fome-Cuf, 46
Bivona Fome Cuff tracheostomy tubes, diameter of, 123
Bivona Fome-Cuf With Talk Attachment tracheostomy tubes, 77
  diameters of, 134

Bivona Hyperflex tracheostomy tubes, 78
  diameters of, 123
Bivona laryngectomy tubes, 93
  diameters of, 134
Bivona Mid-Range Aire-Cuf tracheostomy tubes, 64
  diameters of, 123
Bivona Sleep Apnea tracheostomy tubes, 74–75
  diameters of, 124
Bivona TTS cuff, 46
Bivona TTS tracheostomy tubes, 68–69
  capping of, 186
  diameters of, 124
  positive-pressure ventilation patients with, 197
Bivona Uncuffed tracheostomy tubes, 70
  diameters of, 124
Bjork flap, 29
Blom decannulation plug, 108
Blom tracheostomy tube system, 102–103, 205–207, 334–335
  diameters of, 134
Bronchial hygiene, 163
Bronchial hygiene therapy, tracheostomy tubes with, 329–331
Bronchorrhea, tracheostomy tubes with, 331
Bronchoscope, guidance for PDT with, 31–32

Caps, 106–107
  Bivona, 107
  phonation/cuffless tube with, 186–187
  Shiley, 106
Cartilage
  cricoid, 5, 11
  paired, 11
  pyramidal arytenoids, 6
  thyroid, 10
Cellulitis, 174–175
Child
  airway anatomy of, 13–15
  decannulation in, 319
  PDT contraindicated for, 32
  tracheotomy, 37
Child tracheostomy, 243–263
  bleeding with, 254–255
  changing tube with, 249
  decannulation from, 261–262
    criteria for, 261

inpatient, 261–262
outpatient, 262
developmental issues with, 255–262
activity, 255–256
behavioral, 255–256
language, 256–259
emergency care for, 253
general care for, 248
home care of
physiologic monitoring in, 252–253
resources for, 251–252
humidification for, 250
indications for, 244, 245
infection with, 253–254
language development with, 256–259
children 0–3 months, 256
children 3–6 months, 256–257
children 6–9 months, 257
children 9–12 months, 257
children 12–15 months, 257–258
children 15–36 months, 258
middle/preteen years, 259
preschool/elementary years, 258–259
management in community of, 251–255
medications with, 250–251
pulmonary, 251
outcome with, 244–246
precautions while bathing with, 248–249
procedural steps in care with, 246–255
respiratory distress with, 253
school attending with tube from, 261
shape of stoma with, 254
speaking valve use with, 259–261
contraindications for, 260
suctioning for, 249–250
tube selection for, 246–248
Chronic obstructive pulmonary disease (COPD), 22
Compliance, 162
Complications/emergency procedures, 277–299
anesthesia management, 25
classification of, 277–278
early postoperative, 285–291
external stomal erosion, 288–289
infection, 253–254, 289–290
internal stomal erosion, 288
pneumomediastinum, 290–291
postobstructive pulmonary edema, 291
subcutaneous emphysema, 290

tube displacement/loss of airway, 285–286
tube obstruction, 120, 286–287
emergency child tracheostomy care as, 253
intraoperative, 280–285
air embolism, 283–285
hemorrhage, 280–281
intraoperative fire, 281–283
pneumothorax, 281
late postoperative, 291–299
granuloma formation, 294–295
stomal granulation tissue, 294–295
tracheal stenosis, 296–299
tracheocutaneous fistula, 293–294
tracheoesophageal fistula, 292–293
tracheoinnominate fistula/hemorrhage, 292
tracheomalacia, 295–296
COPD. *See* Chronic obstructive pulmonary disease
Corks, 108
phonation/cuffless tube with, 186–187
Cough
retained secretions, defense mechanism for, 163
strength of, 119–120
poor cough reflex with, 331
Cranial nerves, 10
facial, 10
glossopharyngeal, 10
hypoglossal, 10
trigeminal, 10
vagus, 10
Cricoid cartilage, 5, 11
Cricothyroid ligament, 5
Cricothyroid muscles, 25
Critically ill patient
airway pressures with, 161–162
time to tracheotomy with, 160–161
tracheostomy for, 160–163
work of breathing with, 162–163
Cuff, 42, 43, 45–47
barrel-shaped, 45–46
Bivona Fome-Cuf, 46
Bivona TTS, 46
care of, 216–218
changes at altitude with, 169–172
changes with anesthesia with, 172–173
deflated, 46
evolution of, 45

Cuff *(continued)*
  foam-type, 46
  inflated, 46
  leaks around, 165–169
    cuff inflated but air leaking, 166–167
    cuff inflated but tube small for airway, 166
    cuff not fully inflated, 165
    patient position changes causing, 167
    patient with high PEEP causing, 167–168
    tracheomalacia with, 168–169
  leaks around tube with, 169
  leaks in, 164–169
    algorithm for, 170
  leaks within, 164–165
  low-pressure, 48
  Portex Blue Line, 46
  purpose of, 45
  shapes of, 46
  Shiley SCT, 46
  teardrop-shaped, 46
Cuffed fenestrated tracheostomy tube, 201–203

Decannulation. *See* Downsizing/decannulation
Decannulation plugs, 108
  Blom, 108
  Shiley, 107
  TRACOE, 108
Deglutition, phonation with, 15
Depression, tracheostomy patient home care with, 344–345
Digital occlusion, 183–186
  cuffless or deflated cuff only for, 183
Disconnect wedges, 106
Disposable inner cannulas, 109–110
  Portex Per-Fit, 109
  Shiley DIC, 109
  Shiley SIC, 109
Double-cuffed tracheostomy tubes, 99
Downsizing/decannulation, 303–320
  after, 318–319
  children with, 319
  factors to consider prior to, 304–309
    cannulation times, 306–307
    future artificial airway need, 309
    initial tracheostomy placement reasons, 307–309
    resistance/work of breathing, 304–306
    tube size, 309
  failure with, 319
  protocol for, 311–318
  readiness for, 309–311
Dual-cannula cuffed tracheostomy tubes, 47–54
  Portex DIC, 51
  Portex Flex DIC, 52–53
  Portex Lo-Profile, 54
  Portex Per-Fit, 51
  Shiley DCT, 49
  Shiley LPC, 48
  Shiley PERC, 50
  TRACOE Twist Series, 53–54
Dual-cannula cuffless tracheostomy tubes, 54–61
  Portex DIC Uncuffed, 55
  Portex Flex DIC Uncuffed, 56
  Portex Lo-Profile Uncuffed, 60–61
  Shiley CFS, 57
  Shiley DCFS, 58
  TRACOE Comfort, 60
  TRACOE Twist Cuffless, 59
DuoDERM, 174–175
Dynamic compliance, 162

Eliachar speaking valves, 192
Emergency kit, 211–212
Emergency procedures. *See* Complications/emergency procedures
Emphysema, subcutaneous, 290
Endotracheal intubation
  timing of, 19
  tracheotomy v., 19
Endotracheal tube (ETT), 8
Epiglottis, 4, 9–10
  functional anatomic relevance of, 9–10
  physiology of swallowing with, 9–10
Epiglottitis, 18
ETT. *See* Endotracheal tube
Extra-long tracheostomy tubes, 77–83
  Arcadia Air Cuff Adjustable-Neck Flange, 79
  Bivona Hyperflex, 78
  Portex Blue Line Extra Horizontal Length, 82–83
  Shiley TracheoSoft XLT, 80
  TRACOE Comfort Extra Long, 82
  TRACOE Vario, 81

Facial nerve, 10
Fenestrated tracheostomy tubes, 93–99,
    149–152, 338
  airflow with, 188
  change/placement of, 151–153
  Jackson, 98–99
  phonation with, 187–189
  Portex Blue Line, 96
  Portex Blue Line Ultra, 96
  Portex DIC, 95
  Portex Flex DIC, 95–96
  Portex Lo-Profile, 96
  Shiley, 94–95
  TRACOE Comfort, 98
  TRACOE Twist, 97
Fentanyl, 23, 24
Fire, intraoperative
  management of, 283
  prevention of, 282–283
  tracheostomy complicated by, 281–283
Flap valve, 190
Foam cuff tracheostomy tube, change/
    placement of, 150–151

Glossopharyngeal nerve, 10
Granuloma formation, tracheostomy
    complicated by, 294–295

Heat moisture exchanger, 110
Hemilaryngectomy, 267
  swallowing after, 268
Hemodynamic instability, speaking valves
    use contraindicated by, 196
Hemorrhage
  management of, 280–281
  prevention of, 280
  tracheoinnominate fistula, 292
  tracheostomy complicated by, 280–281
  tracheotomy anesthesia complicated
      by, 25
Holinger laryngectomy tubes, 134
Holinger tracheostomy tubes, 85
  diameters of, 134
Home care, tracheostomy patient,
    232–236
  activities of daily living with, 235–236
  emergency care with, 342
  family members with, 232–233
  managing emergencies with, 234–235
  Medicare reimbursement with,
      342–344

  psychosocial costs with, 344–347
    body image, 346–347
    caregiver burden, 345–346
    depression, 344–345
    quality of life, 345
  rehabilitation/recovery in, 341–347
  suctioning with, 233–234
  teaching for, 233, 341
  tracheostomy care/supplies with,
      341–344
  tracheostomy cleaning with, 341–342
Hood speaking valve, 194
Hood stoma stent, 104–105
Hood T-tube, 230
Humidification
  airway, 227–228
  child tracheostomy with, 250
Hyoid bone, 4, 5
Hypoglossal nerve, 10

IMPACT, 161
Infection
  child tracheostomy with, 253–254
  tracheostomy complicated by, 289–290
Inflammation, 174–175
Inflation line, 42, 45
Infraglottic space, 4
Inspiration, vocal cords position during,
    6–7

Jackson fenestrated tracheostomy tubes,
    98–99
Jackson laryngectomy tubes, 135
Jackson tracheostomy tubes, 84–85
  diameters of, 131

Kisner valve, 190

Laryngectomy
  considerations for patient with,
      265–275
  postoperative care after, 267
  quality of life with, 273–274
  speech after, 270–272
    surgical-prosthetic voice restoration
        for, 270–272
  swallowing after, 268–270
    one-way valve with, 269
    radiographic study of, 268
    tracheostomy with assessment/
        therapy for, 269–270

Laryngectomy (continued)
  types of, 266–267
    hemilaryngectomy, 267
    supraglottic laryngectomy, 266
    total laryngectomy, 196, 267
  ventilator-dependent tracheostomized patients with, 272–273
    breathing with, 272–273
    speech with, 272–273
    swallowing with, 272–273
Laryngectomy tubes, 88–93
  Air-Lon, 134
  Bivona, 93, 134
  diameters of, 134–137
  Holinger, 134
  Jackson, 135
  Martin, 135
  Portex DIC, 89–90, 135
  Provox LaryTube, 91, 136
  Shiley LGT, 89, 136
  Singer, 92, 136
  TRACOE Comfort, 91, 137
  TRACOE Twist, 90, 137
Laryngoscopy, tongue during, 3
Larynx, 5–9, 14
  anatomy of
    anterior view, 5
    arytenoid in, 5
    cricoid cartilage in, 5, 11
    cricothyroid ligament in, 5
    functional relevance, 6–9
    hyoid bone in, 4, 5
    pyramidal arytenoids cartilages in, 6
    recurrent laryngeal nerve in, 6–8
    sagittal view, 5
    thyrohyoid ligament in, 5
    thyroid cartilage in, 5, 10
    vocal cords in, 6–7
Leak speech
  anxiety/discomfort with, 199
  PEEP added for, 199
  phonation for ventilation requiring patients with, 332–334
  phonation with, 198–201
  quality of life improved with, 198
  speaking valve with, 199–201
Lidocaine, open tracheotomy with, 26
Low-pressure cuff (LPC), 48
LPC. See Low-pressure cuff
Luer tracheostomy tubes, 88
  diameters of, 132

Martin laryngectomy tubes, 135
Martin tracheostomy tubes, 87
  diameters of, 132
Mayo Clinic tracheostomy tubes, 87
  diameters of, 132
Mechanical ventilation
  airway pressures with, 161–162
  laryngectomy/tracheostomized patients and
    breathing with, 272–273
    speech with, 272–273
    swallowing with, 272–273
  phonation for patients requiring, 333, 334
  time to tracheotomy with, 160–161
  tracheostomy patient on, 160–163
  tracheostomy patients without requiring, 183–196
  tracheostomy patients with requiring, 197–207
  work of breathing with, 162–163
Medicare reimbursement, tracheostomy patient home care, 342–344
Metal tracheostomy tubes, 41, 83–88, 130
  cleaning of, 216
  Holinger, 85
  Jackson, 84–85
  Luer, 88
  Martin, 87
  Mayo Clinic, 87
  Tucker, 86
Mini-tracheostomy tubes, 101
Montgomery cannula, 105
Montgomery Safe-T-Tubes, 100–101
Montgomery speaking valve, 190–192
Montgomery Ventrach, 192–193
Moore tracheostomy tubes, 73
  diameters of, 124
Mouth, 2–3
  functional anatomic relevance of, 3

Nasal mucosa, 2
Neck flange, 45
Neck plate. See Neck flange
Nomori ventilator talking tracheostomy tube, 205
Nose, 2
  functional anatomic relevance of, 2
Nutrition, 232
Nylon tracheostomy tubes, cleaning of, 216

Obese patients, PDT contraindicated for, 32
Obstructive sleep apnea (OSA), size of
  pharynx with, 5, 14
Obturator, 44–45
Olympic tracheostomy button, 103–104
Olympic Trach Talk, 191
Open tracheotomy, 26–30
  Bjork flap in, 29
  horizontal incision for, 27
  incision with spreaders for, 28
  initial incision for, 27–28
  landmarks for, 26, 27
  lidocaine used in, 26
  palpation of neck landmarks at start of, 26
  patient positioning for, 26–27
  pretracheal fascia dissected in, 28
  setting for, 26
  thyroid gland in, 28
  thyroid isthmus exposure in, 27, 29
  tracheal ring removal, 28–30
  tracheotomy dilator used in, 29
  vertical incision for, 27
Oral care, 229
Oropharyngeal muscle, 3
OSA. *See* Obstructive sleep apnea

Paired cartilage, 11
Paranasal sinuses, 2
Passy-Muir speaking valves, 191–192
PDT. *See* Percutaneous dilational
  tracheotomy
Peak pressure, 161–162
Pediatric airway anatomy, 13–15
Pediatric tracheotomy, 37
  landmarks with, 37
  nylon traction sutures in, 37
  tube position in, 37
PEEP. *See* Positive end-expiratory
  pressure
Percutaneous dilational tracheotomy (PDT),
  30–37
  bronchoscopic guidance with, 31–32
  contraindications to, 32
    children, 32
    obese patients, 32
  criteria for, 32
  guidewire insertion in, 32, 34–36
  history of, 30–31
  insertion of needle in, 32–33
  patient positioning for, 32
  Seldinger technique with, 30

PFT. *See* Pulmonary function tests
Pharynx, 3–5
  anatomy of
    functional relevance, 3–5
    oropharyngeal muscle in, 3
  gas exchange with, 4
  OSA with, 5, 14
  pathogens with, 4
Phonation
  algorithm for, 186
  deglutition with, 15
  larynx with, 14
  methods for, 183, 185
    capping/corking/plugging for, 186–187
    cuffed fenestrated tracheostomy tube
      for, 201–203
    cuffless fenestrated tracheostomy
      tube for, 187–189
    digital occlusion for, 183–186
    leak speech for, 198–201, 332–333
    speaking valves for, 189–196
    talking tracheostomy tube for,
      203–207
  tracheostomy with, 181–207
    patients requiring continuous
      mechanical ventilation, 197–207
    patients with intermittent positive
      pressure ventilation, 196–197
    patients without mechanical
      ventilation, 183–196
    requirements for success
      during, 182–183
    risk of aspiration with, 182
    voice restoration principles
      for, 181–183
  tube choice with, 144–145
  ventilation requiring patients with,
    331–335
    leak speech with, 332–334
    mechanical ventilator adjustment for,
      333, 334
    tracheostomy tubes characteristics
      with, 335
  vocal cords position during, 6–7
Pilot balloon, 43, 45
Pistoning, 169
Plateau pressure, 161–162
Plugs
  Blom, 108
  decannulation, 106–108
  phonation/cuffless tube with, 186–187

Plugs *(continued)*
   Shiley, 107
   TRACOE, 108
Pneumomediastinum, tracheostomy complicated by, 290–291
Pneumothorax
   management of, 281
   prevention of, 281
   tracheostomy complicated by, 281
   tracheotomy anesthesia complicated by, 25
Portex Blue Line Extra Horizontal Length tracheostomy tubes, 82–83
   diameters of, 126
Portex Blue Line fenestrated tracheostomy tubes, 96
Portex Blue Line tracheostomy tubes, 46, 62
   diameters of, 125
Portex Blue Line Trach Talk tracheostomy tubes, 76
   diameters of, 133
Portex Blue Line Ultra fenestrated tracheostomy tubes, 96
   diameters of, 127
Portex Blue Line Ultra Suctionaid tracheostomy tubes, 83
   diameters of, 127
Portex Blue Line Ultra tracheostomy tubes, 63
   diameters of, 126
Portex Blue Line Ultra Uncuffed tracheostomy tubes, 72–73
Portex Blue Line Uncuffed tracheostomy tubes, 72
Portex DIC fenestrated tracheostomy tubes, 95
   diameters of, 125
Portex DIC laryngectomy tubes, 89–90
   diameters of, 135
Portex DIC tracheostomy tubes, 51–52
   diameters of, 124
Portex Flex DIC fenestrated tracheostomy tubes, 95–96
   diameters of, 125
Portex Flex DIC tracheostomy tubes, 52–53
   diameters of, 125
Portex Lo-Profile fenestrated tracheostomy tubes, 96
   diameters of, 127
Portex Lo-Profile tracheostomy tubes, 54
   diameters of, 127

Portex Mini-Trach II, 101
Portex Per-fit inner cannula, 109
Portex Per-fit tracheostomy tubes, 51
   diameters of, 126
Positive end-expiratory pressure (PEEP), 21–22
   cuff leaks with high, 167–168
   leak speech with added, 199
Positive-pressure ventilation
   phonation for patients requiring, 331–335
      leak speech with, 332–334
      mechanical ventilator adjustment for, 333, 334
      tracheostomy tubes characteristics with, 335
   tracheostomy for patients requiring intermittent, 196–197
      Arcadia CTS with, 197
      Bivona TTS with, 197
   tracheostomy tube choice with, 117–118
Pressure differences, 12
Project IMPACT, 161
Propofol, 23, 24
Provox LaryTube laryngectomy tubes, 93
   diameters of, 135
Pulmonary disease, speaking valves use contraindicated by severe, 196
Pulmonary edema, postobstructive, tracheostomy complicated by, 291
Pulmonary function tests (PFT), 22
Pyramidal arytenoids cartilage, 6

Quality of life
   laryngectomy with, 273–274
   tracheostomy patient home care with, 345

Railroad method, 149–150
Recurrent laryngeal nerve (RLN), 6–8
Rehabilitation/recovery, 323–347
   acute rehabilitation, 324–329
      airway placement indications in, 325
      airway protection need evaluation for, 325–326
      qualifying for, 324
      suctioning need evaluation for, 326–329
      tracheostomy tube choice in, 325
   adapting tube choice to plans for, 329–331
      bronchial hygiene therapy in, 329–331
      bronchorrhea in, 331
      strong cough but poor cough reflex in, 331
   clinical follow-up for, 347

discharge disposition with, 323–324
discharge to home in, 339–340
   checklist for, 340
   planning for, 340
home care for, 341–347
   body image with, 346–347
   caregiver burden with, 345–346
   depression with, 344–345
   emergency care with, 342
   Medicare reimbursement with, 342–344
   psychosocial costs with, 344–347
   quality of life with, 345
   teaching points with, 341
   tracheostomy care/supplies with, 341–344
   tracheostomy cleaning with, 341–342
phonation for ventilation requiring patients in, 331–335
   leak speech with, 332–334
   mechanical ventilator adjustment for, 333, 334
   tracheostomy tubes characteristics with, 335
tracheostomy tube transitioning in, 337–339
   cuffless tubes with, 338
   downsizing with, 338
   fenestrated tubes with, 338
   one-way valves with, 338–339
   TTS tubes with, 338
upper airway obstruction relief evaluation for, 335–337
   soft tissue in, 336
   tracheostomy tube in, 336
Respiratory distress, child tracheostomy with, 253
Respiratory system. *See also* Airway
pressure differences across, 12
Retained secretions, 163–164
RLN. *See* Recurrent laryngeal nerve
Rocuronium, 23

Saline lavage, 226–227
SCCM. *See* Society of Critical Care Medicine
Secretions
   retained, 163–164
   tracheostomy reasons related to, 309
Secretions, mobilization of, 221–228
   airway humidification in, 227–228
   mobility in, 228
   suctioning for, 221–227
      bleeding with, 224

      depth of, 224
      frequency of, 222
      hyperinflation with, 224
      open v. closed system of, 224–225
      oxygenation with, 223–224
      saline instillation/lavage with, 226–227
      size of suction catheter with, 222–223
Seldinger technique, 30
Shikani-French valve, 192–194
Shiley cap, 106
Shiley DCT tracheostomy tubes, 49
   diameters of, 127, 129
Shiley decannulation plug, 107
Shiley fenestrated tracheostomy tubes, 94–95
   diameters of, 128
Shiley LGT laryngectomy tubes, 89
   diameters of, 136
Shiley LPC tracheostomy tubes, 48
Shiley PERC tracheostomy tubes, 50
   diameters of, 129
Shiley Phonate Speaking valve, 190, 193
Shiley SCT cuff, 46
Shiley SCT tracheostomy tubes, 61
   diameters of, 129
Shiley TracheoSoft XLT tracheostomy tubes, 80
   diameters of, 129
Silicone tracheostomy tubes, cleaning of, 216
Singer laryngectomy tubes, 92
   diameters of, 136
Single-cannula cuffed tracheostomy tubes, 61–69
   Arcadia Foam Cuff, 67
   Arcadia Silicone Air Cuff, 65
   Arcadia Silicone CTS Cuff, 69
   Bivona Fome-Cuf, 66–67
   Bivona Mid-Range Aire-Cuf, 64
   Bivona TTS, 68–69
   Portex Blue Line, 62
   Portex Blue Line Ultra, 63
   Shiley SCT, 61
Single-cannula cuffless tracheostomy tubes, 69–75
   Air-Lon Tracheostomy Tube and Inhalation Set, 70–71
   Arcadia Silicone Cuffless, 74
   Bivona Sleep Apnea, 74–75
   Bivona Uncuffed, 70
   Moore, 73
   Portex Blue Line Ultra Uncuffed, 72–73
   Portex Blue Line Uncuffed, 72
   TRACOE Comfort, 71

Society of Critical Care Medicine (SCCM), 161
Speaking tracheostomy tubes, 334
Speaking valves, 199–201
  airflow with, 189–190
  child tracheostomy with, 259–261
    contraindications for, 260
  clinical use of, 193–196
  contraindications for, 196
    aspiration risk, 196
    hemodynamic instability, 196
    pulmonary disease, 196
    total laryngectomy, 196
    vocal cord paralysis, 196
  early piston-type, 190
    flap valve, 190
    Toremalm valve, 190
  effect on aspiration of, 195–196
  Eliachar, 192
  Hood, 194
  Kisner, 190
  Montgomery, 190–192
  Montgomery Ventrach, 192–193
  Olympic Trach Talk, 191
  Passy-Muir, 191–192
  phonation with, 189–196
  secretions decreased with use of, 196
  Shikani-French, 192–194
  Shiley Phonate, 190, 193
  Tucker, 193, 195
  types of, 191
Speech. *See also* Leak speech
  after laryngectomy, 270–272
  surgical-prosthetic voice restoration for, 270–272
  ventilator-dependent patients with, 272–273
Static compliance, 162
Sternal notch, 25
Stomal erosion, 173–174
  external, tracheostomy complicated by, 288–289
  internal, tracheostomy complicated by, 288
Stomal granulation tissue
  management of, 295
  prevention of, 295
  tracheostomy complicated by, 294–295
Stoma maintenance devices, 103–105
  tracheal cannula, 104
  tracheostomy button and stoma stent, 103–104

Stoma stent, 103–105
Stroke, 337
Subcutaneous emphysema, tracheostomy complicated by, 290
Succinylcholine, 23
Suctioning, 221–227
  bleeding with, 224
  child tracheostomy, 249–250
  depth of, 224
  frequency of, 222
  hyperinflation with, 224
  open v. closed system of, 224–225
  oxygenation with, 223–224
  patient home care with, 233–234
  rehabilitation need based on evaluation of, 326–329
  saline instillation/lavage with, 226–227
  size of suction catheter with, 222–223
  T-tubes, 231
Supraglottic laryngectomy, 266
  swallowing after, 268
Swallowing
  airway protection with, 120
  after laryngectomy, 268–270
  neural regulation of, 10
  phases of, 9–10
    esophageal phase, 10
    oral preparatory phase, 9
    oral transport phase, 9
    pharyngeal phase, 9
  physiology of, 9–10
  tracheostomy reasons related to, 308–309
  ventilator-dependent patient with, 272–273

Talking tracheostomy tubes, 75–77
  Bivona Fome-Cuf With Talk Attachment, 77
  Blom tracheostomy tube system, 205–207
  diameters of, 133
  Nomori ventilator, 205
  phonation with, 203–207
  Portex Blue Line Trach Talk, 76
  TRACOE Twist With Air Supply Line, 76
TCF. *See* Tracheocutaneous fistula
TEF. *See* Tracheoesophageal fistula
TEP. *See* Tracheoesophageal puncture
Thyrohyoid ligament, 5
Thyroid cartilage, 5, 10

Thyroid gland, 26
Tongue, 3
    functional anatomic relevance of, 3
    during laryngoscopy, 3
Toremalm valve, 190
Total laryngectomy, 267
    speaking valves use contraindicated by, 196
    surgical-prosthetic voice restoration for, 270–272
    swallowing after, 268
Trachea, 11–13
    tracheostomy button fitting with, 155
Tracheal cannula, 104
Tracheal stenosis
    management of, 299
    prevention of, 297–299
    tracheostomy complicated by, 296–299
Tracheocutaneous fistula (TCF)
    management of, 293–294
    prevention of, 293
    tracheostomy complicated by, 293–294
Tracheoesophageal fistula (TEF)
    management of, 293
    prevention of, 293
    tracheostomy complicated by, 292–293
Tracheoesophageal puncture (TEP), 270–272
Tracheoinnominate fistula
    management of, 292
    prevention of, 292
    tracheostomy complicated by, 292
Tracheomalacia
    cuff leak with, 168–169
    management of, 296
    prevention of, 296
    repositioning of tracheostomy tubes with, 118
    tracheostomy complicated by, 295–296
Tracheostomy. *See also* Complications/emergency procedures
    home care/supplies for, 341–344
        cleaning with, 341–342
    patients requiring continuous mechanical ventilation, 197–207
        cuffed fenestrated tracheostomy tube for, 201–203
        leak speech for, 198–201
        talking tracheostomy tube for, 203–207
    patients with intermittent positive pressure ventilation, 196–197
    patients without mechanical ventilation, 183–196
        capping/corking/plugging for, 186–187
        cuffless fenestrated tracheostomy tube for, 187–189
        digital occlusion for, 183–186
        speaking valves for, 189–196
    phonation with, 181–207
        methods for, 183
        requirements for successful, 182–183
        risk of aspiration, 182
    reasons for, 307–309
        obstruction, 307–308
        protection, 308–309
        secretions, 309
        swallowing function, 308–309
        ventilation, 307
        VOPS acronym, 307
    voice restoration with, 181–183
        emotional experience of, 182
        requirements for, 182–183
        risk of aspiration, 182
Tracheostomy button, 103–105
    fitting, 154–156
    length determination for, 154
    Olympic, 104
    posterior angle of trachea with, 155
    purpose of, 154
Tracheostomy patient, 159–178
    care of, 211–236
        activities of daily living in, 235–236
        continuous v. intermittent feedings in, 232
        home emergencies in, 234–235
        mobilization of secretions for, 221–228
        nutrition in, 232
        oral care for, 229
        other tracheal appliance care with, 229–232
        patient at home in, 232–236
        tracheal cannula in, 231–232
        T-tube in, 229–231
        tube maintenance for, 211–221
    cellulitis with, 174–175
    complex wounds with, 173–175
    critically ill patient on mechanical ventilation as, 160–163
        airway pressures with, 161–162
        time to tracheotomy with, 160–161
        work of breathing with, 162–163
    cuff changes at altitude with, 169–172

Tracheostomy patient *(continued)*
  cuff changes with anesthesia with, 172–173
  cuff leaks with, 164–169
    around cuff, 165–169
    around tube, 169
    within cuff, 164–165
  defective tubes with, 177
  discharge disposition with, 323–324
  inflammation with, 174–175
  laryngectomy with ventilator-dependent, 272–273
    breathing with, 272–273
    speech with, 272–273
    swallowing with, 272–273
  missing part with, 177–178
  mobilization of secretions for, 221–228
    airway humidification in, 227–228
    mobility in, 228
    suctioning, 221–227
  pistoning with, 169
  research of experience of, 175–177
    communication, 176
    discomfort, 176
    eating, 176–177
    suctioning, 176
  retained secretions with, 163–164
  stomal erosion with, 173–174
  tube maintenance in care of, 211–221
    care of inner cannula with, 213–214
    care of stoma with, 219–221
    care of tube cuff in, 216–218
    changing tube in, 218–219
    cleaning inner cannula with, 214–216
    emergency supplies for, 211–212
    securing tube in, 212–213
Tracheostomy-securing devices, 111
Tracheostomy tubes, 41–112
  accessories/products with, 103–112
    antidisconnect device, 110
    caps, 106–107
    corks or stoppers, 108
    decannulation plugs, 108
    disconnect wedges, 106
    disposable/spare inner cannulas, 109–110
    heat moisture exchanger, 111
    speaking valves, 103
    stoma maintenance devices, 103–105
    tracheostomy-securing devices, 111
    ventilator adapters, 111

  with additional suction channel, 83
  Blom tracheostomy tube system, 102–103, 133, 205–207
  bronchial hygiene therapy with, 329–331
  bronchorrhea with, 331
  change of, 145–154
    bedside, 147
    benzodiazepine for, 146
    child tracheostomy, 249
    classic method for, 148–149
    cuff deflation with, 147
    deep subglottic suctioning with, 147
    fenestrated tracheostomy tube, 151–153
    foam cuff tracheostomy tube, 150–151
    hemodynamically unstable patient with, 146–147
    nonstandard tube placement in, 150–153
    patient anxiety with, 146
    patient cooperation for, 146
    patient positioning with, 147
    railroad method for, 149–150
    stoma examination with, 148–149
    supplies for, 146–147
    survey of chief residents regarding, 145–146
    tube exchanger technique for, 149–150
  characteristics for ventilation requiring patients of, 335
    dual- v. single-cannula, 335
    ease of changing, 335
    size, 335
  child attending school with, 261
  child, selection of, 246–248
  cough strength/reflex with choice of, 331
  cuffed v. uncuffed choice of, 117–120
    airway protection in, 119–120
    mental status in, 120
    positive-pressure ventilation in, 117–118
    transitioning with, 338
  custom-designed, 101–102
  defective, 177
  diameters of
    adult, 122–132
    neonatal and pediatric, 137–143
  double-cuffed, 99
  dual-cannula cuffless, 54–61
    Portex DIC Uncuffed, 55
    Portex Flex DIC Uncuffed, 56
    Portex Lo-Profile Uncuffed, 60–61

Shiley CFS, 57
Shiley DCFS, 58
TRACOE Comfort, 60
TRACOE Twist Cuffless, 59
dual- v. single-cannula choice for, 120–121
   secretions and tube obstructions in, 120
   suctioning in, 121
   ventilation requiring patients with, 335
extra-long, 77–83
   Arcadia Air Cuff Adjustable-Neck Flange, 79
   Bivona Hyperflex, 78
   Portex Blue Line Extra Horizontal Length, 82–83
   Shiley TracheoSoft XLT, 80
   TRACOE Comfort Extra Long, 82
   TRACOE Vario, 81
fenestrated, 93–99, 149–152, 338
   phonation with, 187–189
   Portex Blue Line Fenestrated, 96
   Portex Blue Line Ultra Fenestrated, 96
   Portex DIC Fenestrated, 95
   Portex Flex DIC Fenestrated, 95–96
   Portex Lo-Profile Fenestrated, 96
   Shiley Fenestrated, 94–95
   TRACOE Comfort Fenestrated, 98
   TRACOE Twist Fenestrated, 97
fitting/changing of, 115–155
   assessing resistance with, 116–117
   child in, 249
   choosing best tube construction with, 143–144
   choosing best tube length with, 144
   choosing cuffed/uncuffed tube with, 117–120
   choosing dual/single-cannula tube with, 120–121
   choosing tube size with, 121–141
   considerations with, 115–116
   goals before, 115–116
   matching tube shape and airway with, 144–145
   patient care with, 218–219
   phonation with tube choice in, 144–145
   questions for planning, 115–116
laryngectomy tubes, 88–93
   Bivona Laryngectomy, 93
   Portex DIC Laryngectomy, 89–90
   Provox LaryTube, 93
   Shiley LGT, 89
   Singer Laryngectomy, 92
   TRACOE Comfort Laryngectomy, 91
   TRACOE Twist Laryngectomy, 90
maintenance of, 211–221
   care of inner cannula with, 213–214
   care of stoma with, 219–221
   care of tube cuff in, 216–218
   cleaning inner cannula with, 214–216
material of, 41
   polyurethane, 41
   polyvinyl chloride, 41
   silicone, 41
   silver, 41
   stainless steel, 41
metal, 41, 83–88, 130
   cleaning of, 216
   Holinger, 85
   Jackson, 84–85
   Luer, 88
   Martin, 87
   Mayo Clinic, 87
   Tucker, 86
mini, 101
missing part with, 177–178
new products, 102–103
Nomori ventilator talking, 205
nonstandard, 150–153
   fenestrated tracheostomy tube, 151–153
   foam cuff tracheostomy tube, 150–151
obstruction of, 120, 286–287
parts of, 42–47
   balloon valve, 42
   cuff, 42, 43, 45–47
   inflation line, 42, 45
   inner cannula, 42, 44
   neck flange, 42, 45
   obturator, 42, 44–45
   outer cannula, 42, 43
   pilot balloon, 42, 45
phonation with capping/corking/plugging of, 186–187
pistoning with, 169
rehabilitation need based on choice of, 325, 329–331
related supplies for, 112
   bibs, 112
   grid or mesh screens, 112
   scarves or ascots, 112

Tracheostomy tubes *(continued)*
   shower protections devices, 112
   tube spacers, 112
  securing, 212–213
  single-cannula cuffed, 61–69
   Arcadia Foam Cuff, 67
   Arcadia Silicone Air Cuff, 65
   Arcadia Silicone CTS Cuff, 69
   Bivona Fome Cuf, 66–67
   Bivona Mid-Range Aire-Cuf, 64
   Bivona TTS, 68–69
   Portex Blue Line, 62
   Portex Blue Line Ultra, 63
   Shiley SCT, 61
  single-cannula cuffless, 69–75
   Air-Lon Tracheostomy Tube and Inhalation Set, 70–71
   Arcadia Silicone Cuffless, 74
   Bivona Sleep Apnea, 74–75
   Bivona Uncuffed, 70
   Moore, 73
   Portex Blue Line Ultra Uncuffed, 72–73
   Portex Blue Line Uncuffed, 72
   TRACOE Comfort, 71
  size of, 121–141
   adult, 122–132
   airflow in, 143
   Air-Lon, 122
   Arcadia adjustable-neck flange, 122
   Arcadia Foam Cuff, 122
   Arcadia Silicone Air Cuff, 122
   Arcadia Silicone CTS Cuff, 123
   Arcadia Silicone Cuffless, 122
   Bivona Fome Cuf, 123
   Bivona Fome-Cuf With Talk Attachment, 133
   Bivona Hyperflex, 123
   Bivona Mid-Range Aire-Cuf, 123
   Bivona Sleep Apnea, 124
   Bivona TTS, 124
   Bivona Uncuffed, 124
   Blom tracheostomy tube system, 133
   decannulation dependent on, 309
   Holinger, 134
   Jackson, 131
   Luer, 132
   Martin, 132
   Mayo Clinic, 132
   Moore, 124
   neonatal and pediatric, 137–143
   Portex Blue Line, 125
   Portex Blue Line Extra Horizontal Length, 126
   Portex Blue Line Trach Talk, 133
   Portex Blue Line Ultra, 126
   Portex Blue Line Ultra fenestrated, 127
   Portex Blue Line Ultra Suctionaid, 127
   Portex DIC, 124
   Portex DIC fenestrated, 125
   Portex Flex DIC, 125
   Portex Flex DIC fenestrated, 125
   Portex Lo-Profile, 127
   Portex Lo-Profile fenestrated, 127
   Portex Per-Fit, 126
   Shiley DCT, 127, 129
   Shiley fenestrated, 128
   Shiley PERC, 129
   Shiley SCT, 128
   Shiley TracheoSoft XLT, 129
   Talking, 133
   TRACOE Comfort, 130
   TRACOE Comfort Extra Long, 130
   TRACOE Twist Series, 129
   TRACOE Twist With Air Supply Line, 134
   TRACOE Vario, 130
   Tucker, 131
  sizing of, 43–44
  speaking, 334
  special use, 75
  standard dual-cannula cuffed, 47–54
   Portex DIC, 51–52
   Portex Flex DIC, 52–53
   Portex Lo-Profile, 54
   Portex Per-fit, 51
   Shiley DCT, 49
   Shiley LPC, 48
   Shiley PERC, 50
   TRACOE Twist Series, 53–54
  talking, 75–77
   Bivona Fome-Cuf With Talk Attachment, 77
   Portex Blue Line Trach Talk, 76
   TRACOE Twist With Air Supply Line, 76
  tracheomalacia and repositioning of, 118
  transitioning, 337–339
   cuffless tubes with, 338
   downsizing with, 338
   fenestrated tubes with, 338
   one-way valves with, 338–339
   TTS tubes with, 338

T-tubes, 99–101
upper airway obstruction evaluation of, 336
voice, 334
Tracheotomy. *See also* Open tracheotomy; Percutaneous dilational tracheotomy
  anesthesia management for, 21–25
    complications with, 25
    emergence in, 25
    equipment in, 22–23
    induction in, 23
    maintenance in, 23–25
    monitoring in, 23
    premedication in, 22
    preoperative evaluation in, 21–22
    technique in, 22
  checklist for bedside, 23
  endotracheal intubation v., 19
  indications for, 18–19
    laryngotracheal trauma, 19
    severe angioneurotic edema, 19
    upper aero-digestive tract neoplasm, 19
  postoperative care with, 37–38
  preoperative management for, 20–21
  procedure, 17–38
  surgical technique for, 25–38
    anatomy of, 25–26
    open tracheotomy, 26–30
    pediatric tracheotomy, 37
    percutaneous dilational tracheotomy, 30–37
  timing of, 19–20
Tracheotomy dilator, 29
TRACOE Comfort Extra Long tracheostomy tubes, 82
  diameters of, 130
TRACOE Comfort fenestrated tracheostomy tubes, 98
TRACOE Comfort laryngectomy tubes, 91
TRACOE Comfort tracheostomy tubes, 71
  diameters of, 130

TRACOE decannulation plug, 108
TRACOE Twist fenestrated tracheostomy tubes, 97
TRACOE Twist laryngectomy tubes, 90
  diameters of, 137
TRACOE Twist Series tracheostomy tubes, 53–54
  diameters of, 129
TRACOE Twist With Air Supply Line tracheostomy tubes, 76
  diameters of, 134
TRACOE Vario tracheostomy tubes, 81
  diameters of, 130
Transpulmonary pressure, 12
Traumatic brain injury, 337
Trigeminal nerve, 10
T-tubes, 99–101
  care of, 229–231
  Hood, 230
  suctioning, 231
Tube displacement/loss of airway, tracheostomy complicated by, 285–286
Tube exchanger technique, 149–150
Tube obstruction, tracheostomy complicated by, 120, 286–287
Tucker tracheostomy tubes, 86
  diameters of, 131
Tucker valve, 193, 195

Vagus nerve, 10
VC. *See* Vocal cords
Ventilator adapters, 111
Vocal cord paralysis, 18
  speaking valves use contraindicated by, 196
Vocal cords (VC), phonation and inspiration with position of, 6–7
Voice restoration, 181–183. *See also* Phonation
  risk of aspiration with, 182
Voice tracheostomy tube, 334